Emerging Therapies Targeting the Pathophysiology of Sickle Cell Disease

Editor

ELLIOTT P. VICHINSKY

HEMATOLOGY/ONCOLOGY CLINICS OF NORTH AMERICA

www.hemonc.theclinics.com

Consulting Editors
GEORGE P. CANELLOS
H. FRANKLIN BUNN

April 2014 • Volume 28 • Number 2

ELSEVIER

1600 John F. Kennedy Boulevard • Suite 1800 • Philadelphia, Pennsylvania, 19103-2899

http://www.theclinics.com

HEMATOLOGY/ONCOLOGY CLINICS OF NORTH AMERICA Volume 28, Number 2
April 2014 ISSN 0889-8588, ISBN 13: 978-0-323-28999-3

Editor: Jessica McCool
Developmental Editor: Donald Mumford

Hematology/Oncology Clinics (ISSN 0889-8588) is published bimonthly by Elsevier Inc., 360 Park Avenue South, New York, NY 10010-1710. Months of issue are February, April, June, August, October, and December. Business and Editorial Offices: 1600 John F. Kennedy Blvd., Ste. 1800, Philadelphia, PA 19103—2899. Customer Service Office: 3251 Riverport Lane, Maryland Heights, MO 63043. Periodicals postage paid at New York, NY and at additional mailing offices. Subscription prices are $385.00 per year (domestic individuals), $633.00 per year (domestic institutions), $190.00 per year (domestic students/residents), $440.00 per year (Canadian individuals), $783.00 per year (Canadian institutions) $520.00 per year (international individuals), $783.00 per year (international institutions), and $255.00 per year (international and Canadian students/residents). International air speed delivery is included in all *Clinics* subscription prices. All prices are subject to change without notice. **POSTMASTER:** Send address changes to *Hematology/Oncology Clinics of North America*, Elsevier Health Sciences Division, Subscription Customer Service, 3251 Riverport Lane, Maryland Heights, MO 63043. Customer Service (orders, claims, online, change of address): Elsevier Health Sciences Division, Subscription Customer Service, 3251 Riverport Lane, Maryland Heights, MO 63043. Tel: 1-800-654-2452 (U.S. and Canada); 314-447-8871 (outside U.S. and Canada). Fax: 314-447-8029. E-mail: journalscustomerservice-usa@elsevier.com (for print support); journalsonlinesupport-usa@elsevier.com (for online support).

Reprints. For copies of 100 or more, of articles in this publication, please contact the Commercial Reprints Department, Elsevier Inc., 360 Park Avenue South, New York, New York 10010-1710; Tel.: 212-633-3874, Fax: 212-633-3820, E-mail: reprints@elsevier.com.

Hematology/Oncology Clinics of North America is covered in *MEDLINE/PubMed (Index Medicus), EMBASE/ Excerpta Medica, and BIOSIS.*

Printed in the United States of America.

Contributors

CONSULTING EDITORS

GEORGE P. CANELLOS, MD
William Rosenberg Professor of Medicine, Department of Medical Oncology, Dana-Farber Cancer Institute, Boston, Massachusetts

H. FRANKLIN BUNN, MD
Professor of Medicine, Division of Hematology, Brigham and Women's Hospital, Harvard Medical School, Boston, Massachusetts

EDITOR

ELLIOTT P. VICHINSKY, MD
Professor of Pediatrics, University of California San Francisco; Medical Director, Hematology/Oncology, Children's Hospital and Research Center Oakland, Oakland, California

AUTHORS

LAURA BREDA, PhD
Research Associate and Associate Professor of Genetic Medicine, Department of Pediatrics, Hematology-Oncology, Weill Cornell Medical College, New York, New York

SHANMUGANATHAN CHANDRAKASAN, MD
Fellow, Divisions of Hematology, Oncology and Bone Marrow Transplant, Cancer and Blood Disease Institute (CBDI), Cincinnati Children's Hospital Medical Center (CCHMC), Cincinnati, Ohio

STEPHEN H. EMBURY, MD
Emeritus Professor of Medicine, University of California San Francisco School of Medicine; Chief Executive Officer, Vanguard Therapeutics, Inc, Half Moon Bay, California

DOUGLAS V. FALLER, MD, PhD
Karin Grunebaum Professor and Director, Cancer Center, Boston University School of Medicine, Boston, Massachusetts

EITAN FIBACH, PhD
Department of Hematology, Hadassah–Hebrew University Medical Center, Ein-Kerem, Jerusalem, Israel

JOSHUA J. FIELD, MD, MS
Investigator, Blood Research Institute, BloodCenter of Wisconsin; Associate Professor, Department of Medicine, Medical College of Wisconsin, Milwaukee, Wisconsin

MARK D. FLEMING, MD, DPhil
Pathologist-in-Chief, S. Burt Wolbach Professor of Pathology, Department of Pathology, Boston Children's Hospital, Harvard Medical School, Boston, Massachusetts

ROBERT P. HEBBEL, MD
Regents Professor and Clark Professor; Director, Vascular Biology Center, Division of Hematology-Oncology-Transplantation, Department of Medicine, University of Minnesota Medical School, Minneapolis, Minnesota

CAROLYN C. HOPPE, MD
Associate Hematologist, Department of Hematology-Oncology, Children's Hospital & Research Center Oakland, Oakland, California

GREGORY J. KATO, MD
Professor of Medicine and Director of Sickle Cell Center of Excellence, Division of Hematology-Oncology, Department of Medicine, Heart, Lung, Blood and Vascular Medicine Institute, University of Pittsburgh, Pittsburgh, Pennsylvania

ABDULLAH KUTLAR, MD
Professor of Medicine and Director, Department of Medicine, Sickle Cell Center, Georgia Regents University, Augusta, Georgia

FRANS A. KUYPERS, PhD
Senior Scientist, Children's Hospital Oakland Research Institute, Oakland, California

JOEL LINDEN, PhD
Professor, Inflammation Biology, La Jolla Institute for Allergy and Immunology, La Jolla, California

PUNAM MALIK, MD
Professor of Pediatrics, Program Leader, Hematology and Gene Therapy, Director, Cincinnati Sickle Cell Program; Division of Experimental Hematology/Cancer Biology; Division of Hematology, Cincinnati Children's Research Foundation, Cancer and Blood Institute (CBDI), Cincinnati Children's Hospital Medical Center (CCHMC), Cincinnati, Ohio

CLAUDIA R. MORRIS, MD, FAAP
Associate Professor of Pediatrics and Emergency Medicine, Division of Emergency Medicine, Department of Pediatrics, Emory-Children's Center for Cystic Fibrosis and Airways Disease Research, Emory University School of Medicine, Atlanta, Georgia

DAVID G. NATHAN, MD
President Emeritus, Department of Pediatric Oncology, Dana-Farber Cancer Institute; Professor of Pediatrics, Division of Pediatric Hematology and Oncology, Boston Children's Hospital; Department of Pediatrics, Harvard Medical School, Boston, Massachusetts

BETTY S. PACE, MD
Professor and Chair, Department of Pediatrics and Biochemistry and Molecular Biology, Georgia Regents University, Augusta, Georgia

ZAHRA PAKBAZ, MD
Division of Hematology Oncology, Davis School of Medicine, Sacramento, California

SUSAN P. PERRINE, MD
Professor and Director Hemoglobinopathy-Thalassemia Research Unit, Cancer Center, Department of Medicine, Pediatrics, Pharmacology and Experimental Therapeutics, Boston University School of Medicine, Boston, Massachusetts

ELIEZER A. RACHMILEWITZ, MD
Wolfson Medical Center, Holon, Israel

STEFANO RIVELLA, PhD
Departments of Pediatrics, Hematology-Oncology and Cell and Developmental Biology, Weill Cornell Medical College, New York, New York

MARTIN K. SAFO, PhD
Associate Professor, Department of Medicinal Chemistry, Institute for Structural Biology and Drug Discovery, School of Pharmacy, Virginia Commonwealth University, Richmond, Virginia

PAUL J. SCHMIDT, PhD
Instructor, Department of Pathology, Boston Children's Hospital, Harvard Medical School, Boston, Massachusetts

MARILYN J. TELEN, MD
Wellcome Professor of Medicine, Division of Hematology, Department of Medicine and Duke Comprehensive Sickle Cell Center, Durham, North Carolina

TED WUN, MD
Division of Hematology Oncology, Davis School of Medicine; UC Davis Clinical and Translational Sciences Center, VA Northern California Health Care System, Sacramento, California

Contents

> Different pathways lead from the simple point mutation in hemoglobin to the membrane changes that characterize the altered interaction of the sickle red blood cell with its environment, including endothelial cells, white blood cells, and platelets. Polymerization and oxidation-induced damage to both lipid and protein components of the red cell membrane, as well as the generation of bioreactive membrane material (microparticles), has a profound effect on all tissues and organs, and defines the vasculopathy of the patient with sickle cell disease.

> Ischemia-reperfusion (I/R) physiology, also called reperfusion injury, instigates vascular and tissue injury in human disease states. This review describes why sickle cell anemia should be conceptualized in this fashion and how I/R physiology explains the genesis of characteristic aspects of vascular pathobiology and clinical disease in sickle cell anemia. The nature of I/R and its relevance to sickle cell anemia are discussed, with an emphasis on the acute chest syndrome, endothelial dysfunction with aberrant vasoregulation, circle of Willis vasculopathy, and inflammatory pain. Viewing sickle disease from this perspective elucidates defining pathophysiology and identifies a host of novel potential therapeutic targets.

> After nearly two decades of struggle, gene therapy for hemoglobinopathies using vectors carrying β or γ-globin gene has finally reached the clinical doorsteps. This was made possible by advances made in our understanding of critical regulatory elements required for high level of globin gene expression and improved gene transfer vectors and methodologies. Development of gene editing technologies and reprogramming somatic cells for regenerative medicine holds the promise of genetic correction of hemoglobinopathies in the future. This article will review the state of the field and the upcoming technologies that will allow genetic therapeutic correction of hemoglobinopathies.

has demonstrated beneficial effects. Activation of $A_{2A}Rs$ decreases inflammation with SCD by blocking activation of invariant natural killer T cells. Decreased inflammation may reduce the severity of vasoocclusive crises. Adenosine signaling through the adenosine A_{2B} receptor ($A_{2B}R$) may be detrimental in SCD. Whether adenosine signaling predominantly occurs through $A_{2A}Rs$ or $A_{2B}Rs$ may depend on differing levels of adenosine and disease state (steady state versus crisis). There may be opportunities to develop novel therapeutic approaches targeting $A_{2A}Rs$ and/or $A_{2B}Rs$ for patients with SCD.

Low global arginine bioavailability (GAB) is associated with numerous complications of SCD including early mortality. Mechanisms of arginine dysregulation involve a complex paradigm of excess activity of the arginine-consuming enzyme arginase, elevated levels of asymmetric dimethylarginine, altered intracellular arginine transport, and nitric oxide synthase dysfunction. Restoration of GAB through exogenous supplementation is therefore, a promising therapeutic target. Studies of arginine therapy demonstrate efficacy in treating patients with leg ulcers, pulmonary hypertension risk, and pain. Co-administration with hydroxyurea increases levels of nitrite and fetal hemoglobin. Addressing the alterations in the arginine metabolome may result in new strategies for treatment of SCD.

P-selectin on endothelial cell surfaces is central to impaired microvascular blood flow in sickle cell disease (SCD). Restoration of blood flow is expected to provide therapeutic benefit for SCD patients, whatever the mechanism of action of the treatment. Long-term oral administration of a P-selectin–blocking agent potentially improves blood flow and averts acute painful vasoocclusive crises in patients with SCD. This review focuses on the pathophysiology of the impairment of microvascular blood flow in SCD with an emphasis on the role of P-selectin and summarizes the status of development of antiselectin therapies as a means of improving microvascular flow.

The pathophysiology of vasoocclusion is thought to involve a wide variety of adhesive interactions involving erythrocytes, leukocytes, and the endothelium. Selectins are expressed by leukocytes, platelets, and the endothelium, among other tissues. They contribute to a wide variety of physiologically important cell-cell interactions, including adhesion of all types of blood cells to the endothelium. In vitro, in vivo, and early-phase clinical studies suggest that E-selectin and pan-selectin inhibitors may be promising new therapeutic agents for the treatment of vasoocclusion in sickle cell disease.

Recent studies suggest that sickle cell disease (SCD) is a hypercoagulable state contributing to vasoocclusive events in the microcirculation, resulting in acute and chronic sickle cell–related organ damage. In this article, we review the existing evidence for contribution of hemostatic system perturbation to SCD pathophysiology. We also review the data showing increased risk of thromboembolic events, particularly newer information on the incidence of venous thromboembolism. Finally, the potential role of platelet inhibitors and anticoagulants in SCD is briefly reviewed.

Use of new compound such as inhibitors of JAK2 or transforming growth factor β-like molecules might soon revolutionize the treatment of β-thalassemia and related disorders. However, this situation requires careful optimization, noting the potential for off-target immune suppression for JAK2 inhibitors and the lack of mechanistic insights for the use of the ligand trap soluble molecules that sequester ligands of activin receptor IIA and B.

In this article, the authors discuss new approaches to treating iron overload diseases using hepcidin mimetics or by modulating endogenous hepcidin expression. In particular, the authors discuss lipid nanoparticle encapsulated siRNA and antisense oligonucleotide–mediated inhibition of TMPRSS6, an upstream regulator of hepcidin, and treatment with transferrin or hepcidin mimetics, including the recently described *minihepcidins*. In each case, in animal models of β-thalassemia, not only do the interventions affect iron absorption but they also act as disease-modifying agents that ameliorate the ineffective erythropoiesis.

HEMATOLOGY/ONCOLOGY
CLINICS OF NORTH AMERICA

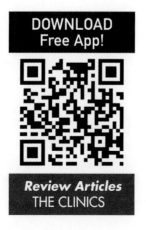

**DOWNLOAD
Free App!**

Review Articles
THE CLINICS

NOW AVAILABLE FOR YOUR iPhone and iPad

Preface

Emerging Therapy in Hemoglobinopathies: Lessons from the Past and Optimism for the Future

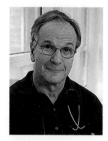

Elliott P. Vichinsky, MD
Editor

Hemoglobinopathies are a worldwide public health problem. Millions of people are affected, with over 400,000 annual births of new cases. Major, recent advances in understanding the complex pathophysiology of hemoglobinopathies have led to the development of several promising therapeutic options. This issue reviews these bench-to-bedside discoveries.[1]

The investigation of these disorders has always provided a unique window to understand basic biology and disease pathophysiology. Yet these molecular and biologic discoveries have had limited clinical impact on the hemoglobinopathy population. Supportive care, transfusion therapy, and hydroxyurea remain the only available therapies for most patients, and these options have not changed in decades. As a clinician and investigator, I am optimistic that the accomplishments described within this issue will result in decreased morbidity and improved quality of life for the patient population. However, it is important to view these discoveries in a historical context to understand the scientific chain of events that led us to these advances and the disappointment of earlier, promising therapeutic discoveries that did not achieve efficacy for the medical and patient community.

Historically, clinical symptoms of hemoglobinopathies appear to be mentioned in Hippocratic writings and have long been observed in African tribal histories. Centuries ago, the diseases were given onomatopoeic names that indicate severe pain and suffering.[2] The African medical literature of the 1870s referred to a disease called "ogbanjes" ("children who come and go") because of the high infant mortality rate with this

Hematol Oncol Clin N Am 28 (2014) xiii–xviii
http://dx.doi.org/10.1016/j.hoc.2014.01.001
0889-8588/14/$ – see front matter © 2014 Elsevier Inc. All rights reserved.

syndrome.[3] In 1910, Drs Herrick and Irons described the sickle cell erythrocyte in the peripheral smear of Dr Noel, a dental student from Granada.[4] This was rapidly followed by the work of Emmel and Hahn, who demonstrated that sickling was an oxygen-dependent phenomenon.[5] In 1934, Drs Diggs and Ching concluded that the symptoms of sickle cell disease were caused by occlusion of the microvasculature.[6] Sherman, in 1940, noted that polymerization was a key factor in the sickling process and secondary vascular obstruction.[7] A decade later Singer and Singer observed this polymerization was inhibited in the presence of fetal hemoglobin.[8] This was followed by Hofrichter and Eaton, who found that the delay time for the initiation of deoxy-hemoglobin-S polymerization was dependent on hemoglobin S concentration and the transit time of red cells.[9]

Sickle cell was classified as the first molecular disease by Pauling and colleagues[10] in 1949, who concluded from their electrophoretic studies that the basic pathology was due to a change in the amino acid structure of hemoglobin. Ingram then identified that sickle hemoglobin differed from normal hemoglobin by a single amino acid substitution of valine for glutamic acid, utilizing the newly developed fingerprinting technique to identify amino acid changes.[11] In the early 1970s, recombinant DNA technology resulted in nucleic acid sequencing showing there was an A → T DNA change in the sickle hemoglobin DNA, which changes the glutamine codon to valine.[12]

In 1980, the understanding that sickle cell disease is a complex vasculopathy was initiated by the seminal work of Hebbel and colleagues,[13] who wrote that sickled red cells abnormally adhere to endothelium and correlate with disease severity. These observations led to the central role of ischemia reperfusion injury and inflammation in sickle cell disease pathology. In 2002, Reiter and colleagues[14] noted that nitric oxide depletion in sickle cell disease is induced by free hemoglobin and amplifies the vasculopathy.

Critical advances in the pathophysiology of thalassemia and iron regulation were occurring concomitantly to discoveries in sickle cell disease. Weatherall and colleagues[15] utilized quantitative methods of hemoglobin synthesis to determine that defective and imbalanced globin synthesis were an essential part of the pathophysiology in the thalassemia syndromes. Finch and Sturgeon,[16] in studying iron and erythrokinetics in patients, demonstrated that marked ineffective erythropoiesis is a hallmark of thalassemia and is responsible for marrow expansion and increased iron absorption regardless of body iron stores. In 1978, Hershko and colleagues[17] described the toxic non-transferrin-bound fraction of plasma iron, which leads to iron-induced free radical damage. In 2001, Park and colleagues[18] discovered the peptide *hepcidin*, which drives the increased gastrointestinal iron absorption in thalassemia.

In the last 50 years, several promising therapies have been proposed based on biologic discoveries. In the 1970s, anti-sickling agents designed to impair polymerization by altering hemoglobin ligands entered clinical trials. *Urea*, initially claimed to decrease sickling, was ineffective in clinical trials and may have increased morbidity.[19] *Cyanate*, which appeared to increase oxygen affinity, resulted in severe neurologic toxicity.[20] Many other anti-sickling agents designed to alter noncovalent and covalent ligands were clinically ineffective. These were followed by clinical trials with membrane-active drugs designed to increase cell hydration. Initial studies with the antidiuretic hormone DDAVP were encouraging, but were discontinued due to lack of efficacy and toxicity.[21] *Cetiedil* induced significant improvement in red cell deformability and hydration by inhibiting the Gardos pathway. Initial clinical observations were positive, but definitive pharmaceutical trials were never undertaken.[22] Several other membrane-active agents were initiated. A novel Gardos channel inhibitor, *senicapoc*, significantly increased hemoglobin levels and improved red cell deformability, but increased pain in phase III trials resulted in its abrupt abandonment.[23] The results of these trials support the theory of different subphenotypes of sickle cell disease with the possibility of drug-induced phenotypic shifts.[24] Agents that alter red cell rheology and vascular flow entered clinical studies in the early 1980s. *Pluronic F-68* (poloxamer 188), a nonionic copolymer surfactant, showed promise in phase II trials for acute pain but was disappointing in phase III trials, with a benefit seen only in a subpopulation of children—again suggesting that drug response may be not be the same in all populations.[25]

The only successful FDA-approved pharmacologic approach to sickling has been in fetal hemoglobin induction. Following the seminal observations by DeSimone and colleagues[26,27] that *5-azacytidine* therapy increases hemoglobin F, multiple clinical trials were undertaken with different agents. 5-Azacytidine increased hemoglobin in both thalassemia and sickle cell patients. Its utilization was abandoned because of mutagenic and carcinogenic risks. Initially, it was thought to activate hemoglobin F synthesis by increased gamma gene expression by affecting methylation. However, several studies with multiple S-phase cytoxic drugs showed a similar hemoglobin F response. It was concluded that hemoglobin F was indirectly increased due to alteration of erythroid progenitor kinetics. *Hydroxyurea*, the least toxic, orally available agent underwent the most clinical studies, leading to its eventual FDA approval for use in adults with sickle cell disease.[28] Exciting work with *butyrate* and other histone deacetylase inhibitors in the mid-1980s suggested they would be efficacious. However, clinical trials were less encouraging possibly due to drug metabolism and/or inhibition of erythropoiesis.[29] Stimulation of fetal hemoglobin synthesis by erythropoietin has been demonstrated for decades, but the modest response and potential toxicity have prevented larger trials.[30]

The biologic advances in sickle cell disease and therapeutic options described in this issue grew out of the scientific foundation described above. The first two articles give an overview of the evolving understanding of the pathophysiology. Dr Kuypers discusses the red cell membrane changes—including increased phosphatidyl serine (PS) exposure—that result in the sickle cell initiating a red cell vasculopathy. He briefly discusses potential therapies to address membrane alterations such as D-annexin binding to PS surfaces. Dr Hebbel provides an insightful discussion of how ischemia reperfusion injury is most likely responsible for much of the clinical syndrome of sickle cell disease, and he reviews the therapeutic options for ischemic reperfusion injury.

Therapeutic interventions can attack sickle cell pathology from the primary mutation to its downstream effects such as inflammation and thrombosis. Drs Chandrakasan and Malik discuss the advances in gene transfer vector technology and self-inactivating *lentivirus* that have resulted in the initial pilot success in thalassemia. They review recent discoveries that will improve clinical options, including gene editing technology, newer vectors, and induced pleuripotent stem cells.

The re-emergence of research interest in the causal relationship between decreased oxygen affinity of hemoglobin S and increased polymerization has resulted in promising pilot clinical studies with hemoglobin modifiers that increase oxygen affinity. Dr Safo and Dr Kato review the pathophysiologic effects resulting from sickle red cells exposed to low oxygen affinity and relevant therapeutic approaches, including the investigations with the aldehyde Aes-1035-HMF.

For several decades, increasing fetal hemoglobin has been a major focus in the treatment of hemoglobinopathies. Except for hydroxyurea, which received FDA approval 20 years ago, there remains no other commercially available hemoglobin

F inducer. Drs Perrine, Pace, and Fowler review the history of hemoglobin F therapeutics and the recent advances in the understanding of fetal hemoglobin regulation. They discuss the new generation of noncytotoxic hemoglobin F inducers, including short-chain fatty acids, low-dose decitabine tetrahydrouridine, benserazide, as well as combinations with epigenetic modifiers and agents that increase translation. Dr Fibach and Dr Rachmilewitz review the effects of erythropoietin administration on hemoglobin F production as well as erythropoiesis, iron utilization, and oxidative stress. They discuss potential trials of erythropoietin alone or in combination with new emerging therapies.

Sickle cell disease is now considered an acute and chronic inflammatory condition. Dr Hoppe summarizes the in vitro and in vivo studies indicating the importance of inflammation in the development of its vasculopathy. Her article provides an overview of the cellular mechanisms involved in the inflammatory response and therapeutic agents that target these pathways. Discussion of key pathways involving adenosine signaling, nitric oxide/arginine dysregulation, selectins, and coagulation is expanded in individual articles. Drs Field, Nathan, and Linden review the important beneficial and detrimental effects of adenosine signaling in SCD pathophysiology. They discuss the anti-inflammatory effect of adenosine resulting from decreased activation of invariant NKT cells mediated by the adenosine A_{2A} receptor and the proinflammatory response to binding with the adenosine A_{2B} receptor. The in vitro and clinical studies with adenosine therapeutics are reviewed, including $A_{2A}R$ agonist regadenoson, and $A_{2B}R$ antagonist pegylated -ADA. Dr Morris reviews the recent studies that demonstrate arginine metabolomics and the dysregulation of nitric oxide hemostasis that plays an important role in the pathophysiology of sickle cell disease. The clinical benefit of arginine supplementation alone or with hydroxyurea in the treatment of leg ulcers, pulmonary hypertension, priapism, and pain is discussed.

Vaso-occlusion and impaired microvascular flow characterize the pathophysiology of sickle cell disease. The adhesive interactions involving erythrocytes, the endothelium, leukocytes, and platelets are central to this process. Selectins are adhesive receptors expressed on these cells that initiate the adhesive interactions. There are multiple species of selectins involved in this process. Drs Kultar and Embury discuss the key role of endothelial P-selectin-mediated cell adhesion as an initiator of abnormal blood flow in sickle cell disease. The authors reviewed the beneficial effects observed in pilot studies with P-selectin blocking agents, including pentosan polysulfate sodium. Dr Telen provides an informative review of the importance of E- and L-selectin in sickle cell disease pathology. GMI1070, a small carbohydrate molecule that binds to selectins—particularly E-selectin, is discussed in detail with highlights of the successful early trials. Dr Pakbaz and Dr Wun highlight the contribution of hemostatic abnormalities in the process of vaso-occlusion and impaired microvascular flow. They review the data showing increased risk of thromboembolic events, the potential role of platelet inhibitors, and anticoagulants.

The issue concludes with recent advances in understanding pathways that modulate erythropoiesis and iron physiology. Drs Rivella and Breda discuss the important role that JAK2 activity has in stress erythropoiesis and the potential therapeutic benefits of JAK2 inhibitors. They discuss the effects of activin signaling in hematopoiesis and the therapeutic strategies targeting deregulation of activin signaling—including clinical studies with ACE/RAP-011 and ACE536. Drs Schmidt and Fleming review the advances in understanding the hepcidin-ferroportin iron regulatory axis. They discuss new approaches to treating iron overload diseases utilizing hepcidin mimetics or by altering endogenous heparin expression. They highlight lipid nanoparticle encapsulated siRNA and antisense oligonucleotide ASO-mediated inhibition of TMPRSS6, and mini-hepcidin therapy. In β-thalassemia intermedia, they discuss the murine model results with transferrin therapy and hepcidin up-regulation.

Elliott P. Vichinsky, MD
Children's Hospital and Research Center Oakland
747 52nd Street
Oakland, CA 94609, USA

E-mail address:
evichinsky@mail.cho.org

REFERENCES

1. Piel FB, Hay SI, Gupta S, et al. Global burden of sickle cell anaemia in children under five, 2010-2050: modeling based on demographics, excess mortality, and interventions. PLoS Med 2013;10(7):e1001484.
2. Konotey-Ahulu FID. Hereditary qualitative and quantitative erythrocyte defects in Ghana: an historical and geographical survey. Ghana Med J 1968;7:188–9.
3. Asakitikpi AE. Born to Die: The Ogbanje Phenomenon and its Implication on Childhood Mortality in Southern Nigeria. Anthropologist 2008;10(1):59–63.
4. Savitt TL, Goldberg MF. Herrick's 1910 case report of sickle cell anemia. The rest of the story. JAMA 1989;261(2):266–71.
5. Emmel VE. A study of erythrocytes in a case of severe anemia with elongated and sickle-shaped red blood corpuscles. Arch Intern Med 1917;20:586–98.
6. Diggs LW, Ching RE. Pathology of sickle cell anemia. South Med J 1934;27: 839–45.
7. Sherman IJ. The sickling phenomenon, with special reference to the differentiation of sickle cell anemia from the sickle cell trait. Bull Johns Hopkins Hosp 1940;67:309–24.
8. Singer K, Singer L. The gelling phenomenon of sickle cell hemoglobin: its biological and diagnostic significance. Blood 1953;8:1008–23.
9. Hofrichter J, Ross PD, Eaton WA. Kinetics and mechanism of deoxyhemoglobin S gelation: a new approach to understanding sickle cell disease. Proc Natl Acad Sci USA 1974;71:4864–8.
10. Pauling L, Itano H, Singer SJ, et al. Sickle cell anemia: a molecular disease. Science 1949;14:279–84.
11. Ingram VM. A specific chemical difference between the globins of normal human and sickle-cell anemia haemoglobin. Nature 1956;178:792–4.
12. Marotta CA, Wilson JT, Forget BG, et al. Human β-globin messenger RNA III. Nucleotide sequences derived from complementary DNA. J Biol Chem 1977; 252:5040–51.
13. Hebbel RP, Boogaerts MA, Eaton JW, et al. Erythrocyte adherence to endothelium in sickle-cell anemia. A possible determinant of disease severity. N Engl J Med 1980;302(18):992–5.
14. Reiter CD, Wang X, Tanus-Santos JE, et al. Cell-free hemoglobin limits nitric oxide bioavailability in sickle-cell disease. Nat Med 2002;8(12):1383–9.
15. Weatherall DJ, Clegg JB, Naughton MA. Globin synthesis in thalassaemia: an in vitro study. Nature 1965;208(5015):1061–5.
16. Finch CA, Sturgeon P. Erythrokinetics in Cooley's anemia. Blood 1957;12(1): 64–73.

17. Hershko C, Graham G, Bates GW, et al. Non-specific serum iron in thalassaemia: an abnormal serum iron fraction of potential toxicity. Br J Haematol 1978;40(2): 255–63.
18. Park CH, Valore EV, Waring AJ, et al. Hepcidin, a urinary antimicrobial peptide synthesized in the liver. J Biol Chem 2001;276(11):7806–10.
19. Treatment of sickle cell crisis with urea in invert sugar. JAMA 1974;228(9):1125–8.
20. Langer EE, Stamatoyannopoulos G, Hlastala MP, et al. Extracorporeal treatment with cyanate in sickle cell disease: preliminary observations in four patients. J Lab Clin Med 1976;87(3):462–74.
21. Charache S, Moyer MA, Walker WG. Treatment of acute sickle cell crises with a vasopressin analogue. Am J Hematol 1983;15(4):315–9.
22. Benjamin LJ, Berkowitz LR, Orringer E, et al. A collaborative, double-blind ran-domized study of cetiedil citrate in sickle cell crisis. Blood 1986;67(5):1442–7.
23. Ataga KI, Reid M, Ballas SK, et al. ICAS-17043-10 Investigators. Improvements in haemolysis and indicators of erythrocyte survival do not correlate with acute vaso-occlusive crises in patients with sickle cell disease: a phase III randomized, placebo-controlled, double-blind study of the Gardos channel blocker senicapoc (ICA-17043). Br J Haematol 2011;153(1):92–104.
24. Castro OL, Gordeuk VR, Gladwin MT, et al. Senicapoc trial results support the ex-istence of different sub-phenotypes of sickle cell disease with possible drug-induced phenotypic shifts. Br J Haematol 2011;155(5):636–8.
25. Orringer EP, Casella JF, Ataga KI, et al. Purified poloxamer 188 for treatment of acute vaso-occlusive crisis of sickle cell disease: a randomized controlled trial. JAMA 2001;286(17):2099–106.
26. DeSimone J, Heller P, Hall L, et al. 5-Azacytidine stimulates fetal hemoglobin syn-thesis in anemic baboons. Proc Natl Acad Sci USA 1982;79(14):4428–31.
27. Ley TJ, DeSimone J, Noguchi CT, et al. 5-Azacytidine increases gamma-globin synthesis and reduces the proportion of dense cells in patients with sickle cell anemia. Blood 1983;62(2):370–80.
28. Charache S, Terrin ML, Moore RD, et al. Effect of hydroxyurea on the frequency of painful crises in sickle cell anemia. Investigators of the Multicenter Study of Hydroxyurea in Sickle Cell Anemia. N Engl J Med 1995;332(20):1317–22.
29. Perrine SP, Ginder GD, Faller DV, et al. A short-term trial of butyrate to stimulate fetal-globin-gene expression in the beta-globin disorders. N Engl J Med 1993; 328(2):81–6.
30. Al-Khatti A, Veith RW, Papayannopoulou T, et al. Stimulation of fetal hemoglobin synthesis by erythropoietin in baboons. N Engl J Med 1987;317(7):415–20.

Dedication

I would like to dedicate this book to Sir David Weatherall. David is the best scientist and clinician-teacher I've ever met. He makes the clinician want to be a scientist, and the scientist want to be a clinician.

Elliott P. Vichinsky, MD
Medical Director, Hematology/Oncology
Children's Hospital & Research Center Oakland
747 52nd Street, Oakland, CA 94609, USA

E-mail address:
evichinsky@mail.cho.org

Hematol Oncol Clin N Am 28 (2014) xix
http://dx.doi.org/10.1016/j.hoc.2014.01.002
0889-8588/14/$ – see front matter © 2014 Published by Elsevier Inc.

Hemoglobin S Polymerization and Red Cell Membrane Changes

Frans A. Kuypers, PhD

KEYWORDS

- Polymerization • Oxidative damage • Membrane lipids • Microparticles

KEY POINTS

- Although the pathophysiology of sickle cell disease may be uniquely related to the polymerization of sickle hemoglobin under low oxygen conditions, it has become apparent that many factors are involved in the vasculopathy that characterizes this disorder affecting millions of individuals worldwide.
- The altered red blood cell (RBC) membrane plays an important role in the dysfunctional interactions of the sickle RBC with other blood cells and vascular endothelium, and leads to premature recognition and removal, an imbalance in hemostasis, vaso-occlusive events, and intravascular hemolysis, and may be involved in acute chest syndrome.
- The complex, well-orchestrated RBC membrane phospholipid organization is apparently lost in subpopulations of RBC during erythropoiesis as well as in the circulation. Increased oxidant stress may play an important role in the inability of the RBC to maintain composition and asymmetry in phospholipid molecular species, but the mechanisms that lead to phosphatidylserine (PS) exposure are poorly understood.
- This lack of knowledge is in part due to the incomplete characterization of the proteins involved in the maintenance of phospholipid asymmetry in the RBC, as well as the complexity of studying a complete plasma membrane in which several protein entities act in synchronization with each other and are governed by protein-protein and protein-lipid interactions.
- The purification and/or expression of the proteins thought to be involved in membrane organization in well-defined lipid bilayers, their 3-dimensional structural modeling, and detailed functional characterization may lead to a better understanding of their individual functions and their interaction with other entities in the bilayer.
- This knowledge will also lead to a better understanding of how the function of these proteins is impaired or altered in leading to PS exposure in hemoglobinopathies, and to a definition of the molecular underpinnings of this complex pathophysiology.

INTRODUCTION

It has been 100 years since Herrick published the first medical case report of the anemia describing abnormal shapes of red blood cells (RBCs) and gave sickle cell anemia its name.[1] In 1949, Pauling and Itano[2] defined the underlying molecular reason by identifying hemoglobin S (HbS), and defined sickle cell anemia as the first

Children's Hospital Oakland Research Institute, 5700 Martin Luther King Jr. Way, Oakland, CA 94609, USA
E-mail address: fkuypers@chori.org

Hematol Oncol Clin N Am 28 (2014) 155–179
http://dx.doi.org/10.1016/j.hoc.2013.12.002
0889-8588/14/$ – see front matter © 2014 Elsevier Inc. All rights reserved.

hemonc.theclinics.com

"molecular disease." The last 60 years have resulted in an increasingly coherent detailed molecular-level description of the pathophysiology of sickle cell disease (SCD). While great progress has been made in describing the basic disease process that accounts for hemolytic anemia and the obstructive events underlying vaso-occlusive events (VOE), many questions remain. The simple mutation in the β6 location of globin has a profound effect on all tissues and organs in the SCD patient, and because the vasculopathy affects a large variety of physiologic mechanisms, the varied genetic background of individual patients makes prediction of the clinical severity highly complex. However, it assuredly starts with the mutated hemoglobin (Hb) and the changes in the membrane that result from it. Hb is a complex molecule that undergoes conformational changes in response to oxygen, and is affected by environmental changes, allosteric effectors, and mutations. The polymerization of deoxy HbS, which forms long fibers inside the RBC, leads to the typical distorted sickle RBC (SRBC) morphology that was noted by Herrick. Together with changes in cytosol, which result from the relatively unstable pro-oxidant character of HbS,[3] the morphology and ability of the SRBC to deform are affected. Both the mechanical stress on the RBC membrane and oxidation-induced damage affect both lipid and protein components of the RBC membrane and alter the interaction of the SRBC with its environment, including endothelial cells, white blood cells, and platelets, and leads to the loss of bioactive membrane material (particles). A loss of normal ion permeability of the SRBC membrane leads to an altered hydration status of the cell. In turn this affects polymerization, and an altered cytosolic calcium status affects a variety of processes, which will affect the plasma membrane and lead to apoptosis during erythropoiesis, in addition to hemolysis and early removal of the adult SRBC. While different pathways may lead from the simple point mutation in hemoglobin to the membrane alterations, the changes in the SRBC membrane and the downstream effects on its environment result in the vasculopathy that characterizes the disease.

POLYMERIZATION

As the predominant cell type, the RBC largely determines the rheologic and hemodynamic behavior of blood. The intricate mechanisms that govern the interaction of the RBC membrane skeleton with membrane proteins and the lipid bilayer[4,5] provide the ability of the RBC to deform under shear stress in the circulation and regain its typical shape as a biconcave disk. In SCD, mechanically fragile, poorly deformable RBCs contribute to impaired blood flow and other pathophysiologic aspects of the disease.[6,7] Formation of hemoglobin polymers in the SRBC negatively affect the RBC's ability to maintain its normal morphology, and it has long been considered that the radical shape change of the SRBC under low oxygen leads to the inability of the SRBC to properly deform and pass though the microvasculature, leading to VOE.[8–11] In addition to the change in shape, HbS polymer formation will cause mechanical stress on the RBC membrane, resulting in membrane changes as well as loss of membrane material, evidenced by the increased circulating RBC-derived microparticles (MPs). The kinetics of HbS polymerization are affected by the presence of normal Hb (HbA) or fetal Hb (HbF). Although sickle cell trait individuals (HbAS) can experience VOE, this is a rare event and seems related to extreme dehydration or low oxygen tension as experienced at higher altitudes. The replacement of 50% of HbS by HbA slows polymerization by approximately 100-fold.[12] Increased levels of gammaglobulin ameliorate the severity of SCD because HbF can effectively replace HbS and lower the rate of polymerization, providing a treatment protocol by reversing the

Hb switch that occurs before birth. The success of hydroxyurea (HU) treatment is mainly based on increasing HbF levels,[13] but the understanding of the molecular mechanism of globin switching is still unclear. In addition to HbF modulation,[14] HU has been implicated in affecting several different genes,[15] the SRBC proteome,[16] and other mechanisms including adhesion,[17–19] phosphatidylserine (PS) exposure,[20] and fatty acid metabolism.[21] Given the central role of HbS polymerization, several approaches aimed at affecting gammaglobulin production have been explored, including the use of decitabine, butyrate, lenalidomide, and pomalidomide (see later discussion). Increased understanding of the factors that regulate gammaglobulin expression provides potential novel approaches, such as the recently identified chromatin factor Friend of Prmt1 (FOP), a critical modulator of gammaglobulin gene expression.[22] Of importance, the complex genetic background of the sickle cell patient that seems to affect the clinical course of the disease has also led to the identification of specific single-nucleotide polymorphisms (SNPs) related to the expression of HbF.[23–26] The repressor BCL11A,[27–31] in particular, seems important in defining the response to hydroxyurea treatment.[32] Because the state of RBC hydration links directly to polymerization, drugs have been tested that decrease intracellular HbS concentration by increasing total cell volume by modulating membrane ion-exchange channels, such as the Gardos Channels and the KCL Cotransporter. These compounds include magnesium pidolate,[33] imidazole antimycotics, arginine, and Senicapoc. In addition to the types of Hb that make up the Hb mixture in the SRBC, the rate of polymerization is strongly affected by the interface between the 2 α/β dimers, exposed in the deoxy state. Factors that modulate this interaction will affect polymerization; the excessive amount of heme[34] released in SRBCs[35] is one of these factors. Free heme at micromolar concentrations induces strong attraction between the hemoglobin molecules,[36] and drastically increases rates of nucleation and polymer fiber growth.[37] In addition to the rate of polymerization, it is also important that modulation of the kinetics of depolymerization is essential to achieve full dissolution of polymers in the lungs or resolution of VOE. Conditions whereby residual HbS polymers exist facilitate repolymerization and thus may be related to abnormality.[38] Because deoxygenation drives the polymerization of HbS, mutations that affect the oxygen-binding equilibrium will likely affect the sickling process. A small number of these mutations occur in 3 predicted druggable binding pockets that might be exploited to directly inhibit polymerization.[39] Compounds that modulate oxygen affinity are tested for their efficacy to increase oxygen affinity and decrease HbS polymerization (see later discussion). Although some studies have been promising in a transgenic sickle animal model, there is a paucity of data from human studies. A promising antisickling agent is yet to be established.[40] In addition, mechanisms that are normally physiologically active in modulating oxygen affinity are exploited. Such mechanisms include hypoxia-mediated elevated adenosine signaling[41] (see later discussion). In addition to polymerization under low oxygen, it has to be taken into account that the oxygenation state of the RBC affects many aspects of RBC metabolism, owing to the interaction of (deoxygenated) Hb and membrane components. Band 3, an integral membrane protein linked to the spectrin/actin cytoskeleton, preferentially binds to deoxygenated Hb at its N-terminus, and affects the association between band 3 and the underlying RBC cytoskeleton.[42] This process affects the generation of adenosine triphosphate (ATP), hydrogenated nicotine adenine dinucleotide (NADH), 2,3-diphosphoglycerate (DPG), and NADH phosphate (NADPH) as the result of competition between deoxyhemoglobin and key Embden-Meyerhof pathway enzymes for binding to the cytoplasmic domain of band 3. In oxygenated RBCs, NADPH generation maximizes glutathione-based antioxidant systems through the hexose monophosphate pathway. A constrained hexose monophosphate pathway flux, caused by| an abnormal oxygen-dependent association of sickle hemoglobin with the RBC membrane, interferes with the regulation of NADPH. This reduced resilience to NADPH, and glutathione recycling and oxidative stress, is manifested by membrane protein oxidation and membrane fragility, suggesting that hypoxia may influence the SCD phenotype[43] independent of polymerization.

EFFECTS OF HBS ON MEMBRANES

The presence of HbS results in many changes in the SRBC cytosol and its membrane, including an altered proteomic[44,45] or metabolomics profile,[46] redox status, altered ion transport,[47] changed adhesive properties[48] (see later discussion), and loss of membrane lipid asymmetry, resulting in PS exposure. Metabolic signatures of specialized circulating hematopoietic cells using liquid chromatography–mass spectrometry based metabolite profiling reveal that RBC and SRBC metabolomes display major differences in glycolysis, glutathione, ascorbate metabolism, and metabolites associated with membrane turnover. In addition, the amounts of metabolites derived from the urea cycle and nitric oxide metabolism that partly take place within RBCs seem different.[49] In part this is related to factors that maintain the redox status and oxygen affinity.

A complicating factor is that SRBCs form a highly heterogeneous population, and membranes are altered differently in subpopulations of RBCs, which makes it extremely difficult to link clinical observations or membrane changes to the average SRBC. The SRBC population includes a wide range of young-deformable to rigid-irreversible SRBCs, as well as cells with different states of hydration. The RBC membrane is endowed with a large variety of ion channels. Although the physiologic role of several of these channels remains unclear and inactive in the resting cell, when activated experimentally these ion channels can lead to a very high single-cell conductance and potentially induce disorders, with the major risks of rapid dehydration and dissipation of gradients.[50] The presence of circulating dense RBCs is important in SCD-related clinical manifestations, but the large range of densities in SRBCs indicates that the membrane alterations that lead to permeability changes of the SRBC vary significantly from cell to cell. The SRBC population exhibits heterogeneous adhesive behavior attributable to the diverse cell morphologies and membrane properties. More adhesive SRBCs interact with the vascular endothelium and trap irreversible sickle cells (ISCs); similarly, adherent leukocytes may also trap ISCs resulting in vaso-occlusion in small and even larger vessels.[51] Although the presence of only a small percentage of PS-exposing cells may sound less important, the prothrombotic PS-exposing surface that these SRBCs provide is very significant in comparison with, for example, the total number of platelets in the circulation.

Furthermore, it is difficult to separate the effects of polymerization from the other changes induced by HbS, including oxidant stress. Oxidant stress will alter the RBC membrane such that additional mechanical stress will result in much larger changes.[52] The altered cytosolic composition of the SRBC leads to several downstream effects. For example, the loss of proper calcium homeostasis in SRBCs will affect several pathways. Ca^{2+} is a universal signaling molecule involved in regulating cell cycle and fate, cell metabolism and structural integrity, and cell motility and volume. Like other cells, erythroid cells, during development and in the circulation, rely on Ca^{2+}-dependent signaling. Intracellular Ca^{2+} levels in the circulating human RBCs take part not only in controlling biophysical properties such as membrane composition, volume, and rheologic properties, but also physiologic parameters such as metabolic activity, redox state, PS exposure, and cell clearance.[53–55]

OXIDATIVE STRESS

A common denominator in the alterations in the SRBC and the damage to the RBC membrane is the well-recognized increased HbS auto-oxidation and Fenton chemistry reactions catalyzed by denatured heme moieties bound to the RBC membrane, further enhanced by NADPH oxidase, which is regulated by protein kinase C, Rac guanosine triphosphatase, and intracellular Ca^{2+} signaling within the sickle RBC[56] (see later discussion). The extremely high level of oxidant stress in SRBC[3] or thalassemic RBC[57–59] leads to higher levels of damage and premature aging of these cells. Footprints of increased oxidant damage such as methemoglobin (MetHb), lipid peroxidation products, or altered protein thiol status, are found in both thalassemic RBCs and SRBCs. The main function of the RBC, oxygen transport, requires a special skill set to deal with the oxidant stress that results from this activity. The continuous process of Hb oxygenation and deoxygenation is accompanied by transient and reversible changes in heme iron redox state from the ferrous (Fe^{2+}) to the ferric (Fe^{3+}) state, with small amounts of superoxide being produced in the process.[60] A complex system of antioxidants and enzymes aims to protect the RBC from oxidant-induced damage. These agents include enzymes such as superoxide dismutase, catalase, thiol-active reagents (glutathione, peroxyredoxin, ergothionine), lipid antioxidants (vitamin E), and enzyme systems that can regenerate oxidized compounds using RBC metabolism, as well as systems that can repair lipid and protein damage. The latter are important, as the RBC is unable to generate new protein and lipid, and despite the antioxidant systems in place, damage to lipids and proteins does occur. These oxidant-induced alterations in structure and function of the RBC need to be repaired, and the inability to do so will lead to the demise of the cell and is in part responsible for the limited life span of the RBC. Superoxide generated by hemoglobin is transformed to hydrogen peroxide (H_2O_2) by superoxide dismutase and subsequently reduced by catalase to water.[61] Superoxide can cause the formation of ferric methemoglobin (metHb), which in turn is reduced back to its oxygen-binding ferrous state by metHb reductase.[60] One percent to 2% of the hemoglobin exists as metHb[60] in normal cells, which in turn is the starting point of the enzymatic reaction that leads to the formation of hemoglobin peroxidase. In the presence of H_2O_2, metHb act as peroxidase and catalyzes the 2-electron reduction of H_2O_2 to water from oxidizing other biological cosubstrates (DNA, lipids, and proteins) in the process. During this process, H_2O_2 (or lipid hydroperoxide) oxidizes ferric heme to perferryl heme and forms a protein-centered radical.[62] The catalytic redox cycling between the perferryl and ferric heme makes a potent peroxide-fueled radical generator. Both perferryl and the protein-centered radicals are highly reactive, like hydroxyl radicals, and are capable of oxidizing biological macromolecules.[63–65] Several thiol-based antioxidant systems are well described in the literature while others are less well studied. The primary defense against heme peroxidase activity is the efficient removal of H_2O_2. In addition to the catalase activity,[61] peroxiredoxin II (Prx II) is a noncatalytic scavenger of H_2O_2, which at 250 μM is the second or third most abundant protein expressed in RBCs. Prx II is the principal protein responsible for detoxifying endogenously generated H_2O_2, but during the course of peroxidation the catalytic cysteine residue of Prx II becomes overoxidized and must be regenerated in a thioredoxin-dependent manner.[60,66] The rate of Prx II regeneration is slow and limits its efficiency in scavenging peroxides at higher concentrations. Consistent with the importance in RBC biology, Prx II knockout mice are anemic and exhibit an elevated rate of RBC turnover, and experience higher rate of oxidative damage. Ergothioneine (ergo), a thiol antioxidant, is predominantly synthesized in fungal organisms[67] and is the second most abundant RBC thiol compound.[68] However, the reasons for this abundance in hematopoietic tissues has not been investigated. Interestingly HbS, which increases Hb pro-oxidant activity, selectively depletes ergo over glutathione, suggesting that ergo has a specialized glutathione-independent function in protecting RBCs against pro-oxidative hemoglobin. Humans lack the capacity to synthesize ergo, but the presence of a highly efficient ergo transporter (Organic Cation Transporter Na Dependent 1; OCTN1) ensures its accumulation and retention across different tissues and cell types.[69,70] Because ergo is derived strictly from diet, it may potentially be an essential (or conditionally essential) dietary micronutrient. At physiologic pH, ergo exists primarily as a thione and acts as a weak antioxidant. Therefore, it is unlikely that its primary role would be its radical scavenging ability.[71] Its weak redox activity also minimizes its pro-oxidant interactions with transition metals[72] and protein-SH moieties. Therefore, cells can accumulate ergo in large quantities without toxicity. It seems logical to assume that ergo is a specialized antioxidant for protecting maturing hematopoietic cells and mature RBCs. A major part of its pro-oxidative potential involves its ability to act as a pseudoperoxidase in the presence of peroxides. High expression of the ergo transporter in hematopoietic precursor cells[69,70] relative to other major tissues, and increased expression in maturing erythroid cells that produce high levels of hemoglobin, corroborate the hypothesis of a critical antioxidant role of ergo during hematopoiesis and in determining the health of mature RBCs. The ability to deal with oxidant stress is compromised and challenged in SCD, resulting in an unbalanced redox state, an altered thiol redox metabolism, and protein and lipid damage. In addition to the altered redox status inside the RBC, the increased levels of hemolysis observed in SCD, as well as iron overload resulting from anemia and transfusion therapy, adds to the oxidant-induced tissue damage. Plasma proteins such as hemopexin[73] and haptoglobin[74] bind to cell-free heme and hemoglobin, and minimize their toxicity. In addition, the prompt induction of the heme-catabolizing enzyme, heme oxygenase-1, during oxidative stress conditions allows cells to attenuate heme stress by degrading excess heme to bilirubin and carbon monoxide gas.[35,75] An antioxidant system specifically designed for inhibiting heme peroxidase activity has not been clearly identified. This factor seems particularly important, as hemoglobin peroxidase is a potent catalyst for damage following hemolysis observed in SCD. In addition to SCD,[76] nonspecific tissue damage from heme/hemoprotein peroxidase activity has been detected in conditions such as myocardial infarcts[77] and cerebral hemorrhage.[65] In all of these cases, myoglobin or hemoglobin released from dying tissues or the RBCs act as peroxidase and initiate nonspecific oxidation of proteins, lipids, and DNA. This mechanism is further illustrated by the presence of myoglobin/hemoglobin cross-linked products in biological fluids (plasma and cerebral spinal fluids) following rhabdomyolysis (muscle damage) or subarachnoid hemorrhage.[63,77,78] These cross-linked products can only be created when protein-centered radicals are formed during myoglobin/hemoglobin peroxidase reactions. In Alzheimer disease, high levels of β-amyloid in the brain can bind tightly to heme[79–81] and act as a peroxidase, causing damage to surrounding neurons in the presence of excess hydrogen peroxide,[82,83] and hemoglobin peroxidase activity has been shown to exacerbate atherogenesis by promoting plaque lipid oxidation and endothelial cell damage.[84] Although these conditions may not seem to be related to the sickle cell mutation, it has to be considered that the multiorgan damage typical of SCD has components that are closely related, and it needs to be considered that treatment regimens used for these disorders may also be applicable to SCD.

MICROPARTICLES

MPs[85] are submicron membrane vesicles or "membrane dust," shed by compromised cells including RBCs. MPs have been described as biomarkers in various vascular diseases, including SCD, and have been associated with an increased risk of thrombosis. Although decline of HbF coincided with an increase in circulating MPs, treatment with hydroxyurea showed lower concentrations of total MPs shed by platelets and RBCs.[86] The increased level of MPs in SCD is linked to intravascular hemolysis, as shown by the correlation between levels of MPs and plasma Hb. In addition, subpopulations of RBCs expressing PS were associated with MPs, and HU treatment decreased these parameters in comparison with untreated controls.[87] Band 3, an integral membrane protein linked to the spectrin/actin cytoskeleton, preferentially binds to deoxygenated Hb at its N-terminus, and affects the association between band 3 and the underlying RBC cytoskeleton.[42] The displacement of ankyrin from band 3 leads to release of the spectrin/actin cytoskeleton from the membrane, and is able to promote unwanted membrane vesiculation and the formation of RBC-derived MPs. The cytoplasmic domain of band 3 serves as a center of RBC membrane organization and constitutes the major substrate of RBC tyrosine kinases. Tyrosine phosphorylation of band 3 is induced by several physiologic stimuli, including malaria parasite invasion, cell shrinkage, normal cell aging, and oxidant stress such as occurs in SCD. Oxidative insult, and band 3 oligomers that result, contribute to the adhesive nature of SRBCs with regard to endothelial cells.[88] Because release of band 3 from its ankyrin and adducin linkages to the cytoskeleton can facilitate changes in multiple membrane properties, tyrosine phosphorylation of band 3 is argued to enable adaptive changes in RBC biology that permit the cell to respond to stress.[89]

In addition to stress from the inside of the SRBC, external factors also have been implicated in the formation of this membrane dust. Thrombospondin 1 (TSP1) triggered rapid RBC conversion into echinocytes in vitro, followed by MP shedding. In a sickle mouse model, TSP1 led to the formation of PS, stimulating MPs and initiating vaso-occlusions within minutes. These events could be countered by cloaking the PS-positive surfaces with annexin-V[90] (PS on the membrane surface of RBCs is discussed in more detail later). The expression of PS on circulating MPs plays an important role in the etiology of the hypercoagulable state of SCD, as well as in the reduced life span of RBCs and adhesive interactions between RBCs and endothelium.

MEMBRANE LIPID

The lipid bilayer of the RBC is likely the best studied mammalian plasma bilayer, and has revealed a highly complex and dynamic system whereby a diverse compilation of molecules are continuously renewed, move rapidly in the plane and across the bilayer in a highly orchestrated fashion, providing the membrane proteins a proper environment and maintaining a proper barrier that separates cytosol from the cell's environment. This system is altered in subpopulations of the SRBC population, leading to altered membrane surface characteristics and permeability. In turn this leads to the large variation in cellular hydration, interaction with other blood cells, and early demise of the SRBC. During the early stages of erythropoiesis, the more than 250 molecular species of glycerophospholipid and sphingomyelin (SM)[91] that form the structural backbone of the lipid bilayer if the RBC are synthesized de novo. Although it can be expected that these molecular species are remodeled by deacylation and reacylation during the various stages of RBC development, virtually no data on these processes during erythropoiesis are available. In the last stage of RBC development, a portion of the membrane lipid bilayer during enucleation is lost and the reticulocyte is born.

Further remodeling in the circulation results in additional loss of membrane material, and the adult RBC starts its life. The glycerophospholipid molecular species (phosphatidylcholine [PC], phosphatidylethanolamine [PE], and PS) together with SM and cholesterol, make up most of the plasma membrane lipids. Their rapid movement in the plane of the bilayer is highly organized and leads to areas that are enriched in specific phospholipid molecular species. These areas or microdomains provide a specific environment for membrane proteins to regulate the traffic of ions and signals across the bilayer. Across the bilayer lipids are highly asymmetrically distributed, with the aminophospholipids mainly (PE) or exclusively (PS) in the inner leaflet of the bilayer and the choline phospholipids (PC, SM) mainly in the outer leaflet. The mature mammalian RBC lacks internal organelles and is incapable of de novo lipid synthesis. Nevertheless, a very dynamic system maintains the overall composition and organization of the membrane during the life of the adult RBC. Lipid molecules are continuously renewed. Fatty acids are rapidly taken up from plasma and incorporated into phospholipids. Despite this rapid phospholipid turnover, and the continuous changes in the substrate pool (plasma fatty acids, determined by diet), the molecular species composition of RBC is remarkably constant. This stability indicates a highly selective system within which several components act in synchronization; it thus seems appropriate to hypothesize that the activities of these proteins are regulated by lipid-protein and/or protein-protein interactions in the membrane that "sense" the need for the generation of certain molecular species or the need for lipid (re-)distribution in the plane and across the bilayer. The mechanisms for these interactions are largely unknown, in part because many of the membrane proteins involved are poorly characterized. Similarly, whereas the exposure of PS on the surface of both adult RBC and RBC precursors is well recognized as an important contributor to SCD pathology, the mechanisms that lead to this exposure are still poorly defined.

LIPID TURNOVER

The turnover of membrane fatty acyl groups and the redistribution of phospholipids across the bilayer is in part the result of the basic function of the RBC, the transport of oxygen, as already indicated. The high levels of reactive oxygen species (ROS) lead to damage of the polyunsaturated acyl groups in the different phospholipid classes despite the presence of a network of antioxidant systems. This aspect is particularly important when either antioxidants are compromised or, as is the case in SCD, when more ROS are generated. The polyunsaturated fatty acids in the phospholipids are prime targets for alterations in oxygen radicals. When oxygen reacts with the double bonds, it introduces a polar entity in the apolar chains. This breach in the normal membrane structure is recognized by phospholipases,[92] which hydrolyze the ester bond and generate lysophospholipids, starting a repair process.[93] Several proteins involved in the deacylation/reacylation mechanism (the so-called Lands pathway[94]) have been identified, including acyl–coenzyme A (CoA) synthetases, acyl-CoA binding proteins, and acyl-CoA transferases.[95–98] The acyl-CoA synthetase ACSL6 in the membrane of the adult RBC activates fatty acids taken up from plasma by ligation of the fatty acid to CoA at the expense of ATP.[98] Subsequently the acyl-CoA is transferred to lysophospholipid by members of the elusive lysophospholipid acyl-CoA acyltransferase (LPLAT) family. Different members of the LPLAT family have preferences for the different phospholipid headgroups, and different proteins may be responsible for the reacylation of lysophosphatidylcholine (LPC), lysophosphatidylethanolamine (LPE), and lysophosphatidylserine (LPS). The protein that reacylates LPC to PC in the RBC membrane was recently identified,[99] and was shown to be sensitive to both calcium and oxidant stress.[100] Oxidant damage is random in nature, and the phospholipid repair system should be able to replace the damaged phospholipid in the complex phospholipid pool with the same molecular species to maintain the bilayer structure. This process requires the ability to reacylate lysophospholipids using specific fatty acids from a substrate pool that changes depending on diet. The mechanisms that govern this well-regulated repair system are not known. Transbilayer movement is coupled with this reacylation process. The reacylation takes place in the inner monolayer, and proper redistribution of the molecular species is required, involving the proteins that transport phospholipids across the bilayer. Therefore, it is logical to assume that the redistribution of these phospholipid species across the bilayer, when they are generated at the inner leaflet, is also a specific process. A rapid translocation from inner to outer monolayer of newly synthesized PC but not PE is observed, suggesting a selective, protein-mediated, outward translocation of newly synthesized PC.[101] The proteins involved in this repair process are themselves vulnerable to oxidant damage. Because the adult RBC is not able to replace damaged proteins, this may lead to the inability to properly repair damaged phospholipids, a dysfunction of the membrane, and demise of the cell.

LIPID ASYMMETRY

The difference in phospholipid composition between the 2 leaflets of the mammalian RBC plasma membrane bilayer was first reported more than 3 decades ago[102,103] This asymmetric transbilayer organization in the membrane of the RBC was originally regarded as a static distribution across the bilayer, generated during erythropoiesis and maintained during the life of the cell, in part by the interaction between PS and spectrin.[104–107] Therefore, HbS polymerization and its mechanical stress on the membrane was thought to result in local loss of asymmetry. In 1984 it was shown that the asymmetric transbilayer distribution is the result of a dynamic and ATP-dependent transport process.[108] The removal of virtually all of the PS from the surface of the plasma membrane seems typical for normal mammalian cells.[109] The ATP-driven transbilayer movement in the RBC is specific for the PE and PS. The outside-to-inside movement, or flip of aminophospholipid in one direction and the flop of another molecule in the reverse to compensate, may involve a "floppase" or proteins such as the multidrug resistance class of transporters.[110,111] This redistribution will be affected by the rapid turnover of phospholipids in the RBC membrane. The incorporation of new fatty acids at the inner monolayer and movement of these species to the outer monolayer links transbilayer movement with the network of proteins involved in the maintenance of the RBC phospholipid composition. The presence of ATP8A1 was reported in adult RBCs and the mRNA in RBC precursors,[112] and confirmed by 2 recently published full-scale RBC proteome studies.[113,114] When ATP8A1 is expressed in yeast vesicles,[115] it acts as an aminophospholipid activated P-ATPase, which can be inhibited by similar factors that affect transbilayer movement in RBCs and is able to transport PS across a bilayer.[115]

PS EXPOSURE IN RBCS

The loss of the asymmetric distribution of phospholipids across the bilayer, and in particular the exposure of PS on the surface of the cell, is an important starting point in many physiologic processes, including the regulation of blood coagulation[116] and the recognition and removal of apoptotic cells.[117] Dying cells, with few exceptions,[109,118] trigger cellular events that result in PS appearing on the cell surface. This PS exposure typically occurs during the last stage of the life of a cell, and triggers phagocyte docking and subsequent engulfment and degradation of the apoptotic cell.[109,119–121] PS externalization is critical to this process, as its absence results in impaired recognition and clearance of apoptotic debris, which can lead to inflammatory and autoimmune responses.[122,123] The appearance of PS at the apoptotic cell surface has been reported to be regulated by specific intracellular signaling events including mitochondrial stress, changes in cytosolic calcium,[124] oxygen radicals, cytochrome c release, caspase activation, and DNA fragmentation.[125] Similarly to apoptosis, PS is exposed in RBC when phospholipids are scrambled across the bilayer. Several in vitro conditions can lead to RBC PS exposure[126] and PS-exposing RBCs in vivo are found in SCD.[127] The underlying mechanism for this scrambling process and exposure of PS is not clear. It involves both a dysfunction of the flippase and increased transbilayer movement defined as phospholipid scrambling. Dielectric breakdown of the RBC membrane[128,129] will increase transbilayer movement, and the incorporation of the calcium ionophore A23187 in the presence of Ca^{2+}[130] to scramble membrane phospholipids is well established. Exposure of PS on the surface induced by the increase in cytosolic calcium could involve a complex of phosphatidylinositol 4,5-bisphosphate (PIP_2) and Ca^{2+},[131] but other factors have been shown to play a role.[132] Ubiquitous RBC membrane proteins such as the anion exchanger band 3 (AE1) are reported to be involved in the movement of phospholipids across the membrane.[133–137] Together, many factors may affect phospholipid movement across the RBC bilayer, and it has been difficult to clearly define a specific floppase or scramblase that is activated under conditions that lead to the exposure of PS.

PS EXPOSURE IN SCD

In SCD and thalassemia, the exposure of PS on the RBC surface is highly amplified. In early studies, phospholipase treatment of RBC samples from sickle cell patients indicated a loss of phospholipid asymmetry related to the sickling process.[138,139] It was thought that the separation of the membrane skeleton from the lipid bilayer in areas as the result of hemoglobin polymerization led to a rapid transbilayer movement and the exposure of PS[140] in all sickled cells. Using flow cytometry and PS-labeling techniques, it has become clear that subpopulations of SRBCs expose PS.[141–144] Most of the RBCs do not expose PS, and seem to be able to maintain their phospholipid asymmetry. Moreover, the size of the PS-exposing subpopulation varies largely from patient to patient. Although some patients do not seem to exhibit PS-exposing cells to a higher extent than controls, the presence of 10% of PS-exposing cells has been reported in the circulation of SCD patients.

The presence of these PS-exposing RBCs in the circulation may be a hallmark of premature aging of the RBCs and may be related to the anemia in these patients. The life span of RBCs in SCD is significantly shorter than the RBC survival in normal humans. Exposure of PS leads to recognition and removal of apoptotic cells in other tissues, and similarly, PS-exposing RBCs will be removed from the circulation. Interestingly these cells can be observed in the peripheral blood, thus indicating that PS-exposing RBCs are being generated in such high numbers that the normal processes to remove these PS-exposing cells are compromised, or simply unable to keep up. The compromised spleen function in sickle cell patients[145] may play an important role in the inability of the body to remove these cells from the circulation. This finding seems underscored by the fact that PS-exposing cells are specifically found in thalassemia patients who are splenectomized.[143,146] In addition to PS-exposing RBCs in the peripheral blood, RBC precursors are present in bone marrow, which, similar to nonviable cells in other tissues, trigger apoptotic processes.

This process leads to the exposure of PS, and removal by macrophages. Particularly in thalassemia, erythropoiesis in bone marrow is marked by high levels of apoptosis or ineffective erythropoiesis.[58,59] The presence of PS-exposing RBCs indicates the inability to maintain proper membrane organization, related to the network of phospholipid maintenance mechanisms as indicated earlier. Several of these processes occur simultaneously to maintain the proper phospholipid organization. Dysfunction of one or several of these mechanisms is, therefore, linked and can be related to the pathologic status. When RBCs from sickle cell patients are analyzed a large diversity in RBC density is observed, and SRBCs exhibit a wide range of PS externalization depending on the age and density of the cells,[147] this density being correlated with a decreased rate of PS movement.[148] The difference in density in subpopulations of SRBCs points to the inability of cells to maintain a proper ion balance across the membrane. Calcium-calmodulin was reported to be involved in PS exposure in SRBCs.[149] Membrane ion transporters will be affected by the lipid organization of the membrane bilayer, which in turn may be linked to the altered phospholipid molecular species organization in these density-separated fractions. Because all RBCs are exposed to the same fatty acid substrates, a difference in phospholipid composition suggests a different phospholipid turnover, in turn suggesting alterations in the enzymes involved in the Lands pathway as described earlier. The exposure of PS on SRBC subpopulations is well established and the pathologic consequences of these cells are well recognized,[127] although the underlying cause remains unclear. Initiation of scrambling by loading RBC with calcium leads ultimately to the exposure of PS, a process that is greatly accelerated when the cells are pretreated with sulfhydryl reagents such as N-ethylmaleimide (NEM). On the other hand, NEM treatment or oxidant damage inhibits flippase activity but does not lead to rapid PS exposure in vitro unless scrambling is also initiated.[150] This finding suggests an efficient competition between the inward movement of PS and calcium-induced phospholipid scrambling, despite the rapid ATP decrease in the RBCs under these conditions and the inhibitory effect of calcium on the Mg-ATP–dependent ATP8A1. These data suggest that PS exposure becomes apparent in a short period of time only when both the inward movement is blocked and scrambling is initiated. The common denominator in PS-exposing SRBCs seems to be the inability to move PS from the outer to the inner monolayer.[150] This apparent slower inward movement of PS can result from both a decreased inward movement of PS (lower activity of the aminophospholipid translocase) and a rapid scrambling (a return movement of PS from inner to outer monolayer). Measurements using intact RBC report on the transbilayer movement and distribution at steady state of the entire system, and not on the activity of a particular protein. In other words, these measurements describe the ability of the cell to maintain phospholipid asymmetry and do not describe the activity of a specific protein in the red cell membrane. Fluorescently labeled PC is not transported by an ATP-dependent mechanism. Hence a rapid redistribution of PC across the bilayer suggests increased phospholipid scrambling in PS-exposing cells. The measurement of movement of both fluorescently labeled PS and PC suggests that inward movement in SRBCs is inhibited and that this, together with an increase in scrambling, leads to PS exposure. As indicated earlier, both proteins and lipids are altered by oxidant damage during the life of the RBC. In normal RBCs thiol modification can alter transbilayer movement of aminophospholipid across the RBC bilayer,[151–153] and similarly, movement is affected by oxidant stress. Normal or sickle murine RBCs that are temporarily depleted of ATP show a significant difference in their ability to restore PS asymmetry when ATP is restored, which is correlated with oxidant stress,[151] suggesting that the flippase is irreversibly oxidatively damaged in subpopulations of SRBCs. Oxidant stress is random in nature, and many avenues may lead to an inhibition or alteration of the RBC flippase, ultimately leading to the inability of the RBC to maintain its phospholipid asymmetry. The mechanisms by which sulfhydryl reactive compounds and oxidant modifications act on the different isoforms of the ATP8A1 are poorly understood. The subpopulation of RBCs that exposes PS in SCD show an inhibited transbilayer movement of PS,[150] and the inhibition by NEM points at 1 or more cysteines being vulnerable to oxidative damage, but other oxidative modifications cannot be excluded from playing a role in the inhibition of the flippase. ATP8A1 has 21 cysteines, all of which, based on sequence homology with other P-ATPases, are likely to be located in the RBC cytosol. It is currently not known which of these residues are involved in sulfhydryl bridges or are potentially vulnerable to modifications. In an intact RBC NEM affects many different proteins, and a direct relation between ATPase activity transport and NEM modification is difficult to make. At this point no direct proof is available on the oxidative modification of the flippase in SRBCs, in part because of the lack of detailed information on this protein, or the involvement (and dysregulation) of other components in the maintenance of phospholipid asymmetry. In a yeast vesicle system, the phosphorylation of the aspartate residue, essential to the phosphate cycle of P-ATPases, seems to be related to NEM modification of ATP8A1.[115] Whereas both PS and PE are actively transported by ATP-dependent processes, RBC storage studies have shown that PE transbilayer movement in RBCs can be compromised while PS is still actively transported.[154] These data suggest that inactivation of the flippase may not be an all-or-nothing process and, because 2 isoforms have been identified in RBCs,[112] these forms may be differently affected. Sickle cell patients have a very diverse presentation of clinical pathology despite all of them having the same mutation in the β locus of hemoglobin. Similarly, the number of PS-exposing RBCs in the circulation varies significantly. The highly increased erythropoiesis may affect the expression of the different isoforms of ATP8A1. Several efforts are under way to link the clinical data in this patient population to differences in genetic background. These studies may also shed some light on the expression of ATP8A1 or the relevance of SNPs in the gene for ATP8A1. In sickle cell patients, specific SNPs have been identified as being related to the expression of HbF,[23–26] in particular the repressor BCL11A,[27–31] and/or to a positive response to hydroxyurea treatment.[32] It cannot be excluded that abnormal regulation of erythroid-specific genes observed in SCD, including the modulation of treatment regimen aimed at gammaglobulin production, could also affect the expression of the isoforms of ATP8A1 as well as flippase activity or specificity.

Together the maintenance of composition and organization of the plasma membrane phospholipids are closely connected, and a loss of function in any of these components can be expected to lead to a loss of membrane viability and a relationship with the pathology of SCD.

Overall, a complex picture emerges of phospholipid movement, kinetics, and distribution for the different molecular species across the RBC bilayer. Nevertheless, the phospholipid headgroup distribution at equilibrium is well maintained during the life of the RBC.

CONSEQUENCES OF PS EXPOSURE

The presence of PS-exposing RBC in the circulation or during erythropoiesis has many pathologic consequences. The rapid removal of PS-exposing erythroid cells (in either marrow or peripheral blood) plays a role in anemia, as macrophages recognize and remove these cells.[55,141] This normal process whereby RBCs are removed from the circulation is referred to as eryptosis.[126] The greatly increased level of PS exposure in SCD seems in part responsible for the reduced RBC life span in both sickle cell patients and transgenic mice. This increased cell-cell interaction is not limited to RBC–white blood cell contacts. Interactions between (PS-exposing) RBCs and vascular endothelium results in endothelial dysfunction and is related to vaso-occlusive events.[144] Hydroxyurea treatment, used in a significant number of sickle cell patients, seems to attenuate activated neutrophil-mediated PS exposure in SRBCs and adhesion to pulmonary vascular endothelium.[20] The exposure of PS is essential in platelet activation. However, a docking surface for hemostatic factors is unwarranted in RBCs, and leads to an imbalance in hemostasis[155,156] (see earlier discussion). Prothrombotic levels of coagulation factors in sickle cell patients may be related to PS exposure and may play an important role in pathology.[157,158]

The ineffective removal of PS-exposing cells can have many other consequences for vascular function. Subpopulations of PS-exposing RBCs in SCD are exposed to secretory phospholipase A2, an inflammatory lipid mediator that is elevated in sickle cell plasma.[159] Whereas this enzyme does not break down normal RBCs, it will hydro-lyze phospholipids in PS-exposing RBCs[160,161] and hemolyze the PS-exposing RBCs. The delayed hemolytic transfusion reaction in SCD patients can occur in the absence of detectable antibody and may be related to PS-exposing RBCs,[162] and PS exposure could be triggered by plasma from these patients. The combination of elevated secretory phospholipase A2 and increasing amounts of PS-exposing RBCs could be clinically relevant under these conditions. Hemolysis has been correlated with a dysregulated arginine and nitric oxide metabolism, and vascular dysfunction.[163–165] In addition to hemolysis, phospholipid hydrolysis by phospholipase A2 will generate phospholipid breakdown products that affect endothelial function and in turn may be related to acute chest syndrome.[159] In RBCs that have lost their ability to maintain phospholipid asymmetry and expose PS, a phospholipase D is activated[166] to generate phosphatidic acid from PC. The relatively high levels of phosphatidic acid in PS-exposing cells will lead to the formation of lysophosphatidic acid (LPA), a powerful lipid mediator, involved in a myriad of signal transduction pathways including vascular dysfunction.[161] Annexin A5, an intracellular protein abundantly present in endothelial cells and platelets, exhibits high affinity for PS and has been shown to inhibit several of these PS-mediated pathophysiologic processes. SCD patients have elevated plasma levels of annexin A5- and PS-exposing MPs, the levels of which vary during crisis, but it is not clear how annexin A5 may modulate PS-related pathophysiologic processes in SCD.[167] Novel compounds such as Di-annexin[160] bind to PS surfaces, and have been effective in coagulation[168] and ischemia/reperfusion events,[169,170] and should be considered as a possible way to cloak PS-exposing cells in SCD and avoid the downstream negative effects.

SUMMARY

In 1949, Linus Pauling identified sickle cell anemia as the first molecular disease.[2] Although the pathophysiology of SCD may be uniquely related to the polymerization of sickle Hb under low oxygen conditions, it has become apparent that many factors are involved in the vasculopathy that characterizes this disorder affecting millions of individuals worldwide. The altered RBC membrane plays an important role in the dysfunctional interactions of the SRBC with other blood cells and vascular endothelium, and leads to premature recognition and removal, an imbalance in hemostasis, vaso-occlusive events, and intravascular hemolysis, and may be involved in acute chest syndrome (**Fig. 1**). The complex, well-orchestrated RBC membrane

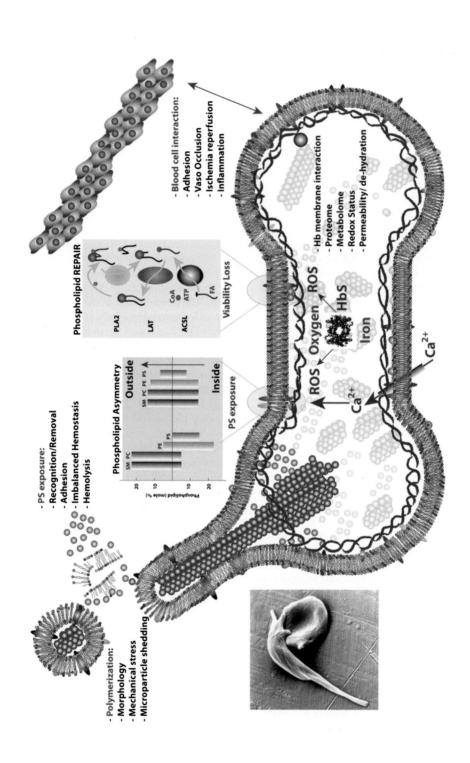

Fig. 1. Hemoglobin S and red cell membrane changes. Polymerization of sickle hemoglobin under low oxygen tension changes red cell morphology, separates the lipid bilayer from the membrane skeleton, puts mechanical stress on the membrane, and results in the shedding of PS exposing microparticles. The unstable character of sickle hemoglobin increases oxidant stress, alters the metabolome and proteome, changes the redox status of the cytosol, and damages membrane lipids and proteins. Oxidized lipids are recognized and hydrolyzed by phospholipase (PLA2). Fatty acid from plasma is activated to acylCoA by acylCoa synthetase (ACSL) and used by lysophospholipid acylCoA transferase (LAT) to reacylate the lysophospholipid. Damage to this repair system results in impaired repair, membrane viability is lost, and the sickle red cell membrane takes a central role in adhesion, vaso occlusion, ischemia reperfusion, and inflammatory processes. The increase of cytosolic calcium and oxidant stress leads to apoptotic plasma membrane processes including the loss of phospholipid asymmetry. PS exposure results in recognition and removal of the sickle red blood cell, increased adhesion, imbalanced hemostasis and hemolysis. All these processes contribute to the vasculopathy that characterizes sickle cell disease.

phospholipid organization is apparently lost in subpopulations of RBC during erythropoiesis as well as in the circulation. Increased oxidant stress may play an important role in the inability of the RBC to maintain composition and asymmetry of phospholipid molecular species, but the mechanisms that lead to PS exposure are poorly understood. This lack of knowledge is in part due to the incomplete characterization of the proteins involved in the maintenance of phospholipid asymmetry in the RBC, as well as the complexity of studying a complete plasma membrane wherein several protein entities act in synchronization with each other and are governed by protein-protein and protein-lipid interactions. The purification and/or expression of the proteins thought to be involved in membrane organization in well-defined lipid bilayers, their 3-dimensional structural modeling, and their detailed functional characterization may lead to a better understanding of their individual functions as well as their interaction with other entities in the bilayer. This knowledge will also lead to a better understanding of how the function of these proteins is impaired or altered in leading to PS exposure in hemoglobinopathies, and to a definition of the molecular underpinnings of this complex pathophysiology.

REFERENCES

1. Herrick JB. Peculiar elongated and sickle-shaped red blood corpuscles in a case of severe anemia. 1910. Yale J Biol Med 2001;74(3):179–84.
2. Pauling L, Itano HA, et al. Sickle cell anemia a molecular disease. Science 1949; 110(2865):543–8.
3. Hebbel RP. The sickle erythrocyte in double jeopardy: autoxidation and iron decompartmentalization. Semin Hematol 1990;27(1):51–69.
4. Mohandas N, An X. New insights into function of red cell membrane proteins and their interaction with spectrin-based membrane skeleton. Transfus Clin Biol 2006;13(1–2):29–30. http://dx.doi.org/10.1016/j.tracli.2006.02.017.
5. Tse WT, Lux SE. Red blood cell membrane disorders. Br J Haematol 1999; 104(1):2–13.
6. Martorana MC, Mojoli G, Cianciulli P, et al. Sickle cell anaemia: haemorheological aspects. Ann Ist Super Sanita 2007;43(2):164–70.
7. Athanassiou G, Moutzouri A, Kourakli A, et al. Effect of hydroxyurea on the deformability of the red blood cell membrane in patients with sickle cell anemia. Clin Hemorheol Microcirc 2006;35(1–2):291–5.

8. Vekilov PG. Sickle-cell haemoglobin polymerization: is it the primary pathogenic event of sickle-cell anaemia? Br J Haematol 2007;139(2):173–84. http://dx.doi. org/10.1111/j.1365-2141.2007.06794.

9. Knee KM, Roden CK, Flory MR, et al. The role of beta93 Cys in the inhibition of Hb S fiber formation. Biophys Chem 2007;127(3):181–93. http://dx.doi.org/10. 1016/j.bpc.2007.02.002.

10. Aprelev A, Weng W, Zakharov M, et al. Metastable polymerization of sickle hemoglobin in droplets. J Mol Biol 2007;369(5):1170–4. http://dx.doi.org/10.1016/j. jmb.2007.04.030.

11. Srinivasulu S, Perumalsamy K, Upadhya R, et al. Pair-wise interactions of polymerization inhibitory contact site mutations of hemoglobin-S. Protein J 2006; 25(7–8):503–16. http://dx.doi.org/10.1007/s10930-006-9034-3.

12. Rotter M, Yosmanovich D, Briehl RW, et al. Nucleation of sickle hemoglobin mixed with hemoglobin A: experimental and theoretical studies of hybrid-forming mixtures. Biophys J 2011;101(11):2790–7. http://dx.doi.org/10.1016/j. bpj.2011.10.027.

13. Wang WC. The pharmacotherapy of sickle cell disease. Expert Opin Pharmacother 2008;9(17):3069–82. http://dx.doi.org/10.1517/14656560802519878.

14. Coleman E, Inusa B. Sickle cell anemia: targeting the role of fetal hemoglobin in therapy. Clin Pediatr 2007;46(5):386–91. http://dx.doi.org/ 10.1177/0009922806297751.

15. Moreira LS, de Andrade TG, Albuquerque DM, et al. Identification of differentially expressed genes induced by hydroxyurea in reticulocytes from sickle cell anaemia patients. Clin Exp Pharmacol Physiol 2008;35(5–6):651–5. http:// dx.doi.org/10.1111/j.1440-1681.2007.04861.

16. Ghatpande SS, Choudhary PK, Quinn CT, et al. Pharmaco-proteomic study of hydroxyurea-induced modifications in the sickle red blood cell membrane proteome. Exp Biol Med 2008;233(12):1510–7. http://dx.doi.org/10.3181/0805-S-149.

17. Johnson C, Telen MJ. Adhesion molecules and hydroxyurea in the pathophysiology of sickle cell disease. Haematologica 2008;93(4):481–5. http://dx.doi.org/ 10.3324/haematol.12734.

18. Cartron JP, Elion J. Erythroid adhesion molecules in sickle cell disease: effect of hydroxyurea. Transfus Clin Biol 2008;15(1–2):39–50. http://dx.doi.org/10.1016/j. tracli.2008.05.001.

19. Styles LA, Lubin B, Vichinsky E, et al. Decrease of very late activation antigen-4 and CD36 on reticulocytes in sickle cell patients treated with hydroxyurea. Blood 1997;89(7):2554–9.

20. Haynes J Jr, Obiako B, Hester RB, et al. Hydroxyurea attenuates activated neutrophil-mediated sickle erythrocyte membrane phosphatidylserine exposure and adhesion to pulmonary vascular endothelium. Am J Physiol Heart Circ Physiol 2008;294(1):H379–85. http://dx.doi.org/10.1152/ajpheart.01068.2007.

21. Daak AA, Ghebremeskel K, Elbashir MI, et al. Hydroxyurea therapy mobilises arachidonic acid from inner cell membrane aminophospholipids in patients with homozygous sickle cell disease. J Lipids 2011;2011:718014. http://dx. doi.org/10.1155/2011/718014.

22. van Dijk TB, Gillemans N, Pourfarzad F, et al. Fetal globin expression is regulated by Friend of Prmt1. Blood 2010;116(20):4349–52. http://dx.doi.org/10. 1182/blood-2010-03-274399.

23. Chen Z, Luo HY, Basran RK, et al. A T-to-G transversion at nucleotide -567 upstream of HBG2 in a GATA-1 binding motif is associated with elevated hemoglobin F. Mol Cell Biol 2008;28(13):4386–93.

24. Lettre G, Sankaran VG, Bezerra MA, et al. DNA polymorphisms at the BCL11A, HBS1L-MYB, and beta-globin loci associate with fetal hemoglobin levels and pain crises in sickle cell disease. Proc Natl Acad Sci U S A 2008;105(33): 11869–74.

25. Sebastiani P, Wang L, Nolan VG, et al. Fetal hemoglobin in sickle cell anemia: Bayesian modeling of genetic associations. Am J Hematol 2008;83(3):189–95. http://dx.doi.org/10.1002/ajh.21048.

26. Uda M, Galanello R, Sanna S, et al. Genome-wide association study shows BCL11A associated with persistent fetal hemoglobin and amelioration of the phenotype of beta-thalassemia. Proc Natl Acad Sci U S A 2008;105(5):1620–5.

27. Menzel S, Garner C, Gut I, et al. A QTL influencing F cell production maps to a gene encoding a zinc-finger protein on chromosome 2p15. Nat Genet 2007; 39(10):1197–9.

28. Saiki Y, Yamazaki Y, Yoshida M, et al. Human EVI9, a homologue of the mouse myeloid leukemia gene, is expressed in the hematopoietic progenitors and down-regulated during myeloid differentiation of HL60 cells. Genomics 2000; 70(3):387–91.

29. Sankaran VG, Menne TF, Xu J, et al. Human fetal hemoglobin expression is regulated by the developmental stage-specific repressor BCL11A. Science 2008;322(5909):1839–42.

30. Sedgewick AE, Timofeev N, Sebastiani P, et al. BCL11A is a major HbF quantitative trait locus in three different populations with beta-hemoglobinopathies. Blood Cells Mol Dis 2008;41(3):255–8.

31. Senawong T, Peterson VJ, Leid M. BCL11A-dependent recruitment of SIRT1 to a promoter template in mammalian cells results in histone deacetylation and transcriptional repression. Arch Biochem Biophys 2005;434(2):316–25.

32. Ma Q, Wyszynski DF, Farrell JJ, et al. Fetal hemoglobin in sickle cell anemia: genetic determinants of response to hydroxyurea. Pharmacogenomics J 2007; 7(6):386–94.

33. Hankins JS, Wynn LW, Brugnara C, et al. Phase I study of magnesium pidolate in combination with hydroxycarbamide for children with sickle cell anaemia. Br J Haematol 2008;140(1):80–5. http://dx.doi.org/10.1111/j.1365-2141.2007.06884.

34. Nagababu E, Fabry ME, Nagel RL, et al. Heme degradation and oxidative stress in murine models for hemoglobinopathies: thalassemia, sickle cell disease and hemoglobin C disease. Blood Cells Mol Dis 2008;41(1):60–6. http://dx.doi.org/ 10.1016/j.bcmd.2007.12.003.

35. Takahashi T, Shimizu H, Morimatsu H, et al. Heme oxygenase-1: a fundamental guardian against oxidative tissue injuries in acute inflammation. Mini Rev Med Chem 2007;7(7):745–53.

36. Pan W, Uzunova VV, Vekilov PG. Free heme in micromolar amounts enhances the attraction between sickle cell hemoglobin molecules. Biopolymers 2009; 91(12):1108–16. http://dx.doi.org/10.1002/bip.21191.

37. Uzunova VV, Pan W, Galkin O, et al. Free heme and the polymerization of sickle cell hemoglobin. Biophys J 2010;99(6):1976–85. http://dx.doi.org/10.1016/j.bpj. 2010.07.024.

38. Wang JC, Kwong S, Ferrone FA, et al. Fiber depolymerization: fracture, fragments, vanishing times, and stochastics in sickle hemoglobin. Biophys J 2009;96(2):655–70. http://dx.doi.org/10.1016/j.bpj.2008.04.001.

39. Weinkam P, Sali A. Mapping polymerization and allostery of hemoglobin S using point mutations. J Phys Chem B 2013;117(42):13058–68. http://dx.doi.org/10. 1021/jp4025156.

40. Dash BP, Archana Y, Satapathy N, et al. Search for antisickling agents from plants. Pharmacogn Rev 2013;7(13):53–60. http://dx.doi.org/10.4103/0973-7847.112849.

41. Zhang Y, Xia Y. Adenosine signaling in normal and sickle erythrocytes and beyond. Microbes Infect 2012;14(10):863–73. http://dx.doi.org/10.1016/j.micinf.2012.05.005.

42. Stefanovic M, Puchulu-Campanella E, Kodippili G, et al. Oxygen regulates the band 3-ankyrin bridge in the human erythrocyte membrane. Biochem J 2013; 449(1):143–50. http://dx.doi.org/10.1042/BJ20120869.

43. Rogers SC, Ross JG, d'Avignon A, et al. Sickle hemoglobin disturbs normal coupling among erythrocyte O2 content, glycolysis, and antioxidant capacity. Blood 2013;121(9):1651–62. http://dx.doi.org/10.1182/blood-2012-02-414037.

44. Goodman SR, Daescu O, Kakhniashvili DG, et al. The proteomics and interactomics of human erythrocytes. Exp Biol Med 2013;238(5):509–18. http://dx.doi.org/10.1177/1535370213488474.

45. Biondani A, Turrini F, Carta F, et al. Heat-shock protein-27, -70 and peroxiredoxin-II show molecular chaperone function in sickle red cells: evidence from transgenic sickle cell mouse model. Proteomics Clin Appl 2008;2(5): 706–19. http://dx.doi.org/10.1002/prca.200780058.

46. Kaore SN, Amane HS, Kaore NM. Citrulline: pharmacological perspectives and its role as an emerging biomarker in future. Fundam Clin Pharmacol 2013;27(1): 35–50. http://dx.doi.org/10.1111/j.1472-8206.2012.01059.

47. Ellory JC, Robinson HC, Browning JA, et al. Abnormal permeability pathways in human red blood cells. Blood Cells Mol Dis 2007;39(1):1–6. http://dx.doi.org/10.1016/j.bcmd.2007.02.011.

48. Raghupathy R, Billett HH. Promising therapies in sickle cell disease. Cardiovasc Hematol Disord Drug Targets 2009;9(1):1–8.

49. Darghouth D, Koehl B, Junot C, et al. Metabolomic analysis of normal and sickle cell erythrocytes. Transfus Clin Biol 2010;17(3):148–50. http://dx.doi.org/10.1016/j.tracli.2010.06.011.

50. Thomas SL, Bouyer G, Cueff A, et al. Ion channels in human red blood cell membrane: actors or relics? Blood Cells Mol Dis 2011;46(4):261–5. http://dx.doi.org/10.1016/j.bcmd.2011.02.007.

51. Lei H, Karniadakis GE. Probing vasoocclusion phenomena in sickle cell anemia via mesoscopic simulations. Proc Natl Acad Sci U S A 2013;110(28):11326–30. http://dx.doi.org/10.1073/pnas.1221297110.

52. Hebbel RP, Mohandas N. Reversible deformation-dependent erythrocyte cation leak. Extreme sensitivity conferred by minimal peroxidation. Biophys J 1991; 60(3):712–5. http://dx.doi.org/10.1016/S0006-3495(91)82100-2.

53. Bogdanova A, Makhro A, Wang J, et al. Calcium in red blood cells-a perilous balance. Int J Mol Sci 2013;14(5):9848–72. http://dx.doi.org/10.3390/ijms14059848.

54. Vandorpe DH, Xu C, Shmukler BE, et al. Hypoxia activates a Ca^{2+}-permeable cation conductance sensitive to carbon monoxide and to GsMTx-4 in human and mouse sickle erythrocytes. PloS one 2010;5(1):e8732. http://dx.doi.org/10.1371/journal.pone.0008732.

55. Kuypers FA, de Jong K. The role of phosphatidylserine in recognition and removal of erythrocytes. Cell Mol Biol 2004;50(2):147–58.

56. George A, Pushkaran S, Konstantinidis DG, et al. Erythrocyte NADPH oxidase activity modulated by Rac GTPases, PKC, and plasma cytokines contributes to oxidative stress in sickle cell disease. Blood 2013;121(11):2099–107. http://dx.doi.org/10.1182/blood-2012-07-441188.

57. Fibach E, Rachmilewitz E. The role of oxidative stress in hemolytic anemia. Curr Mol Med 2008;8(7):609–19.
58. Schrier SL. Thalassemia: pathophysiology of red cell changes. Annu Rev Med 1994;45:211–8.
59. Schrier SL. Pathophysiology of thalassemia. Curr Opin Hematol 2002;9(2): 123–6.
60. Johnson RM, Goyette G Jr, Ravindranath Y, et al. Hemoglobin autoxidation and regulation of endogenous H_2O_2 levels in erythrocytes. Free Radic Biol Med 2005;39(11):1407–17. http://dx.doi.org/10.1016/j.freeradbiomed. 2005.07.002.
61. Scott MD, Lubin BH, Zuo L, et al. Erythrocyte defense against hydrogen peroxide: preeminent importance of catalase. J Lab Clin Med 1991;118(1): 7–16.
62. Hiner AN, Raven EL, Thorneley RN, et al. Mechanisms of compound I formation in heme peroxidases. J Inorg Biochem 2002;91(1):27–34.
63. Reeder BJ. The redox activity of hemoglobins: from physiologic functions to pathologic mechanisms. Antioxid Redox Signal 2010;13(7):1087–123. http://dx.doi.org/10.1089/ars.2009.2974.
64. Svistunenko DA, Dunne J, Fryer M, et al. Comparative study of tyrosine radicals in hemoglobin and myoglobins treated with hydrogen peroxide. Biophys J 2002; 83(5):2845–55. http://dx.doi.org/10.1016/S0006-3495(02)75293-4.
65. Reeder BJ, Svistunenko DA, Sharpe MA, et al. Characteristics and mechanism of formation of peroxide-induced heme to protein cross-linking in myoglobin. Biochemistry 2002;41(1):367–75.
66. Low FM, Hampton MB, Peskin AV, et al. Peroxiredoxin 2 functions as a noncatalytic scavenger of low-level hydrogen peroxide in the erythrocyte. Blood 2007; 109(6):2611–7. http://dx.doi.org/10.1182/blood-2006-09-048728.
67. Ey J, Schomig E, Taubert D. Dietary sources and antioxidant effects of ergothioneine. J Agric Food Chem 2007;55(16):6466–74. http://dx.doi.org/10.1021/ jf071328f.
68. Suh JH, Kim R, Yavuz B, et al. Clinical assay of four thiol amino acid redox couples by LC-MS/MS: utility in thalassemia. J Chromatogr B Analyt Technol Biomed Life Sci 2009;877(28):3418–27. http://dx.doi.org/10.1016/j.jchromb.2009. 06.041.
69. Grigat S, Harlfinger S, Pal S, et al. Probing the substrate specificity of the ergothioneine transporter with methimazole, hercynine, and organic cations. Biochem Pharmacol 2007;74(2):309–16. http://dx.doi.org/10.1016/j.bcp.2007.04.015.
70. Grundemann D, Harlfinger S, Golz S, et al. Discovery of the ergothioneine transporter. Proc Natl Acad Sci U S A 2005;102(14):5256–61. http://dx.doi.org/10. 1073/pnas.0408624102.
71. Akanmu D, Cecchini R, Aruoma OI, et al. The antioxidant action of ergothioneine. Arch Biochem Biophys 1991;288(1):10–6.
72. Zhu BZ, Mao L, Fan RM, et al. Ergothioneine prevents copper-induced oxidative damage to DNA and protein by forming a redox-inactive ergothioneine-copper complex. Chem Res Toxicol 2011;24(1):30–4. http://dx.doi.org/10. 1021/tx100214t.
73. Robinson SR, Dang TN, Dringen R, et al. Hemin toxicity: a preventable source of brain damage following hemorrhagic stroke. Redox Rep 2009;14(6):228–35. http://dx.doi.org/10.1179/135100009X12525712409931.
74. Wicher KB, Fries E. Evolutionary aspects of hemoglobin scavengers. Antioxid Redox Signal 2010;12(2):249–59. http://dx.doi.org/10.1089/ars.2009.2760.

75. Xue H, Guo H, Li YC, et al. Heme oxygenase-1 induction by hemin protects liver cells from ischemia/reperfusion injury in cirrhotic rats. World J Gastroenterol 2007;13(40):5384–90.

76. Reeder BJ, Wilson MT. Hemoglobin and myoglobin associated oxidative stress: from molecular mechanisms to disease states. Curr Med Chem 2005;12(23): 2741–51.

77. Galaris D, Eddy L, Arduini A, et al. Mechanisms of reoxygenation injury in myocardial infarction: implications of a myoglobin redox cycle. Biochem Biophys Res Commun 1989;160(3):1162–8.

78. Cassidy RA, Burleson DG, Delgado AV, et al. Effects of heme proteins on nitric oxide levels and cell viability in isolated PMNs: a mechanism of toxicity. J Leukoc Biol 2000;67(3):357–68.

79. Atamna H. Amino acids variations in amyloid-beta peptides, mitochondrial dysfunction, and new therapies for Alzheimer's disease. J Bioenerg Biomembr 2009;41(5):457–64. http://dx.doi.org/10.1007/s10863-009-9246-2.

80. Atamna H, Boyle K. Amyloid-beta peptide binds with heme to form a peroxidase: relationship to the cytopathologies of Alzheimer's disease. Proc Natl Acad Sci U S A 2006;103(9):3381–6. http://dx.doi.org/10.1073/pnas. 0600134103.

81. Atamna H. Heme binding to Amyloid-beta peptide: mechanistic role in Alzheimer's disease. J Alzheimers Dis 2006;10(2–3):255–66.

82. Kosicek M, Malnar M, Goate A, et al. Cholesterol accumulation in Niemann Pick type C (NPC) model cells causes a shift in APP localization to lipid rafts. Biochem Biophys Res Commun 2010;393(3):404–9. http://dx.doi.org/10.1016/j. bbrc.2010.02.007.

83. Burns M, Gaynor K, Olm V, et al. Presenilin redistribution associated with aberrant cholesterol transport enhances beta-amyloid production in vivo. J Neurosci 2003;23(13):5645–9.

84. Nagy E, Eaton JW, Jeney V, et al. Red cells, hemoglobin, heme, iron, and atherogenesis. Arterioscler Thromb Vasc Biol 2010;30(7):1347–53. http://dx.doi.org/ 10.1161/ATVBAHA.110.206433.

85. Piccin A, Murphy WG, Smith OP. Circulating microparticles: pathophysiology and clinical implications. Blood Rev 2007;21(3):157–71. http://dx.doi.org/10. 1016/j.blre.2006.09.001.

86. Nebor D, Romana M, Santiago R, et al. Fetal hemoglobin and hydroxycarbamide modulate both plasma concentration and cellular origin of circulating microparticles in sickle cell anemia children. Haematologica 2013;98(6):862–7. http://dx.doi.org/10.3324/haematol.2012.073619.

87. Westerman M, Pizzey A, Hirschman J, et al. Microvesicles in haemoglobinopathies offer insights into mechanisms of hypercoagulability, haemolysis and the effects of therapy. Br J Haematol 2008;142(1):126–35. http://dx.doi.org/10. 1111/j.1365-2141.2008.07155.x.

88. Villaescusa R, Arce AA, Lalanne-Mistrih ML, et al. Natural antiband 3 antibodies in patients with sickle cell disease. C R Biol 2013;336(3):173–6. http://dx.doi. org/10.1016/j.crvi.2012.09.002.

89. Ferru E, Giger K, Pantaleo A, et al. Regulation of membrane-cytoskeletal interactions by tyrosine phosphorylation of erythrocyte band 3. Blood 2011; 117(22):5998–6006. http://dx.doi.org/10.1182/blood-2010-11-317024.

90. Camus SM, Gausseres B, Bonnin P, et al. Erythrocyte microparticles can induce kidney vaso-occlusions in a murine model of sickle cell disease. Blood 2012; 120(25):5050–8. http://dx.doi.org/10.1182/blood-2012-02-413138.

91. Myher JJ, Kuksis A, Pind S. Molecular species of glycerophospholipids and sphingomyelins of human erythrocytes: improved method of analysis. Lipids 1989;24(5):396–407.
92. van den Berg JJ, Op den Kamp JA, Lubin BH, et al. Conformational changes in oxidized phospholipids and their preferential hydrolysis by phospholipase A2: a monolayer study. Biochemistry 1993;32(18):4962–7.
93. Lubin BH, Kuypers FA. Phospholipid repair in human erythrocytes. 1st edition. New York: Pergamon Press; 1991.
94. Lands WE. Lipid metabolism. Annu Rev Biochem 1965;34:313–46.
95. Fyrst H, Knudsen J, Lubin BH, et al. Detection of AcylCoA binding protein in human red cells and investigation of its role in membrane phospholipid renewal. Biochem J 1995;306:793–9.
96. Malhotra K, Malhotra K, Lubin B, et al. Identification and molecular characterization of acyl-CoA synthetase in human erythrocytes and erythroid precursors. Biochem J 1999;344(1):135–41.
97. Soupene E, Serikov V, Kuypers FA. Characterization of an acyl-coenzyme A binding protein predominantly expressed in human primitive progenitor cells. J Lipid Res 2008;49(5):1103–12.
98. Soupene E, Kuypers FA. Multiple erythroid isoforms of human long-chain acyl-CoA synthetases are produced by switch of the fatty acid gate domains. BMC Mol Biol 2006;7(1):21.
99. Soupene E, Fyrst H, Kuypers FA. Mammalian acyl-CoA:lysophosphatidylcholine acyltransferase enzymes. Proc Natl Acad Sci U S A 2008;105(1):88–93.
100. Soupene E, Kuypers FA. Phosphatidylcholine formation by LPCAT1 is regulated by Ca(2+) and the redox status of the cell. BMC Biochem 2012;13:8. http://dx.doi.org/10.1186/1471-2091-13-8.
101. Andrick C, Broring K, Deuticke B, et al. Fast translocation of phosphatidylcholine to the outer membrane leaflet after its synthesis at the inner membrane surface in human erythrocytes. Biochim Biophys Acta 1991;1064(2):235–41.
102. Bretscher MS. Phosphatidyl-ethanolamine: differential labelling in intact cells and cell ghosts of human erythrocytes by a membrane-impermeable reagent. J Mol Biol 1972;71(3):523–8.
103. Bretscher MS. Asymmetrical lipid bilayer structure for biological membranes. Nature New Biol 1972;236(61):11–2.
104. Haest CW, Deuticke B. Possible relationship between membrane proteins and phospholipid asymmetry in the human erythrocyte membrane. Biochim Biophys Acta 1976;436(2):353–65.
105. Haest CW, Plasa G, Kamp D, et al. Spectrin as a stabilizer of the phospholipid asymmetry in the human erythrocyte membrane. Biochim Biophys Acta 1978;509(1):21–32.
106. Haest CW, Erusalimsky J, Dressler V, et al. Transbilayer mobility of phospholipids in the erythrocyte membrane. Influence of the membrane skeleton. Biomed Biochim Acta 1983;42(11–12):S17–21.
107. Dressler V, Haest CW, Plasa G, et al. Stabilizing factors of phospholipid asymmetry in the erythrocyte membrane. Biochim Biophys Acta 1984;775(2):189–96.
108. Seigneuret M, Devaux PF. ATP-dependent asymmetric distribution of spin-labeled phospholipids in the erythrocyte membrane: relation to shape changes. Proc Natl Acad Sci U S A 1984;81(12):3751–5.
109. Balasubramanian K, Schroit AJ. Aminophospholipid asymmetry: a matter of life and death. Annu Rev Physiol 2003;65:701–34.

110. Dekkers DW, Comfurius P, Schroit AJ, et al. Transbilayer movement of NBD-labeled phospholipids in red blood cell membranes: outward-directed transport by the multidrug resistance protein 1 (MRP1). Biochemistry 1998;37(42):14833–7.

111. Dekkers DW, Comfurius P, van Gool RG, et al. Multidrug resistance protein 1 regulates lipid asymmetry in erythrocyte membranes. Biochem J 2000;350(Pt 2):531–5.

112. Soupene E, Kuypers FA. Identification of an erythroid ATP-dependent amino-phospholipid transporter. Br J Haematol 2006;133(4):436–8. http://dx.doi.org/10.1111/j.1365-2141.2006.06051.x.

113. Pasini EM, Kirkegaard M, Mortensen P, et al. In-depth analysis of the membrane and cytosolic proteome of red blood cells. Blood 2006;108(3):791–801.

114. Pasini EM, Kirkegaard M, Salerno D, et al. Deep coverage mouse red blood cell proteome: a first comparison with the human red blood cell. Mol Cell Proteomics 2008;7(7):1317–30.

115. Soupene E, Utami Kemaladewi D, Kuypers FA. ATP8A1 activity and phosphatidylserine transbilayer movement. J Receptor Ligand Channel Res 2008;1:1–10.

116. Zwaal RF, Comfurius P, Bevers EM. Lipid-protein interactions in blood coagulation. Biochim Biophys Acta 1998;1376(3):433–53.

117. Williamson P, Schlegel RA. Transbilayer phospholipid movement and the clearance of apoptotic cells. Biochim Biophys Acta 2002;1585(2–3):53–63.

118. Elliott JI, Surprenant A, Marelli-Berg FM, et al. Membrane phosphatidylserine distribution as a non-apoptotic signalling mechanism in lymphocytes. Nat Cell Biol 2005;7(8):808–16.

119. Fadok VA, Bratton DL, Rose DM, et al. A receptor for phosphatidylserine-specific clearance of apoptotic cells. Nature 2000;405(6782):85–90.

120. Fadok VA, de Cathelineau A, Daleke DL, et al. Loss of phospholipid asymmetry and surface exposure of phosphatidylserine is required for phagocytosis of apoptotic cells by macrophages and fibroblasts. J Biol Chem 2001;276(2):1071–7.

121. Savill J, Fadok V. Corpse clearance defines the meaning of cell death. Nature 2000;407(6805):784–8.

122. Gaipl US, Voll RE, Sheriff A, et al. Impaired clearance of dying cells in systemic lupus erythematosus. Autoimmun Rev 2005;4(4):189–94.

123. Kuhtreiber WM, Hayashi T, Dale EA, et al. Central role of defective apoptosis in autoimmunity. J Mol Endocrinol 2003;31(3):373–99.

124. Mirnikjoo B, Balasubramanian K, Schroit AJ. Mobilization of lysosomal calcium regulates the externalization of phosphatidylserine during apoptosis. J Biol Chem 2009;284(11):6918–23.

125. Kagan VE, Tyurina YY, Bayir H, et al. The "pro-apoptotic genies" get out of mitochondria: oxidative lipidomics and redox activity of cytochrome c/cardiolipin complexes. Chem Biol Interact 2006;163(1–2):15–28.

126. Foller M, Huber SM, Lang F. Erythrocyte programmed cell death. IUBMB Life 2008;60(10):661–8. http://dx.doi.org/10.1002/iub.106.

127. Kuypers FA. Membrane lipid alterations in hemoglobinopathies. Hematology Am Soc Hematol Educ Program 2007;68–73. http://dx.doi.org/10.1182/asheducation-2007.1.68.

128. Dressler V, Schwister K, Haest CW, et al. Dielectric breakdown of the erythrocyte membrane enhances transbilayer mobility of phospholipids. Biochim Biophys Acta 1983;732(1):304–7.

129. Haest CW, Oslender A, Kamp D. Nonmediated flip-flop of anionic phospholipids and long-chain amphiphiles in the erythrocyte membrane depends on membrane potential. Biochemistry 1997;36(36):10885–91.

130. Henseleit U, Plasa G, Haest C. Effects of divalent cations on lipid flip-flop in the human erythrocyte membrane. Biochim Biophys Acta 1990;1029(1):127–35.

131. Shiffer KA, Rood L, Emerson RK, et al. The effects of phosphatidylinositol diphosphate on phospholipid asymmetry in the human erythrocyte membrane. Biochemistry 1998;37(10):3449–58.

132. Bevers EM, Wiedmer T, Comfurius P, et al. The complex of phosphatidylinositol 4,5-bisphosphate and calcium ions is not responsible for Ca^{2+}-induced loss of phospholipid asymmetry in the human erythrocyte: a study in Scott syndrome, a disorder of calcium-induced phospholipid scrambling. Blood 1995;86(5): 1983–91.

133. Schwichtenhovel C, Deuticke B, Haest CW. Alcohols produce reversible and irreversible acceleration of phospholipid flip-flop in the human erythrocyte membrane. Biochim Biophys Acta 1992;1111(1):35–44.

134. Serra MV, Kamp D, Haest CW. Pathways for flip-flop of mono- and di-anionic phospholipids in the erythrocyte membrane. Biochim Biophys Acta 1996; 1282(2):263–73.

135. Vondenhof A, Oslender A, Deuticke B, et al. Band 3, an accidental flippase for anionic phospholipids? Biochemistry 1994;33(15):4517–20.

136. Kleinhorst A, Oslender A, Haest CW, et al. Band 3-mediated flip-flop and phosphatase-catalyzed cleavage of a long-chain alkyl phosphate anion in the human erythrocyte membrane. J Membr Biol 1998;165(2):111–24.

137. Axelsen KB, Palmgren MG. Inventory of the superfamily of P-type ion pumps in Arabidopsis. Plant Physiol 2001;126(2):696–706.

138. Franck PF, Chiu DT, Op den Kamp JA, et al. Accelerated transbilayer movement of phosphatidylcholine in sickled erythrocytes. A reversible process. J Biol Chem 1983;258(13):8436–42.

139. Lubin B, Chiu D, Bastacky J, et al. Abnormalities in membrane phospholipid organization in sickled erythrocytes. J Clin Invest 1981;67(6):1643–9.

140. Franck PF, Bevers EM, Lubin BH, et al. Uncoupling of the membrane skeleton from the lipid bilayer. The cause of accelerated phospholipid flip-flop leading to an enhanced procoagulant activity of sickled cells. J Clin Invest 1985; 75(1):183–90. http://dx.doi.org/10.1172/JCI111672.

141. de Jong K, Emerson R, Butler H, et al. Short survival of PS exposing red blood cells in murine sickle cell anemia. Blood 2001;98(5):1577–84.

142. Kuypers FA, Lewis RA, Ernst JD, et al. Detection of altered membrane phospholipid asymmetry in subpopulations of human red cells using fluorescently labeled annexin V. Blood 1996;87(3):1179–87.

143. Kuypers FA, Yuan J, Lewis RA, et al. Membrane phospholipid asymmetry in human thalassemia. Blood 1998;91(8):3044–51.

144. Setty BN, Kulkarni S, Stuart MJ. Role of erythrocyte phosphatidylserine in sickle red cell-endothelial adhesion. Blood 2002;99(5):1564–71.

145. Lane PA. The spleen in children. Curr Opin Pediatr 1995;7(1):36–41.

146. Singer ST, Kuypers F, Olivieri N, et al. Fetal haemoglobin augmentation in E/b0 thalassaemia: clinical and haematological outcome. Br J Haematol 2005;131: 378–88.

147. Yasin Z, Witting S, Palascak MB, et al. Phosphatidylserine externalization in sickle red blood cells: associations with cell age, density, and hemoglobin F. Blood 2003;102(1):365–70. http://dx.doi.org/10.1182/blood-2002-11-3416.

148. Blumenfeld N, Zachowski A, Galacteros F, et al. Transmembrane mobility of phospholipids in sickle erythrocytes: effect of deoxygenation on diffusion and asymmetry. Blood 1991;77(4):849–54.

149. Sabina RL, Wandersee NJ, Hillery CA. Ca^{2+}-CaM activation of AMP deaminase contributes to adenine nucleotide dysregulation and phosphatidylserine externalization in human sickle erythrocytes. Br J Haematol 2009;144(3): 434–45.

150. de Jong K, Larkin SK, Styles LA, et al. Characterization of the phosphatidylserine-exposing subpopulation of sickle cells. Blood 2001;98(3):860–7.

151. Banerjee T, Kuypers FA. Reactive oxygen species and phosphatidylserine externalization in murine sickle red cells. Br J Haematol 2004;124(3):391–402.

152. de Jong K, Kuypers FA. Sulphydryl modifications alter scramblase activity in murine sickle cell disease. Br J Haematol 2006;133(4):427–32. http://dx.doi.org/10.1111/j.1365-2141.2006.06045.x.

153. De Jong K, Geldwerth D, Kuypers FA. Oxidative damage does not alter membrane phospholipid asymmetry in human erythrocytes. Biochemistry 1997; 36(22):6768–76.

154. Geldwerth D, Kuypers FA, Bütikofer P, et al. Transbilayer mobility and distribution of red cell phospholipids during storage. J Clin Invest 1993;92:308–14.

155. Cappellini MD. Coagulation in the pathophysiology of hemolytic anemias. Hematology Am Soc Hematol Educ Program 2007;74–8. http://dx.doi.org/10.1182/asheducation-2007.1.74.

156. Zwaal RF, Comfurius P, Bevers EM. Surface exposure of phosphatidylserine in pathological cells. Cell Mol Life Sci 2005;62(9):971–88.

157. Adedeji MO, Cespedes J, Allen K, et al. Pulmonary thrombotic arteriopathy in patients with sickle cell disease. Arch Pathol Lab Med 2001;125(11):1436–41.

158. Marfaing-Koka A, Boyer-Neumann C, Wolf M, et al. Decreased protein S activity in sickle cell disease. Nouv Rev Fr Hematol 1993;35(4):425–30.

159. Kuypers FA, Styles LA. The role of secretory phospholipase A2 in acute chest syndrome. Cell Mol Biol 2004;50(1):87–94.

160. Kuypers FA, Larkin SK, Emeis JJ, et al. Interaction of an annexin V homodimer (Diannexin) with phosphatidylserine on cell surfaces and consequent antithrombotic activity. Thromb Haemost 2007;97(3):478–86.

161. Neidlinger NA, Larkin SK, Bhagat A, et al. Hydrolysis of phosphatidylserine-exposing red blood cells by secretory phospholipase A2 generates lysophosphatidic acid and results in vascular dysfunction. J Biol Chem 2006;281(2): 775–81.

162. Chadebech P, Habibi A, Nzouakou R, et al. Delayed hemolytic transfusion reaction in sickle cell disease patients: evidence of an emerging syndrome with suicidal red blood cell death. Transfusion 2009;49(9):1785–92.

163. Morris CR, Kuypers FA, Kato GJ, et al. Hemolysis-associated pulmonary hypertension in thalassemia. Ann N Y Acad Sci 2005;1054:481–5.

164. Gladwin MT, Kato GJ. Hemolysis-associated hypercoagulability in sickle cell disease: the plot (and blood) thickens! Haematologica 2008;93(1):1–3.

165. Kato GJ, Gladwin MT, Steinberg MH. Deconstructing sickle cell disease: reappraisal of the role of hemolysis in the development of clinical subphenotypes. Blood Rev 2007;21(1):37–47.

166. Bütikofer P, Yee MC, Schott MA, et al. Generation of phosphatidic acid during calcium-loading of human erythrocytes—evidence for a phosphatidylcholine-hydrolyzing phospholipase D. Eur J Biochem 1993;213(1):367–75.

167. van Tits LJ, van Heerde WL, Landburg PP, et al. Plasma annexin A5 and microparticle phosphatidylserine levels are elevated in sickle cell disease and increase further during painful crisis. Biochem Biophys Res Commun 2009; 390(1):161–4. http://dx.doi.org/10.1016/j.bbrc.2009.09.102.

168. Rand ML, Wang H, Pluthero FG, et al. Diannexin, an annexin A5 homodimer, binds phosphatidylserine with high affinity and is a potent inhibitor of platelet-mediated events during thrombus formation. J Thromb Haemost 2012;10(6): 1109–19. http://dx.doi.org/10.1111/j.1538-7836.2012.04716.x.
169. Hale SL, Allison AC, Kloner RA. Diannexin reduces no-reflow after reperfusion in rabbits with large ischemic myocardial risk zones. Cardiovasc Ther 2011;29(4): e42–52. http://dx.doi.org/10.1111/j.1755-5922.2010.00223.x.
170. Wever KE, Wagener FA, Frielink C, et al. Diannexin protects against renal ischemia reperfusion injury and targets phosphatidylserines in ischemic tissue. PloS one 2011;6(8):e24276. http://dx.doi.org/10.1371/journal.pone.0024276.

Ischemia-reperfusion Injury in Sickle Cell Anemia
Relationship to Acute Chest Syndrome, Endothelial Dysfunction, Arterial Vasculopathy, and Inflammatory Pain

Robert P. Hebbel, MD

KEYWORDS

• Ischemia-reperfusion • Sickle • Endothelial dysfunction • Inflammation

KEY POINTS

Disparate clinical features and vascular biological abnormalities characteristic of sickle cell anemia can be explained readily by viewing this disease as an example of ischemia-reperfusion (I/R) injury, which establishes a chronic, systemic inflammatory state.

• In sickle I/R, the triggering ischemia probably occurs in the microvasculature and in a dispersed, multifocal manner.

• Features of sickle I/R are influenced by the multitude of modulating factors present in its uniquely complex milieu.

• Acute chest syndrome may be an example of I/R-induced remote organ injury.

• Other sickle disease features explainable by the I/R character of sickle disease include endothelial dysfunction with aberrant vasoregulation, large vessel vasculopathy, and inflammatory pain.

INTRODUCTION

Ischemia-reperfusion (I/R) physiology, also called reperfusion injury, is a fundamental vascular pathobiological paradigm, which instigates vascular and tissue injury in a variety of human disease states. This review describes why sickle cell anemia should be conceptualized in this fashion and how I/R physiology explains the genesis of characteristic aspects of vascular pathobiology and clinical disease in sickle cell anemia.

Disclosures: Nothing to disclose.
Division of Hematology-Oncology-Transplantation, Department of Medicine, University of Minnesota Medical School, 420 Delaware Street South East, Mayo Mail Code 480, Minneapolis, MN 55455, USA
E-mail address: hebbe001@umn.edu

Hematol Oncol Clin N Am 28 (2014) 181–198
http://dx.doi.org/10.1016/j.hoc.2013.11.005
0889-8588/14/$ – see front matter © 2014 Elsevier Inc. All rights reserved.

For clarity, the nature of I/R generally is presented first, followed by an exposition of the relevance of this information to sickle cell anemia. The clinical complications to be emphasized are the acute chest syndrome (ACS), endothelial dysfunction with aberrant vasoregulation, circle of Willis vasculopathy, and inflammatory pain. Viewing sickle disease from this perspective elucidates defining pathophysiology and identifies a host of novel potential therapeutic targets.

I/R INJURY

The basic concept of I/R is that tissue injury resulting from vascular occlusion occurs in 2 distinct phases. The first is direct ischemia-induced tissue injury or death, determined primarily by severity and duration of blood supply interruption. If occlusion resolves, allowing reperfusion of the previously ischemic area, the accompanying resupply of oxygen triggers a second, inflammatory phase. The latter establishes systemic inflammation and its sequelae, and sometimes results in remote organ injury (ROI) or even multiorgan dysfunction syndrome (MODS). This complex aspect of biomedicine is described by 2 reviews covering different decades of research using experimental animal models of I/R.[1,2] Additional citations are provided here when specific points require emphasis. This review emphasizes features that most clearly are specifically relevant to the sickle disease context.

Initiation of I/R

An occlusion causing ischemia triggers loss of adenosine triphosphate and reciprocal accumulation of hypoxanthine. This process is followed by cytosolic calcium accumulation, mitochondrial dysfunction, cell swelling, and cell death by inflammatory (necrosis) and noninflammatory (autophagy) mechanisms. In parallel, there is a dramatic change in xanthine dehydrogenase (XD), a widely distributed cellular enzyme that is particularly enriched in capillary endothelial cells, hepatocytes, and intestinal enterocytes. During hypoxia, XD is converted to its xanthine oxidase (XO) form, and significant amounts can be released into the blood space. Within minutes of restoration of reperfusion, XO begins using the accumulated hypoxanthine plus newly available oxygen to fuel superoxide radical generation. In turn, this process enables generation of other reactive oxygen species (ROS), events promoted by iron bioavailability. Thus, XO is understood to be largely responsible for the proximate burst of ROS that is believed to initiate the overall I/R process, resulting in I/R injury.[3]

The Further Evolution of I/R

Subsequent events rapidly become complex, with recruitment of an alarming panoply of cellular, vascular, and parenchymal cell processes that follow from I/R initiation. Additional sources of superoxide radical become activated. Blood-borne XO becomes associated with endothelial cell surfaces, thereby establishing superoxide generation at the endothelial surface. Activity of endothelial nicotinamide adenine dinucleotide phosphate (NADPH) oxidase increases, and endothelial dysfunction ensues with uncoupled endothelial nitric oxide synthase (eNOS) (see later discussion). Leukocytes become activated and generate oxidant. Other superoxide sources can contribute as well. Effects of ROS are indirect (caused by peroxide-based disruption of thiol redox status), modulatory (via effects on cell signaling), and damaging. Oxidant stress causes widespread and varied oxidative and nitrosative damage, which can adversely affect virtually all biological molecules.[4]

The ischemic area acquires multiple activated leukocyte types (polymorphonuclear neutrophils [PMN], monocytes, lymphocytes), dominated initially by PMN infiltration.

Sometimes, the concordant endothelial and PMN activation[5] leads to leukocyte-mediated microvascular plugging, which can even precipitate a no-reflow phenomenon, with local expansion of the original area of ischemic injury. Activation of platelets, endothelial cells, tissue resident macrophages, and mast cells initiates elaboration of a host of inflammatory substances that cause local inflammation and injury.

Of these biological mediators, tumor necrosis factor α (TNF-α) is most strongly implicated as a proximate promoter, its principal producers being blood monocytes, tissue resident macrophages, and perivascular mast cells. In turn, TNF-α induces chemokine production, further ROS production, and critical activation of nuclear factor κB (NFκB), the master trigger of inflammatory gene expression.[6] These events occur explosively, because NFκB activation begins within minutes of onset of reperfusion.

Through these mechanisms, various additional inflammatory mediators appear, in particular: platelet activating factor (PAF), leukotriene B_4 (LTB_4), monocyte chemoattractant protein 1 (MCP-1), vascular endothelial growth factor (VEGF), and, in some models, complement component C5a. Toll-like receptor 2 (TLR2) and TLR4 signaling (in leukocytes, endothelial cells, parenchymal cells, mast cells), prompted by classic TLR ligands generated by cell damage, independently initiates inflammatory cytokine responses.[7]

As part of this overall process, activation of mast cell plays a prominent amplification role. Their many activators include superoxide, PAF, and possibly IgE. By secretion or degranulation, mast cells release TNF-α, interleukin 6 (IL-6), and IL-1β, VEGF, LTB_4, PAF, tryptase, histamine, and other agents.[8] Activation of monocytes, tissue macrophages, mast cells, natural killer cells, and other lymphocyte subsets can exert injurious effects on tissues.

Despite the complexity of this spectrum of biological processes and mediators involved in I/R injury, some emerge as thematically dominant (ie, as master triggers and effectors: a proximate burst of superoxide generation, classically via XO activity; early provocation by TNF-α; mediation by endothelial NFκB activation; infiltration by PMN; amplification by mast cells; and probably attempted mitigation by heme oxygenase 1 [HO-1]).[9]

Differential Organ Susceptibilities

Experimental animal studies show that different organs have differing susceptibilities to developing injury if local I/R occurs; these are in descending order of susceptibility: brain; myocardium, kidney, intestine; liver, skeletal muscle; lung. Direct injury from the initial ischemia develops relatively rapidly, but full development of additional local injury from the reperfusion phase can extend over several days. The pace and the severity threshold at which the former versus latter components develop can vary from organ to organ, thus explaining some of the differential susceptibilities.

The susceptibility of the brain derives from its multiple atypical features: the highest metabolic activity; its absolute metabolic requirement for glucose, despite low local storage; and its high polyunsaturated fatty acid content, despite lower levels of antioxidant enzymes.

Conversely, the lung is uniquely resistant to local initiating ischemia because of its abluminal high oxygen availability. When it does occur, I/R within the lung is complicated, because oxygen tensions of blood (bronchial artery) and tissue (alveolus) can vary independently.

Systemic Implications

A key theme of I/R is that it unleashes a systemic inflammatory response, a process potentially so robust as to generate MODS.[10] On reperfusion, activated blood cells, inflammatory mediators, and other endothelial cell perturbing factors enter the circulation and travel to sites remote from the original occlusion. Activated endothelial cells support capture, adhesion, and transmigration of previously activated PMN.[5] Activated platelets can deposit inflammatory chemokines on the endothelial surface.[11]

Endothelial Dysfunction

During these events, endothelial cells attempt to integrate discordant signals into an appropriate response, but the inflammatory onslaught nudges them toward a maladaptive state. Increased activity of endogenous NADPH oxidase shifts oxidant impact away from normal mediation of homeostatic signaling and toward exertion of oxidant stress[12]; newly acquired endothelial surface XO contributes. This situation results in oxidative loss of tetrahydrobiopterin and perhaps of its rate limiting formative enzyme[13]; this process uncouples eNOS, causing it to generate superoxide rather than nitric oxide (NO).

This combination of enhanced oxidative stress plus diminished NO bioavailability is characteristic of endothelial dysfunction, a state that also includes increased vascular permeability and a shift toward prothrombotic and proinflammatory endothelial cell phenotypes. Endothelial cells themselves begin generating inflammation-promoting agents (eg, MCP-1, IL-1, and PAF). The biodeficiency of NO subverts its normal inhibitory effect on platelet activation, leukocyte adhesion, NFκB-mediated transcription, vasoconstriction, superoxide excess, and Weibel-Palade body release of von Willebrand factor and P-selectin.[14] In addition, the inflammatory state triggers degradation of the endothelial glycocalyx, which normally provides husbandry of homeostatic endothelial functions.[15] Thus, systemic endothelial dysfunction involving both conduit and microvascular vessels is a typical feature of I/R injury states.

ROI

As a truly hallmark feature of I/R, it can initiate injurious effects at sites remote from the site of initial ischemia: ROI or even MODS. In experimental models, such potentially catastrophic complications derive from I/R originating in heart, intestine, lung, kidney, muscle, and liver. Features of I/R-induced systemic inflammation that are particularly pathogenic in ROI include deposition of XO on endothelial surfaces and concurrent activation of leukocytes and endothelium.

The lung is the most commonly involved ROI target organ in both experimental and human disease I/R states. Its unusual vulnerability probably derives from its several unique features.[16,17] The pulmonary capillary bed shows sequential arrangement, with a vast endothelial surface area ($\sim$126 m^2 in adult humans). It the first capillary bed exposed to any postischemic blood. Not only is it oxygen rich (supportive of oxidative biology), but normally it is also uniquely highly enriched for blood leukocytes. Further, the leukocyte/endothelial interactions central to the inflammatory process in the lung may take place in these capillaries rather than in postcapillary venules as in other organs.

Ischemic Preconditioning

Short or pulsed minor episodes of I/R insult can initiate cellular survival adaptations that enable cells to forestall injury from a subsequent, more severe ischemic event. Long believed to comprise an adaptive response by individual involved cells, recent data suggest that remote effects may help direct preconditioning.[18] Most animal and human studies of this have been directed at cardiovascular and cerebrovascular ischemia, for which mechanistic details vary. Generally, there is an early preconditioning effect evident only if the interval between the first (potentially preconditioning) brief ischemic event and the subsequent more severe (injurious) ischemic event is less than about 2 hours. If the interval is 24 hours, preconditioning effects are dependent on gene transcription and protein synthesis. Emerging data suggest that preconditioning effects in the brain may be derived from epigenetic changes.[19]

The converse strategy of ischemic postconditioning has also been observed to help protect from I/R injury.[20] Although much less well understood than preconditioning, this strategy would allow an after-the-fact, or at least a during-the-fact, maneuver to spare further tissue injury, an exciting possibility if it is sufficiently tractable to be used in clinical medicine.

I/R IN HUMAN BIOMEDICINE

In human biomedicine, I/R is believed to explain the genesis of vascular and tissue injury in various conditions in which blood supply is interrupted.[21] Examples include myocardial infarction,[22] stroke,[23] organ transplantation, angioplasty and thrombolytic therapy, cardiopulmonary bypass, ischemic acute renal failure, aortic cross-clamping, and vascular insults affecting liver and intestine.[24] In addition, occurrence of nonseptic acute lung injury (ALI) and MODS can derive from underlying I/R occurring in the context of severe traumatic injury. In general, attribution to I/R in these disease states has resulted from recognition that the data attainable from humans are highly consistent with the extensive data collected from experimental animal models of specific vascular events. The perspective that clinical sickle disease also reflects an underlying I/R pathophysiology finds support in both experimental studies of sickle transgenic mice and clinical observations made in humans.

SICKLE MICE AND EXPERIMENTAL I/R

With the exception of sickle studies, experimental animal models typically have used abrupt interruption of the arterial supply to a given organ or segment thereof. This large vessel maneuver recapitulates only a few events in sickle disease (eg, pulmonary infarction, circle of Willis stroke). Yet the lessons derived from such nonsickle studies predict features that have been found to be characteristic of sickle mouse models even at ambient air, without artificially induced hypoxic stress. Multiple aspects of the baseline features of sickle transgenic mice are consistent with an underlying I/R genesis, as shown in **Table 1**.[25–37]

I/R Induction in Sickle Mice

Sickle disease is understood to involve multifocal microvascular occlusions. Investigators have simulated this process by subjecting sickle mice to transient hypoxia, followed by reoxygenation by return to ambient air (hypoxia/reoxygenation [H/R]). This strategy is intended to statistically increase the chance of sickling and occlusion (with location[s] unknown), followed by some resolution thereof, within a defined time window that enables experimental observation.

In the seminal sickle study, mild-phenotype sickle mice (NY1DD) were exposed to transient hypoxia (8% O_2 for 3 hours), which induced a 10-fold increase in number of sickled RBC.[27] In this manner, several sickle models have been studied. On return to ambient air they showed (within the first 2 hours): vascular occlusions (**Fig. 1A**[38]); conversion of XD to XO (see **Fig. 1B**[27]); and increased oxidant generation, including within endothelial cells (see **Fig. 1C**[27], **D**[25]). In accordance with the expected I/R cascade, they developed increased NFκB activation in lung and liver (**Fig. 2A**[27,39]) and, after a delay, increased IL-6 and TNF-α in plasma (see **Fig. 2B**[40]).

Table 1
I/R-like features of unmanipulated sickle mice at ambient air

Leukocytosis	Kaul et al,[37] 2000
↑ Serum amyloid P	Belcher et al,[78] 2003
Oxidant stress	Osarogiagbon et al,[27] 2000 Dasgupta et al,[28] 2006 Aslan et al,[29] 2007
↑ Lipid peroxidation	Dasgupta et al,[28] 2006
↓ Plasma NO_x levels	Dasgupta et al,[28] 2006
↑ NFκB activation	Belcher et al,[26] 2003
↑ Conversion of XD to XO	Osarogiagbon et al,[27] 2000
↑ XO on endothelium	Ou J et al,[30] 2003; Pritchard et al,[90] 2004
↑ White blood cell/endothelial interaction	Kaul et al,[25] 2000
↑ Platelet activation	Polanowska-Grabowska et al,[31] 2010
Endothelial cell activation	Solovey et al,[32] 2001 Solovey et al,[33] 2004 Aufradet et al,[40] 2013 Vinchi et al,[34] 2013
↑ HO-1	Kaul et al,[35] 2008
Aberrant vasoregulation	Nath et al,[36] 2000 Kaul et al,[37] 2000 Aslan and Freeman,[29] 2007 Kaul et al,[35] 2008

Some hours later, pulmonary endothelial cell activation became evident via upregulation of tissue factor[33] and vascular cell adhesion molecule 1 (VCAM-1),[39,40] with increased whole lung messenger RNA for VCAM-1, intercellular adhesion molecule 1 (ICAM-1), IL-1β, endothelin 1, eNOS, and tissue factor.[40] In addition, there was a dramatic increase in (P-selectin–dependent) leukocyte/endothelial interactions, including transmigration (**Fig. 3**A–D[25]) and augmentation of pain behaviors,[41] possibly mediated by mast cell activation.[42]

Thus, the observations made on both unstressed and H/R-stressed sickle mice show the characteristic pattern of I/R pathophysiology previously identified in various nonsickle models. In addition, indirect evidence is found in the consistent beneficial responses of sickle mice to a variety of therapeutics having known efficacy in experimental I/R models (see later discussion). In aggregate, these data from sickle mice show that the vascular occlusive impact of sickle blood mimics other well-defined I/R states.

CLINICAL SICKLE DISEASE AND I/R

Many aspects of clinical sickle disease are consistent with I/R. Yet, the sickle milieu is complex,[43,44] so superimposition of any new event exerting I/R effects would be occurring within a biological context that is already very complicated. Therefore, precise details of I/R pathobiology in sickle disease may show variations on the classical themes established from nonsickle experimental models and disease states that, by comparison, are more simple. Thus, the following discussion does not address the more obvious opportunities for I/R in sickle disease, such as pulmonary infarction and watershed strokes. Rather, the present focus is on several sickle disease complications that are less obviously ascribable to I/R, even although it is highly likely that they are the consequence of I/R pathobiology.

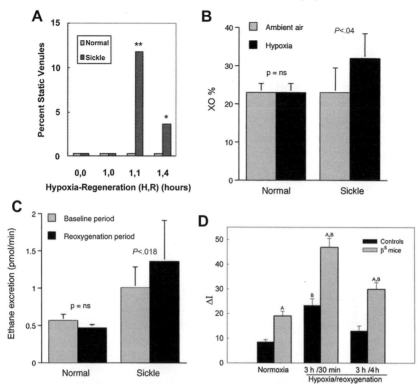

Fig. 1. Onset of I/R injury footprints in mice exposed to H/R. NY1DD sickle mice were examined at ambient air (baseline) and after exposure to hypoxia (3 or 4 hours at 7% or 8% O_2) followed by reoxygenation (H/R) for footprints of I/R injury. (A) Vascular stasis (shown as % of venules that are static) is shown for normal control (*open bars*) versus sickle (*closed bars*) exposed to varying combinations of hypoxia (H) and reoxygenation (R) times (shown in hours, as pairs of H,R times), which included 0 or 1 hour of hypoxia (*left numeral*) and 0, 1, or 4 hours of reoxygenation (*right numeral*). Sickle mice developed robust and maximal stasis after 1 hour H followed by 1 hour R. (B) Proportion of xanthine oxidoreductase in its XO form (expressed as %) is shown for normal control (*left bar pair*) and sickle (*right bar pair*) mice at ambient air (*gray bars*) and after H/R (*black bars*). Only sickle mice showed increased formation of XO in response to H/R. (C) Respiratory excretion of ethane (a maker of biological lipid peroxidation, expressed in pmol/min) is shown for normal control (*left bar pair*) and sickle (*right bar pair*) mice at ambient air (*gray bars*) and after H/R (*black bars*), the later samples collected during the first 50 minutes of the reoxygenation period. Exposure to H/R stress caused increased ethane excretion in the sickle mice. (D) Endothelial cell oxidant stress, detected as fluorescence intensity change (ΔI) of ROS detector dihydrorhodamine in venular endothelial cells in situ in normal control (*black bars*) and sickle (*gray bars*) mice. Mice were examined at ambient air (*left bar pair*) and after 3 hours hypoxia followed by 30 minutes reoxygenation (*middle bar pair*) or 4 hours of reoxygenation (*right bar pair*). ROS generation was higher in sickle mice at all time points, and they showed a more robust increase on exposure to H/R, especially at the earlier reoxygenation time point (30 minutes). A = $P<.0002$ to .0001 for normal versus sickle comparison; B = $P<.05$ compared with respective normal control. (*From* [A] Kalambur VS, Mahaseth H, Bischof JC, et al. Microvascular blood flow and stasis in transgenic sickle mice: utility of a dorsal skin fold chamber for intravital microscopy. Am J Hematol 2004;77(2):121, with permission; and [B, C] Osarogiagbon UR, Choong S, Belcher JD, et al. Reperfusion injury pathophysiology in sickle transgenic mice. Blood 2000;96(1):316;318, with permission; and [D] Kaul DK, Hebbel RP, Hypoxia/reoxygenation causes inflammatory response in transgenic sickle mice but not in normal mice. J Clin Invest 2000;106(3):418, with permission.)

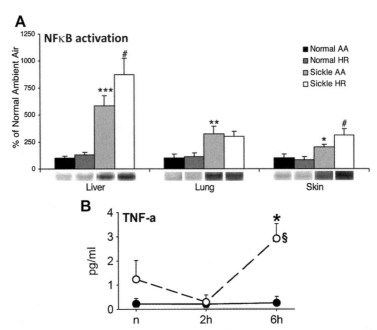

Fig. 2. Evolution of I/R in sickle mice exposed to H/R. (*A*) NFκB activation is expressed as % of that under ambient air conditions for liver, lung, and skin. The mice studied included normal control mice at ambient air (*black bars*) and after H/R exposure (*dark gray bars*), and sickle mice at ambient air (*light gray bars*) and after H/R exposure (*open bars*). Tissues from sickle mice showed increased NFκB activation at baseline, with a further increase in liver and skin after H/R exposure. (*B*) Level of plasma TNF-α level over time (in hours) after H/R exposure for SAD sickle mice (*open symbols*) versus normal control mice (*closed symbols*). Sickle but not normal mice exhibited an increase in TNFα level. (*From* [A] Belcher JD, Mahaseth H, Welch TE, et al. Critical role of endothelial cell activation in hypoxia-induced vasoocclusion in transgenic sickle mice. Am J Physiol Heart Circ Physiol 2005;288(6):H2719, with permission; and [B] Aufradet E, DeSouza G, Bourgeaux V, et al. Hypoxia/reoxygenation stress increases markers of vaso-occlusive crisis in sickle SAD mice. Clin Hemorheol Microcirc 2013;54:303, with permission.)

Cause of Sickle I/R

Fundamentally, the concept of reversible sickling suggests on-and-off occlusive events that, in turn, seem to fulfill the precise requirement for triggering I/R injury. This situation probably occurs from dispersed microvascular occlusions causing multifocal ischemia (eg, as often seen by a multifocal pain pattern with acute vasoocclusive crises). The instability of acute phase reactants in sickle patients between acute events[45–47] shows that subclinical occlusive vents are occurring and resolving often and possibly continuously. The probing consideration of sickle vasoocclusion by Embury is recommended.[48]

Sickle Complexity and the I/R Paradigm

The uniquely complex sickle milieu includes effects from many concurrent, sickling-independent modifiers; some could help mitigate I/R impact, whereas others would enhance organ susceptibility to I/R-mediated injury. Only a few can be noted here.

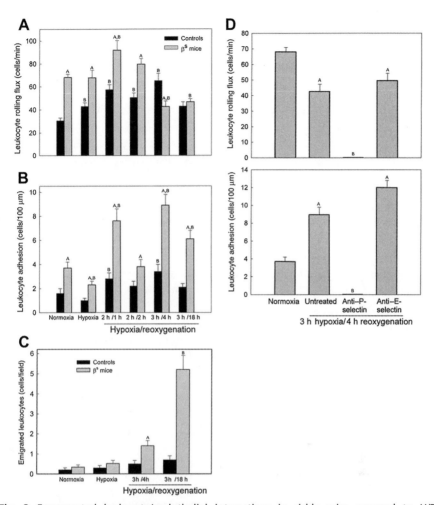

Fig. 3. Exaggerated leukocyte/endothelial interactions in sickle mice exposed to H/R. Abnormal leukocyte interaction with endothelium is shown as (*A*) rolling flux (expressed as cells/min), and (*B*) firm adhesion (expressed as cells/100 μm). A = $P<.01$ to .0001 compared with normal control; B = $P<.05$ compared with respective normoxic control. Abnormal leukocyte interaction with endothelium is shown as (*C*) emigration (expressed as cells/field). A = $P<.01$; B = $P<.0001$ versus corresponding normal controls. In (*A, B, C*) the data are shown for normal control (*black bars*) and sickle (*gray bars*) mice at ambient air (normoxia) and on H/R stress, in various combinations with H applied for 2 to 3 hours and R for 1 to 18 hours. H/R triggers exaggerated leukocyte/endothelial interaction in sickle mice. (*D*) The therapeutic effect of anti-P-selectin, but not anti-E-selectin, is shown for rolling flux (*top*) and firm adhesion (*bottom*), expressed as explained earlier. A = $P<.05$ compared with normoxia values; B = $P<.05$ compared with other groups. These experiments show that only P-selectin blockade inhibited the abnormal leukocyte/endothelia adhesion in sickle mice. (*From* [*A–D*] Kaul DK, Hebbel RP. Hypoxia/reoxygenation causes inflammatory response in transgenic sickle mice but not in normal mice. J Clin Invest 2000;106(3):410;417; with permission.)

Hemolytic anemia

Hemolytic anemia leads to hypoxia, increased wall shear stress in large vessels, and liberation of cell-free hemoglobin (oxidative effects,[4] NO consumption,[49] and free heme-triggered TLR4 signaling effects[50] in endothelial cells and monocyte/macrophages, and possibly in mast cells). Increased erythropoietin can exert cytoprotective effects on nonhematopoietic cells,[51] and the expanded erythroid compartment elaborates placental growth factor, a proximate monocyte activator.[52]

Genetic polymorphisms

Genetic polymorphisms of great variety undoubtedly occur and exert influences. The African *TLR4* haplotype confers an exaggerated inflammatory cytokine response to TLR4 signaling.[53] The decoy chemokine receptor, Duffy antigen, is present on red cells of ~30% of African Americas, who, therefore, may have different chemokine biology from the remainder, who are Duffy negative.[54] Indeed, duffy-negative African Americans tend to show increased severity of ALI (acute lung injury),[55] possibly predicting heterogeneity in severity of sickle ACS episodes.

Epigenetic effects

Epigenetic effects from fetal stressors (maternal tobacco exposure, gestational malnutrition, maternal obesity) can establish harmful effects.

Environmental stressors

Environmental stressors can influence biology (eg, the adverse impact of tobacco smoke on endothelium[56] or the cytoprotective effect of carbon monoxide in ALI).[57]

Sickle preconditioning?

A potentially fascinating aspect of sickle disease is the seeming probability that near-constant on-and-off microvascular occlusions, as a basis for I/R, conversely would exert preconditioning effects. This theory is wholly speculative at present, but it requires research attention, because ability to manipulate preconditioning offers a potential therapeutic intervention.

CLINICAL EXAMPLES OF SICKLE I/R
Clinical Endothelial Dysfunction

Widespread endothelial dysfunction, the consequence of I/R, causes a biodeficiency of NO. Other aspects of inflammation establish upregulation of both vasoconstrictors and non-NO vasodilators. The result is aberrant vasoregulation[58,59] and probably a state of vascular instability.[36] As an example of the latter, the baseline endothelial dysfunction in sickle cell anemia predictably would heighten risk for episodic pulmonary arterial vasoconstriction in the form of exaggerated responses to unrelated potential vasoconstrictors (eg, hypoxia, PAF, incremental hemolytic rate). In turn, this situation may comprise a plausible cause of unexplained sudden death.[60]

ACS

ACS in sickle disease is described as being caused by proximate infection, fat embolism, atelectasis from rib pain, thromboembolism, in situ thrombosis, or vascular occlusion with infarction. However, it is posited here that in some (perhaps even most) cases, ACS is an example of ROI (remote organ injury) resulting from I/R occurring elsewhere. ACS is associated with acute vasoocclusive crisis for ~72% of patients with sickle,[61] and its timing after onset of acute pain mimics the interval between triggering I/R and consequent lung ROI in research models. In general, lung ROI can present with the entire severity spectrum seen in sicke ACS and in nonsickle ALI/acute respiratory distress syndrome (ARDS). Lung ROI is most likely to follow I/R involving the intestine, raising the perplexing question whether ACS events may be derived from small-scale intestinal ischemic episodes occurring (perhaps as only vague abdominal pain) as part of the multifocal acute vasoocclusive crisis.

Sickle ACS is associated with leukocytosis or fat embolism,[61] asthma,[62] and exposure to tobacco smoke.[63] Each of these factors is specifically consistent with sickle disease comprising an underlying ACS diathesis resulting from I/R features.

Leukocytosis reflects inflammation, which can trigger priming of circulating neutrophils so that they have heightened susceptibility to subsequent activating agents,[64] potentially a significant generative factor in lung ROI occurring in I/R states.[65]

Fat embolism, reflecting marrow infarction, possibly offers new substrate for blood phospholipase A_2,[66] thereby liberating free fatty acids that can incite pulmonary edema. The baseline sickle milieu may be unusually conducive to pulmonary edema formation because of the increased levels of various permeability promoters (eg, VEGF, PAF, substance P).

Tobacco exposure causes endothelial cell dysfunction,[56] and even in utero passive exposure is associated with later childhood asthma.[67] So, it seems plausible that the adverse effects of smoke exposure on both vessel wall and airways would increase lung susceptibility to ALI/ACS as ROI from an inciting I/R event.

Asthma association with ACS is particularly intriguing, because both are associated with increased levels of total and allergen-specific IgE.[68] The sickle milieu includes other (allergen-independent) mast cell activators (superoxide, PAF), and one wonders if this total IgE includes hidden cytokinergic IgE.[69] Mast cells may be able to undergo a priminglike change, increasing their susceptibility to later activation.[70] Whether TLR4 signaling effects of heme[50] can exert this effect on mast cells remains to be seen, but TLR4 is implicated in pathogenesis of both ARDS and I/R-induced ROI.[71] A sickle mouse model did show an exaggerated inflammatory response to endotoxin,[72] a classic TLR4 ligand. Thus, ACS susceptibility perhaps could derive from presence of previously primed mast cells, which put the lung at heightened risk for ROI after I/R events.

Arterial Vasculopathy

The relevance of this I/R paradigm as underlying other complications is more speculative because the presumed vector from I/R to consequence is less direct, plus fewer relevant data are available. Yet, the systemic inflammatory state of sickle cell anemia provides a plausible mechanism by which microvascular occlusive disease (the classic sickle paradigm) results in macrovascular vasculopathy (ie, vasculopathic lesions in arteries that themselves are too large to allow occlusion from cell sickling or adhesion). The paradigmatic example of this situation, circle of Willis disease, shows the response of the arterial wall (intimal hyperplasia, smooth muscle cell proliferation, abnormal internal elastic lamina) to inflammation, as seen in atherosclerosis, a less robust inflammatory state than sickle disease. However, in the sickle context, additional stressors probably contribute to development (and location) of lesions. For example, increased growth factor levels (VEGF[73]) and increased wall shear stress[74] would most likely be particularly important in the circle of Willis region.

Inflammatory Pain

The complex pain patterns in sickle cell anemia must include pain driven by inflammatory substances,[75] for which I/R provides mechanistic recruitment of concurrent ischemic and inflammatory pain components. This process would involve neuroimmune linkage with bidirectional positive feedback loops that are effected by inflammatory neuropeptides such as substance P. Sickle mice show hyperalgesia at baseline and substantial augmentation of pain on H/R stress.[41,42] Mast cell activation is implicated as an underlying basis, so the issues discussed earlier (for relationship between vasoocclusion, ACS, and asthma) regarding mast cell susceptibility to activation are also directly relevant to pain. This factor provides, for example, a potential, compelling explanation for the seemingly ballistic development of severe pain after a prodromal phase of acute painful episodes.[75]

IMPLICATIONS OF I/R FOR THERAPEUTICS

Recognition of I/R injury as the underlying basis for the inflammatory state and some major clinical complications of sickle cell anemia immediately identifies a broad spectrum of potential therapeutic targets and agents. The literature on these factors generally is organized in terms of single organ approaches (eg, myocardial, intestinal), more out of interest group focus than for reasons of substantial organ-to-organ differences in pathobiology (although there are some). Some therapeutics for I/R pathobiology that are in the translational research stage have been reviewed recently.[21] Some of these therapeutics attempting pharmacologic simulation of ischemic preconditioning, or alternatively actual preconditioning via exposure to pulsed short ischemic episodes, seem particularly interesting in terms of the sickle context.

In considering I/R-rationalized therapeutics for sickle disease, it seems reasonable, as a general principle, to expect that targets more proximate in the I/R cascade would be more robust. On the other hand, many participants in the I/R cascade were initially discovered because they were targets of narrowly specific interventions that showed surprising efficacy. However, transposition of such insights to sickle cell anemia may not be entirely straightforward, because of the complexity of the sickle milieu, as noted earlier. For example, it would be counterproductive if attempted I/R mitigation impaired those occlusive events that exert preconditioning effects but left unimpeded those that trigger I/R physiology and injury. We have no idea where the border between these 2 potential outcomes might fall in sickle I/R, with its unique genesis via multifocal, small-scale microvascular occlusions than may even occur incessantly.

The spectrum of anti-I/R interventions thus far found to have efficacy for sickle transgenic mice subjected to I/R-initiating H/R stress is delineated in **Table 2**. Thus, disparate therapeutic options have already been identified. Because there is no way to fill in the gap between sickle mouse and sickle human, it seems that careful pilot testing of some of these (and other) approaches is warranted. However, that endeavor requires application of robust pathobiological insight to study design. For example, the therapeutic goal of I/R injury mitigation may require choosing primary study end points that are only surrogate, short-term markers that (it is hoped, but not assuredly) predict beneficial long-term impact. Classic measures related to pain are possibly poor choices as study end points, because they may not be informative vis-à-vis long-term therapeutic impact on the complex biology of I/R, I/R injury, and ROI. Conversely, selection of nonpain I/R makers will be counterproductive if markers are chosen that are too sensitive; some biomarkers of inflammation (eg, C-reactive protein) and endothelial activation (eg, soluble VCAM-1) probably fluctuate too chaotically to be informative in sickle disease.

To aid in maintaining pathobiological perspective while considering I/R-targeted therapeutic approaches to sickle disease, **Fig. 4** is offered to add structure to the fluid landscape created by the complex sickle milieu. For example, it emphasizes whether potential targets are proximate to, distal from, or inherent components of the I/R process.

Two approaches targeting the critical step of inflammation amplification (integral to I/R injury) are being examined: inhibition of invariant natural killer T cells[76] and of mast

Table 2
Successful I/R therapeutics applied to sickle mice for H/R exposure[a]

Category	Agent	Reference
Antioxidants		
XO inhibitor	Allopurinol	27,79
ROS scavengers	Superoxide dismutase and catalase	79
SOD mimetic	Polynitroxyl albumin	80,81
Iron chelators	Didox, trimadox	82
	Vorinostat, tricostatin A	83
Antiinflammatory agents		
Proximate inhibition	Etanercept	89
NFκB inhibitors	Sulfasalzine and others	79,84
Corticosteroid	Dexamethasone	39
Heme oxygenase-I	Gene therapy	85
TLR4 signaling blockade	TAK-242	86
Immunomodulatory targets		
iNKT cell inhibition	Adenosine A2A receptor agonist	76
Mast cell inhibition	Imatinib	42
Adhesion molecule blockade		
Vascular "lubricant"	Poloxoamer 188 (pluronic F-68)	87
Antibody	Anti-P-selectin[b]	25
	Anti-VCAM1 and anti-ICAM1	39
Hemostatic manipulation		
Platelet inhibition	Clopidogrel	31
Inhibit tissue factor expression	Lovastatin	33
	Tricostatin A	83
	eNOS gene therapy	88
	NFκB inhibitors	84
Impact NO and CO biology		
CO delivery	Pegylated CO hemoglobin	78
NO bioavailability	eNOS gene therapy	88
	Arginine supplementation	28
Endothelial sparing		
Statin	Lovastatin	33
Apolipoprotein A-1 mimetic	L-4F	30
HDAC inhibitor	Vorinostat, tricostatin A	83

Abbreviations: HDAC, histone deacetylase; INKT cell, invariant natural killer T cell; SOD, superoxide dismutase.

[a] These studies examined various (and often differing) I/R footprints for improvement by the tested potential therapeutics. Some of these agents exerted beneficial effects on multiple categories of action, especially lovastatin and the histone deacetylase inhibitors.

[b] An E-selectin blocking antibody was ineffective.

cells.[42] These approaches are notable because, in terms of **Fig. 4**, they are located at the arrow that connects I/R and inflammation. Initially, one might think that intervention in sickle pathobiology at this step would be too distal to be effective. However, the amplification step of I/R physiology is critical for the vector leading to ROI, for example. Hence, interference with the immune or immunomodulatory participants[77] in I/R amplification perhaps offers an elegant and straightforward approach.

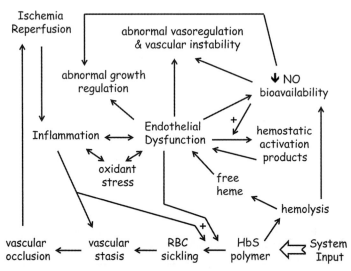

Fig. 4. The role of ischemia/reperfusion physiology in the vascular pathobiology of sickle cell anemia. This hierarchical organization of the checkpoint events in sickle disease pathobiology shows that ischemia/reperfusion physiology Is the central (and perhaps incessant) driver of the disparate injurious biological processes that lead to clinical complications. In that sense, I/R comprises the fundamental linkage between the sickle gene and clinical disease.

A final word of caution: the complexity of the sickle milieu makes predictability difficult, so clinical testing of new therapeutics must be performed with recognition of the probably heightened risk for unintended consequences in the sickle context.

REFERENCES

1. Carden DL, Granger DN. Pathophysiology of ischaemia-reperfusion injury. J Pathol 2000;190:255–66.
2. Kalogeris T, Baines CP, Krenz M, et al. Cell biology of ischemia/reperfusion injury. Int Rev Cell Mol Biol 2012;298:229–317.
3. McCord JM. Oxygen-derived free radicals in postischemic tissue injury. N Engl J Med 1985;312:159–63.
4. Kvietys PR, Granger DN. Role of reactive oxygen and nitrogen species in the vascular responses to inflammation. Free Radic Biol Med 2012;52:556–92.
5. Ley K, Laudanna C, Cybulsky MI, et al. Getting to the site of inflammation: the leukocyte adhesion cascade updated. Nat Rev Immunol 2007;7:678–89.
6. Sun Z, Andersson R. NF-kappaB activation and inhibition: a review. Shock 2002; 18:99–106.
7. Arumugam TV, Okun E, Tang SC, et al. Toll-like receptors in ischemia-reperfusion injury. Shock 2009;32:4–16.
8. Strbian D, Kovanen PT, Karjalainen-Lindsberg ML, et al. An emerging role of mast cells in cerebral ischemia and hemorrhage. Ann Med 2009;41:438–50.
9. Liao YF, Zhu W, Li DP, et al. Heme oxygenase-1 and gut ischemia/reperfusion injury: a short review. World J Gastroenterol 2013;19:3555–61.
10. Bone RC. Sepsis and coagulation. An important link. Chest 1992;101:594–6.
11. Projahn D, Koenen RR. Platelets: key players in vascular inflammation. J Leukoc Biol 2012;92:1167–75.

12. Frey RS, Ushio-Fukai M, Malik AB. NADPH oxidase-dependent signaling in endothelial cells: role in physiology and pathophysiology. Antioxid Redox Signal 2009;11:791–810.
13. Alkaitis MS, Crabtree MJ. Recoupling the cardiac nitric oxide synthases: tetra-hydrobiopterin synthesis and recycling. Curr Heart Fail Rep 2012;9:200–10.
14. Lowenstein CJ, Morrell CN, Yamakuchi M. Regulation of Weibel-Palade body exocytosis. Trends Cardiovasc Med 2005;15:302–8.
15. Lipowsky HH, Gao L, Lescanic A. Shedding of the endothelial glycocalyx in arterioles, capillaries, and venules and its effect on capillary hemodynamics during inflammation. Am J Physiol Heart Circ Physiol 2011;301:H2235–45.
16. Gil J. Organization of microcirculation in the lung. Annu Rev Physiol 1980;42:177–86.
17. Burns AR, Smith CW, Walker DC. Unique structural features that influence neutrophil emigration into the lung. Physiol Rev 2003;83:309–36.
18. Bailey TG, Birk GK, Cable NT, et al. Remote ischemic preconditioning prevents reduction in brachial artery flow-mediated dilation after strenuous exercise. Am J Physiol Heart Circ Physiol 2012;303:H533–8.
19. Thompson JW, Dave KR, Young JI, et al. Ischemic preconditioning alters the epigenetic profile of the brain from ischemic intolerance to ischemic tolerance. Neurotherapeutics 2013;10(4):789–97.
20. Zhao ZQ. Postconditioning in reperfusion injury: a status report (invited review). Cardiovasc Drugs Ther 2010;24:265–79.
21. Eltzschig HK, Eckle T. Ischemia and reperfusion–from mechanism to translation. Nat Med 2011;17:1391–401.
22. Yellon DM, Hausenloy DJ. Myocardial reperfusion injury. N Engl J Med 2007; 357:1121–35.
23. Rodrigo R, Fernandez-Gajardo R, Gutierrez R, et al. Oxidative stress and path-ophysiology of ischemic stroke: novel therapeutic opportunities. CNS Neurol Disord Drug Targets 2013;12:698–714.
24. Vollmar B, Menger MD. Intestinal ischemia/reperfusion: microcirculatory pathol-ogy and functional consequences. Langenbecks Arch Surg 2011;396:13–29.
25. Kaul DK, Hebbel RP. Hypoxia/reoxygenation causes inflammatory response in transgenic sickle mice but not in normal mice. J Clin Invest 2000;106:411–20.
26. Belcher JD, Bryant CJ, Nguyen J, et al. Transgenic sickle mice have vascular inflammation. Blood 2003;101:3953–9.
27. Osarogiagbon UR, Choong S, Belcher JD, et al. Reperfusion injury pathophys-iology in sickle transgenic mice. Blood 2000;96:314–20.
28. Dasgupta T, Hebbel RP, Kaul DK. Protective effect of arginine on oxidative stress in transgenic sickle mouse models. Free Radic Biol Med 2006;41:1771–80.
29. Aslan M, Freeman BA. Redox-dependent impairment of vascular function in sickle cell disease. Free Radic Biol Med 2007;43:1469–83.
30. Ou J, Ou Z, Jones DW, et al. L-4F, an apolipoprotein A-1 mimetic, dramatically improves vasodilation in hypercholesterolemia and sickle cell disease. Circula-tion 2003;107:2337–41.
31. Polanowska-Grabowska R, Wallace K, Field JJ, et al. P-selectin-mediated platelet-neutrophil aggregate formation activates neutrophils in mouse and human sickle cell disease. Arterioscler Thromb Vasc Biol 2010;30:2392–9.
32. Solovey AA, Solovey AN, Harkness J, et al. Modulation of endothelial cell activa-tion in sickle cell disease: a pilot study. Blood 2001;97:1937–41.
33. Solovey A, Kollander R, Shet A, et al. Endothelial cell expression of tissue factor in sickle mice is augmented by hypoxia/reoxygenation and inhibited by lova-statin. Blood 2004;104:840–6.

34. Vinchi F, De Franceschi L, Ghigo A, et al. Hemopexin therapy improves cardiovascular function by preventing heme-induced endothelial toxicity in mouse models of hemolytic diseases. Circulation 2013;127:1317–29.

35. Kaul DK, Zhang X, Dasgupta T, et al. Arginine therapy of transgenic-knockout sickle mice improves microvascular function by reducing non-nitric oxide vasodilators, hemolysis, and oxidative stress. Am J Physiol Heart Circ Physiol 2008;295:H39–47.

36. Nath KA, Shah V, Haggard JJ, et al. Mechanisms of vascular instability in a transgenic mouse model of sickle cell disease. Am J Physiol Regul Integr Comp Physiol 2000;279:R1949–55.

37. Kaul DK, Liu XD, Fabry ME, et al. Impaired nitric oxide-mediated vasodilation in transgenic sickle mouse. Am J Physiol Heart Circ Physiol 2000;278:H1799–806.

38. Kalambur VS, Mahaseth H, Bischof JC, et al. Microvascular blood flow and stasis in transgenic sickle mice: utility of a dorsal skin fold chamber for intravital microscopy. Am J Hematol 2004;77:117–25.

39. Belcher JD, Mahaseth H, Welch TE, et al. Critical role of endothelial cell activation in hypoxia-induced vasoocclusion in transgenic sickle mice. Am J Physiol Heart Circ Physiol 2005;288:H2715–25.

40. Aufradet E, DeSouza G, Bourgeaux V, et al. Hypoxia/reoxygenation stress increases markers of vaso-occlusive crisis in sickle SAD mice. Clin Hemorheol Microcirc 2013;54:297–312.

41. Cain DM, Vang D, Simone DA, et al. Mouse models for studying pain in sickle disease: effects of strain, age, and acuteness. Br J Haematol 2012;156:535–44.

42. Vincent L, Vang D, Nguyen J, et al. Mast cell activation contributes to sickle cell pathobiology and pain. Blood 2013;122(11):1853–62.

43. Hebbel RP, Osarogiagbon R, Kaul D. The endothelial biology of sickle cell disease: inflammation and a chronic vasculopathy. Microcirculation 2004;11:129–51.

44. Hebbel RP, Vercellotti G, Nath KA. A systems biology consideration of the vasculopathy of sickle cell anemia: the need for multi-modality chemo-prophylaxis. Cardiovasc Hematol Disord Drug Targets 2009;9:271–92.

45. Akinola NO, Stevens SM, Franklin IM, et al. Subclinical ischaemic episodes during the steady state of sickle cell anaemia. J Clin Pathol 1992;45:902–6.

46. Singhal A, Doherty JF, Raynes JG, et al. Is there an acute-phase response in steady-state sickle cell disease? Lancet 1993;341:651–3.

47. Stuart J, Stone PC, Akinola NO, et al. Monitoring the acute phase response to vaso-occlusive crisis in sickle cell disease. J Clin Pathol 1994;47:166–9.

48. Embury SH. The not-so-simple process of sickle cell vasoocclusion. Microcirculation 2004;11:101–13.

49. Reiter CD, Wang X, Tanus-Santos JE, et al. Cell-free hemoglobin limits nitric oxide bioavailability in sickle-cell disease. Nat Med 2002;8:1383–9.

50. Figueiredo RT, Fernandez PL, Mourao-Sa DS, et al. Characterization of heme as activator of Toll-like receptor 4. J Biol Chem 2007;282:20221–9.

51. Ogunshola OO, Bogdanova AY. Epo and non-hematopoietic cells: what do we know? Methods Mol Biol 2013;982:13–41.

52. Selvaraj SK, Giri RK, Perelman N, et al. Mechanism of monocyte activation and expression of proinflammatory cytochemokines by placenta growth factor. Blood 2003;102:1515–24.

53. Ferwerda B, McCall MB, Verheijen K, et al. Functional consequences of toll-like receptor 4 polymorphisms. Mol Med 2008;14:346–52.

54. Schnabel RB, Baumert J, Barbalic M, et al. Duffy antigen receptor for chemokines (Darc) polymorphism regulates circulating concentrations of monocyte chemoattractant protein-1 and other inflammatory mediators. Blood 2010;115:5289–99.

55. Kangelaris KN, Sapru A, Calfee CS, et al. The association between a Darc gene polymorphism and clinical outcomes in African American patients with acute lung injury. Chest 2012;141:1160–9.
56. Celermajer DS, Adams MR, Clarkson P, et al. Passive smoking and impaired endothelium-dependent arterial dilatation in healthy young adults. N Engl J Med 1996;334:150–4.
57. Faller S, Hoetzel A. Carbon monoxide in acute lung injury. Curr Pharm Biotechnol 2012;13:777–86.
58. Belhassen L, Pelle G, Sediame S, et al. Endothelial dysfunction in patients with sickle cell disease is related to selective impairment of shear stress-mediated vasodilation. Blood 2001;97:1584–9.
59. Gladwin MT, Schechter AN, Ognibene FP, et al. Divergent nitric oxide bioavailability in men and women with sickle cell disease. Circulation 2003;107:271–8.
60. Hebbel RP. Reconstructing sickle cell disease: a data-based analysis of the "hyperhemolysis paradigm" for pulmonary hypertension from the perspective of evidence-based medicine. Am J Hematol 2011;86:123–54.
61. Vichinsky EP, Neumayr LD, Earles AN, et al. Causes and outcomes of the acute chest syndrome in sickle cell disease. National Acute Chest Syndrome Study Group. N Engl J Med 2000;342:1855–65.
62. Boyd JH, Macklin EA, Strunk RC, et al. Asthma is associated with acute chest syndrome and pain in children with sickle cell anemia. Blood 2006;108:2923–7.
63. Cohen RT, DeBaun MR, Blinder MA, et al. Smoking is associated with an increased risk of acute chest syndrome and pain among adults with sickle cell disease. Blood 2010;115:3852–4.
64. Vercellotti GM, Yin HQ, Gustafson KS, et al. Platelet-activating factor primes neutrophil responses to agonists: role in promoting neutrophil-mediated endothelial damage. Blood 1988;71:1100–7.
65. Moore EE, Moore FA, Franciose RJ, et al. The postischemic gut serves as a priming bed for circulating neutrophils that provoke multiple organ failure. J Trauma 1994;37:881–7.
66. Ballas SK, Files B, Luchtman-Jones L, et al. Secretory phospholipase A2 levels in patients with sickle cell disease and acute chest syndrome. Hemoglobin 2006;30:165–70.
67. Akuete K, Oh SS, Thyne S, et al. Ethnic variability in persistent asthma after in utero tobacco exposure. Pediatrics 2011;128:e623–30.
68. An P, Barron-Casella EA, Strunk RC, et al. Elevation of IgE in children with sickle cell disease is associated with doctor diagnosis of asthma and increased morbidity. J Allergy Clin Immunol 2011;127:1440–6.
69. Bax HJ, Keeble AH, Gould HJ. Cytokinergic IgE action in mast cell activation. Front Immunol 2012;3:229.
70. Sandig H, Bulfone-Paus S. TLR signaling in mast cells: common and unique features. Front Immunol 2012;3:185.
71. Hu R, Xu H, Jiang H, et al. The role of TLR4 in the pathogenesis of indirect acute lung injury. Front Biosci (Landmark Ed) 2013;18:1244–55.
72. Holtzclaw JD, Jack D, Aguayo SM, et al. Enhanced pulmonary and systemic response to endotoxin in transgenic sickle mice. Am J Respir Crit Care Med 2004;169:687–95.
73. Solovey A, Gui L, Ramakrishnan S, et al. Sickle cell anemia as a possible state of enhanced anti-apoptotic tone: survival effect of vascular endothelial growth factor on circulating and unanchored endothelial cells. Blood 1999;93:3824–30.

74. Wei P, Milbauer LC, Enenstein J, et al. Differential endothelial cell gene expression by African Americans versus Caucasian Americans: a possible contribution to health disparity in vascular disease and cancer. BMC Med 2011;9:2.

75. Ballas SK, Gupta K, Adams-Graves P. Sickle cell pain: a critical reappraisal. Blood 2012;120:3647–56.

76. Wallace KL, Linden J. Adenosine A2A receptors induced on iNKT and NK cells reduce pulmonary inflammation and injury in mice with sickle cell disease. Blood 2010;116:5010–20.

77. Ioannou A, Dalle Lucca J, Tsokos GC. Immunopathogenesis of ischemia/reperfusion-associated tissue damage. Clin Immunol 2011;141:3–14.

78. Belcher JD, Young M, Chen C, et al. MP4CO, a pegylated hemoglobin saturated with carbon monoxide is a modulator of HO-1, inflammation and vaso-occlusion in transgenic sickle mice. Blood 2013;122(15):2757–64.

79. Kaul DK, Liu XD, Choong S, et al. Anti-inflammatory therapy ameliorates leukocyte adhesion and microvascular flow abnormalities in transgenic sickle mice. Am J Physiol Heart Circ Physiol 2004;287:H293–301.

80. Mahaseth H, Vercellotti GM, Welch TE, et al. Polynitroxyl albumin inhibits inflammation and vasoocclusion in transgenic sickle mice. J Lab Clin Med 2005;145:204–11.

81. Kaul DK, Liu XD, Zhang X, et al. Inhibition of sickle red cell adhesion and vaso-occlusion in the microcirculation by antioxidants. Am J Physiol Heart Circ Physiol 2006;291:H167–75.

82. Kaul DK, Kollander R, Mahaseth H, et al. Robust vascular protective effect of hydroxamic acid derivatives in a sickle mouse model of inflammation. Microcirculation 2006;13:489–97.

83. Hebbel RP, Vercellotti GM, Pace BS, et al. The HDAC inhibitors trichostatin A and suberoylanilide hydroxamic acid exhibit multiple modalities of benefit for the vascular pathobiology of sickle transgenic mice. Blood 2010;115:2483–90.

84. Kollander R, Solovey A, Milbauer LC, et al. Nuclear factor-kappa B (NFkappaB) component p50 in blood mononuclear cells regulates endothelial tissue factor expression in sickle transgenic mice: implications for the coagulopathy of sickle cell disease. Transl Res 2010;155:170–7.

85. Belcher JD, Vineyard JV, Bruzzone CM, et al. Heme oxygenase-1 gene delivery by Sleeping Beauty inhibits vascular stasis in a murine model of sickle cell disease. J Mol Med (Berl) 2010;88:665–75.

86. Belcher J, Nguyen J, Chen C, et al. Plasma hemoglobin and heme trigger Weibel Palade body exocytosis and vaso-occlusion in transgenic sickle mice. Blood 2011;118:896 [abstract].

87. Smith CM 2nd, Hebbel RP, Tukey DP, et al. Pluronic F-68 reduces the endothelial adherence and improves the rheology of liganded sickle erythrocytes. Blood 1987;69:1631–6.

88. Solovey A, Kollander R, Milbauer LC, et al. Endothelial nitric oxide synthase and nitric oxide regulate endothelial tissue factor expression in vivo in the sickle transgenic mouse. Am J Hematol 2010;85:41–5.

89. Solovey A, Somani A, Chen C, et al. Interference with TNF-alpha using long-term Etanercept in S+SAntilles sickle transgenic mice ameliorates abnormal endothelial activation, vasoocclusion, and pulmonary hypertension including its pulmonary aterial wall remodeling. Blood 2013;122:728 [Abstract].

90. Pritchard KA, Ou J, Ou Z, et al. Hypoxia-induced acute lung injury in murine models of sickle cell disease. Am J Physiol Lung Cell Mol Physiol 2004;286:L705–14.

Gene Therapy for Hemoglobinopathies
The State of the Field and the Future

Shanmuganathan Chandrakasan, MD[a], Punam Malik, MD[b,c],*

KEYWORDS

- Hemoglobinopathy • Thalassemia • Sickle cell disease • Gene therapy

KEY POINTS

- Hemoglobinopathies are the most common genetic defects worldwide. Hematopoietic stem cell (HSC) transplant, although curative, is limited by the availability of matched donors.
- Genetic modification of autologous HSC overcomes the availability of donors (every patient is their own donor) and immunological side effects (graft versus host disease/graft rejection).
- Critical determinants unique to gene therapy for hemoglobinopathies are erythroid-lineage and developmental stage-specific high levels of transgene expression and pretransplant conditioning that will allow 10%–20% gene-modified HSC chimerism.
- Scientific insights into regulation of the globin gene locus and improvements in gene transfer technology have led to development of β-/γ-globin based additive gene therapy a clinical reality.
- Clinical trials with β-/γ-globin lentivirus vectors are now open at multiple sites and transfusion independence following gene therapy has been reported in 1 patient with β-thalassemia.
- Promising new technologies such as induced pluripotent stem cells and genome editing can usher in a new era in the field of gene therapy.

Conflict of Interest: None.
[a] Division of Hematology, Oncology and Bone Marrow Transplant, Cancer and Blood Disease Institute (CBDI), Cincinnati Children's Hospital Medical Center (CCHMC), 3333 Burnet Avenue, Cincinnati, OH 45229, USA; [b] Division of Experimental Hematology/Cancer Biology, Cincinnati Children's Research Foundation, Cancer and Blood Institute (CBDI), Cincinnati Children's Hospital Medical Center (CCHMC), 3333 Burnet Avenue, Cincinnati, OH 45229, USA; [c] Division of Hematology, Cincinnati Children's Research Foundation, Cancer and Blood Institute (CBDI), Cincinnati Children's Hospital Medical Center (CCHMC), 3333 Burnet Avenue, Cincinnati, OH 45229, USA
* Corresponding author. Division of Experimental Hematology and Cancer Biology, Cincinnati Children's Hospital Medical Center, ML 7013, 3333 Burnet Avenue, Cincinnati, OH 45229.
E-mail address: punam.malik@cchmc.org

Hematol Oncol Clin N Am 28 (2014) 199–216
http://dx.doi.org/10.1016/j.hoc.2013.12.003
0889-8588/14/$ – see front matter © 2014 Elsevier Inc. All rights reserved.

hemonc.theclinics.com

INTRODUCTION

Over the last 2 decades significant advances have been made in gene therapy for hemoglobinopathies. Gene therapy has exploited the ability of retrovirus (RV) vectors, which are equipped with the machinery to reverse transcribe their RNA into complementary DNA (cDNA) and integrate this cDNA into the host cell genome to deliver therapeutic genes into cells. Inherited hematopoietic disorders are potentially targetable, because hematopoietic stem cells (HSC) can be readily isolated from bone marrow or mobilized peripheral blood, manipulated ex vivo, and transplanted back using current tools and knowledge of bone marrow transplant technology. The initial vectors used for gene therapy were derived from the murine Moloney leukemia virus (MLV), a simple retrovirus belonging to the γ-retrovirus family, and were termed RV vectors. Despite initial successes in several immunodeficiency disorders, limitations of the RV include their inability to infect the quiescent nondividing HSC, hematopoietic malignancies from inadvertent integration of these vectors near cellular proto-oncogenes, and their activation by the viral promoter enhancer in the vector long terminal repeat (LTR) regions. For hemoglobinopathies, an additional limitation is their inability to carry the large cargo of the globin gene and its regulatory elements, required for high-level expression. These limitations prompted the development of human immunodeficiency virus (HIV)–based vectors. HIV belongs to the lentivirus (LV) family of retroviruses and hence these vectors are termed LV vectors. LV have several advantages for gene therapy for hemoglobinopathies. They differ from RV in their ability to enter an intact nucleus and integrate into nondividing cells, and hence they transduce HSC efficiently. Their self-inactivating (SIN) design, which removes all viral transcriptional machinery, and their ability to carry a large cargo makes them ideally suited for gene therapy for hemoglobinopathies. Since the first use of gene therapy for adenosine deaminase (ADA) deficiency in 1990, generational changes have made the vector design more effective and safe, advanced molecular tools have made it easier to study the insertional effects of gene transfer. Gene therapy has been shown to be effective in correction of many immunodeficiency disorders such as X-linked severe combined immunodeficiency (X-SCID), Wiskott-Aldrich syndrome (WAS), and chronic granulomatous disease (CGD). However, gene therapy for hemoglobinopathies has a unique set of challenges.

Hemoglobinopathies have the additional challenge of requiring high levels of expression of β-/γ-globin genes for therapeutic correction. Identification of critical regulatory elements needed for high expression of β-globin transgene has made gene therapy for β-hemoglobinopathies (sickle cell disease [SCD] and β-thalassemia) a feasible option. More recently, encouraging results from the first successful gene therapy for a patient with hemoglobin E-β-thalassemia in a French trial has opened up gene therapy as a potential definitive treatment option for patients with β-hemoglobinopathies. Trials with different iterations of the β-globin and γ-globin genes in SIN LV to treat thalassemia or SCD are beginning in Italy and 4 centers in the United States (New York, Memphis, TN; Cincinnati, OH; and Los Angeles, CA).

Because expression of increased levels of fetal hemoglobin (HbF) significantly ameliorates the phenotype of both SCD and β-thalassemia, critical elements involved in γ-globin repression in postnatal life have been identified, which has opened up new gene therapy approaches to increase endogenous γ-globin production without the need to add the globin genes and the large locus control region regulatory elements.

Even more promising is the development of gene editing approaches. The design of zinc finger nuclease (ZFN)–mediated repair was the first such approach. This approach was soon superseded by transcription activator–like effector nucleases

(TALENs) and, more recently, by the CRISPR/Cas technology, both facilitating efficient gene editing to correct the genetic defect in situ in cells with high specificity and efficiency. Once this technology is refined, it will allow genetic correction of the β-hemoglobinopathies in situ in HSC, without the need for gene insertion therapy. This article reviews the advances in gene therapy for hemoglobinopathies, with specific reference to β-thalassemia and SCD.

RATIONALE

Disorders of β-globin such as β-thalassemia and SCD are among the most common monogenic defects in the world. Based on World Health Organization worldwide estimates, about 275,000 babies with SCD and 56,000 babies with β-thalassemia are born each year.[1] Improved supportive care has prolonged the survival of these patients. However, there is still significant long-term mortality and morbidity associated with these diseases.

In β-thalassemia, mutations affecting every step in β-globin expression have been reported, from initiation of transcription to posttranslational modification.[2] These defects either result in decreased β-globin production (β^+) or an absence of β-globin production (β^0). The decreased β-globin synthesis in β-thalassemia results in excess of alpha globin, leading to intracellular precipitation of excess unbound alpha globin chains in erythroid precursors.[2] This condition results in red cell membrane damage, early cell death, and ineffective erythropoiesis.[2] At present, lifelong regular transfusions and iron chelation is the mainstay in the management of thalassemia. Despite aggressive iron chelation, iron overload leading to tissue damage and organ toxicity is the leading cause of morbidity and mortality in these patients.[3,4] Inadequate transfusions lead to massive erythroid hyperplasia, extramedullary hematopoiesis, splenomegaly, and failure to thrive.

SCD is caused by a point mutation (A-T) in the sixth codon of the β-globin gene. This genetic defect results in defective β-globin, which polymerizes in the deoxygenated state leading to change in shape of an otherwise round, doughnut-shaped, flexible red blood cell (RBC) into a hook/sickle-shaped, inflexible RBC that obstructs microvessels and has reduced survival from repeated cycles of sickling and unsickling. SCD is characterized clinically by varying degree of anemia, and episodic vaso-occlusive crisis leading to mutiorgan damage and premature death. Medical management options currently available for SCD include supportive management of vaso-occlusive crisis, long-term transfusions to avoid or prevent recurrence of severe complications of SCD such as stroke or acute chest syndrome, and HbF induction with hydroxyurea. Despite improvement in the supportive care, the estimated life expectancy for patients with SCD is significantly foreshortened; the median age at death was 42 years for men and 48 years for women with SCD.[5]

At present, allogeneic hematopoietic stem cell transplant (HCT) is the only established definitive curative option for patients with β-thalassemia and SCD. In both these diseases, the overall survival following matched sibling donor (MSD) HCT is excellent in children, with disease-free survival rates greater than 80%, and a graft failure rate of about 10%.[6,7]

However, most patients do not have a human leucocyte antigen (HLA)-matched sibling. In SCD, it is estimated that less than 14% have a matched sibling and, in the United States,[8] only 30% of African Americans have an identifiable matched unrelated donor (MUD) for HCT (**Fig. 1**). Over the last decade, MUD HCT have increasingly been used for management of thalassemia and SCD.[9] Results from the Italian multicenter trial showed an excellent overall survival and thalassemia-free survival of 97% and

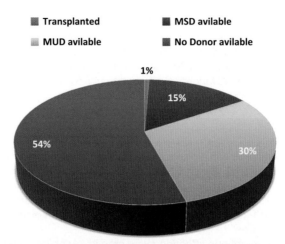

Fig. 1. The frequency of donors and transplants in patients with SCD.

80%, respectively, in low-risk groups. However, in the high-risk groups, the results were less encouraging; overall survival and thalassemia-free survival were considerably lower at 65% and 54%, respectively.[10] Most of this mortality was attributed to grade II to IV graft-versus-host disease (GVHD) or graft failure.[11–13]

In addition, there is poor acceptance of allogeneic HCT as a treatment options among patients with SCD and fewer than 400 transplants have been performed for this disease, because the HCT-related side effects are not acceptable to this patient population (see **Fig. 1**).[14,15] Considering all these limitations with allogeneic HCT, gene transfer using autologous stem cells can potentially cure both thalassemia major and SCD, and could overcome the problems in allogeneic HCT, especially lack of available donors and immunologic side effects such as GVHD or graft rejection.

PREREQUISITES FOR SUCCESSFUL GENE THERAPY IN β-HEMOGLOBINOPATHIES

The following requirements need to be met for successful gene therapy for β-globinopathies:

1. High-efficiency gene transfer and high HSC engraftment
2. Position independent or consistent expression independent of the site of integration
3. High level expression of the β-/γ-globin gene expression
4. Erythroid lineage–specific and developmental stage-specific expression of the transferred β-globin gene
5. Safe expression with little or no risk of insertional mutagenesis/oncogenesis

UNDERSTANDING THE DEVELOPMENTAL SWITCH OF β-GLOBIN AND ITS REGULATION IN POSTNATAL LIFE

In humans, β-like gene cluster is on chromosome 11 and it consists of 5 functional genes: ε, Gγ, Aγ, δ, and β.[2] During different stages of human development, timed switch in expression occurs within this gene cluster. In fetal life, the γ-globin gene (resulting in HbF; α2γ2) is the predominant gene expressed in β-globin locus and β-globin gene expression is repressed. However, after birth, expression of γ-globin gene decreases to negligible levels, with concomitant increase in β-globin expression, which decreases HbF with a corresponding increase in HbA ($\alpha 2 \beta 2$). This process of switching from γ- to β-globin is complex, and it is regulated by multiple transcription factors such as GATA1, BCL11A, KLF1, MYB, and SOX6, and chromatin modification by histone deacetylase 1 and 2 (HDAC 1 and 2).[16,17] The current interest to increase γ-globin expression stems from some important observations. In both SCD and β-thalassemia, hereditary persistence of HbF (HPFH) leads to milder disease phenotype. As a result, pharmacologic measures to induce HbF have resulted in clinical improvement.[18,19] An in-depth understanding of the role of these regulatory elements in γ-globin gene silencing during postnatal life can help design targeted interventions to reactivate endogenous γ-globin expression.[16,17]

The regulation of β-globin is also complex, and elements apart from the β-globin promoter are needed for high levels of expression of the β-globin gene.[20,21] A regulatory element of 40 to 60 Kb upstream of the β-globin gene, known as the locus control region (LCR), is a strong erythroid-specific enhancer that is necessary for high levels of expression of the β-globin gene.[22] The LCR is extremely sensitive to DNase 1 in erythroid cells, with 5 DNase hypersensitive (HS) sites, HS1 to HS5 (**Fig. 2**). Of the 5 HS regions, HS2 was critical for the position independent activity of the LCR, and HS3 was an important determent of its enhancer activity.[23,24] Similar to the LCR for the β-globin locus, HS40, a DNase-hypersensitive site was identified as an alpha globin enhancer 40 Kb upstream of the alpha globin locus acts as an alpha globin enhancer.[25]

INTRODUCTION TO GENE THERAPY

Many viral and nonviral vectors have been tried for gene transfer into cells. Nonviral vectors include plasmids or naked DNA that require physical means such as electroporation to enter cells. The gene transfer efficiency is best with virus vectors, because they have evolved over millions of years to be able to readily enter cells. In addition, physical techniques are too harsh for fragile cells such as HSC. Although nanoparticles that can carry the genetic material in a phospholipid scaffold are a promising proposition, a lot of work is still needed to improve their efficiency and specificity.

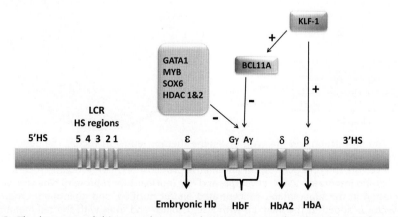

Fig. 2. The human γ-globin gene locus on chromosome 11, showing the ontology of expression of the embryonic, fetal, and adult globin genes, controlled by the LCR. In adult life, the transcription of γ-globin is highly repressed. Some of the major transcription factors involved in the repression of γ-globin are highlighted.

Most of the viral vectors in preclinical studies and in clinical trials are derived from Retroviridae, a family of viruses that can permanently integrate into cellular genomes. Other viral vectors include adenovirus, herpes simplex virus, vaccinia, pox virus, and adeno-associated virus, but lack the integration apparatus. The viruses in the Retroviridae family that are currently used in clinical trials or in advanced preclinical testing include retrovirus (RV), LV, and foamy virus (FV) vectors. These viral vectors are bioengineered viral particles in which the genetic elements needed for pathogenicity and replication are removed and are replaced by the cellular transgene of interest. By using these viral vectors, clinicians could use the viral machinery to enter cells and accomplish the delivery and permanent integration of the transgene of interest into human genome, thus correcting the underlying genetic defect (**Fig. 3**). A synopsis of common terminology used in gene therapy and comparison of different characteristics of the commonly used gene therapy vectors in hemoglobinopathies are given in **Tables 1** and **2** respectively.

RV vectors were the first vectors to be used in clinical trials. The vectors had intact viral LTRs, which contain strong ubiquitous enhancers at either end, with some packaging elements and the transgene of interest (**Fig. 4**). Although these LTR-intact vectors mediated high levels of transgene expression leading to clinical improvement, the success in the trials were soon marred by safety concerns from insertional

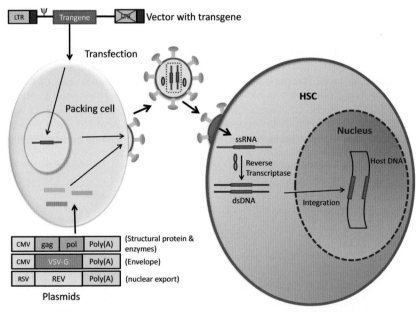

Fig. 3. The production and life cycle of a gene therapy lentivirus vector. The desired viral vectors are made in packaging cells with genetic elements provided separately by different plasmid vectors carrying *gag* (capsid and matrix proteins) and *pol* (protease, reverse transcriptase, and integrase), *VSV-G* envelope, and *Rev* (nuclear export protein). The viral vector is harvested in the supernatant, concentrated and/or purified, and quantified. When the viral vector is added to the medium with HSC, it binds and fuses with the cell membrane of HSC and single-stranded RNA genome is released into the cytoplasm and converted to double-stranded cDNA by the vector reverse transcriptase. The double-stranded DNA forms a preintegration complex that enters the nucleus, where the vector integrase integrates it randomly in the genome of the host cell.

Table 1		
Synopsis of commonly used gene therapy terminology		
Viral vector	Bioengineered genetically disabled viral particles devoid of the components responsible for pathogenic potential but that act as carriers of the therapeutic transgene of interest	
LTR	Long terminal repeats are identical sequences at the ends of RVs: LTR contains U3, R, and U5 regions. The U3 region has strong promoter and enhancer activity and is used by the virus to reverse transcribe and integrate the genetic material into the host genomes	
SIN	Self-inactivating vector design is used to improve safety. Deletion of the U3 region in the 3′ LTR deletes the TATA box and enhancer and abolishes the LTR promoter and enhancer activity. This deletion does not affect vector integration	
Transgene	Human cellular gene (transgene) carried by the vector	
Promoter	Cellular promoter needed for transgene expression	
Enhancer	Cellular enhancers are short segments of DNA that enhance the transcription of the cellular gene, unlike promoters they may not be in close proximity to the gene	
Insulator	Boundary elements flanking the gene cluster of interest; they protect the transgene from silencing by surrounding heterochromatin. Insulators also have enhancer blocking activity	
Process		
Titers	Vectors are made from different plasmid systems in packaging cells. The vector yield or "titer" is measured as the number of particles per milliliter	
Transduction efficiency	Percentage of cells that have been genetically modified by the vector. The higher the transduction (gene transfer) efficiency the better the outcome	
Insertion site	The site in the host chromosome where the vector integrates the transgene with minimal viral elements. The preference of insertion sites vary among different integrating vectors	
Vector copy	Number of transgene/vector copies integrated per cell of interest	

oncogenesis from transactivation of cellular oncogenes by the RV LTR.[26] The lympho-proliferation and leukemia in X-SCID and WAS was ascribed to insertion activation of the LMO2 oncogene.[27,28] In the gene therapy trial for CGD, after initial success, there was silencing of transgene expression caused by methylation of the viral promoter, and myelodysplasia developed with monosomy 7 as a result of insertional activation of ecotropic viral integration site 1 (EVI1/MDS).[29]

Bioengineering of HIV-1 devoid of any pathogenic elements resulted in the development of lentivirus (LV) vectors. Initial studies had established LV vectors as dependable vehicles for high-efficiency gene transfer. Later, a SIN LV vector was constructed by deleting the viral promoter/enhancer in the U3 region of the 3′ LTR, a deletion that gets copied to the 5′ LTR, minimizing transactivation of neighboring cellular promoters and creating an improved safety profile.[30] In addition, several other advantages of LV were noted compared with RV vectors:

1. LV vector can infect quiescent, nondividing cells including HSC, providing an important advantage because long-term HSC are more quiescent than short-term HSC and precursors.[30,31] Gene transfer in long-term quiescent HSC offers a stable long-term correction.
2. Because of higher transduction efficiency, shorter culture time of 24 to 48 hours is need for LV-based vectors compared with more than 72 hours for RV vectors.

Table 2
Properties of gene therapy vectors used in hemoglobinopathies

	Gamma RV Vectors	LV Vectors	FV Vectors
Genus	Retroviridae	Retroviridae	Retroviridae
Viral genome	RNA	RNA	RNA → cDNA
Pathogenicity	Derived from pathogenic murine leukemia virus	Derived from pathogenic HIV virus	Derived from nonpathogenic, nonhuman FV
Cell division requirement	Yes	No	Yes
Packaging limitation	Up to 5 Kb, unstable with large transgene cassettes	Up to 7 Kb	Up to 9 Kb, large transgene cassettes
Transduction efficiency	High in dividing cells	High in dividing and nondividing cells	Efficient entry in dividing and nondividing cells. However, integration occurs in dividing cells
Integration site	Preferentially near transcription start sites (60%–70%)	Preferentially within transcribed genes (60%–70%)	Integration into nongenic regions is preferred approximately 60% of the time. However, integrants that occur in gene-rich regions have the same profile as RV
Safety in clinical trials	Leukemia in X-SCID and WAS trials MDS/monosomy 7 in CGD trial	No overt malignancy seen after 2–6 years Clonal expansion of HMGA2 in one thalassemia patient, that has now decreased	No human clinical data
Experimental genotoxicity data	High risk for insertion oncogenesis	Safer than RV. Safety high with self-inactivating design and use of cellular promoters and enhancers	Safer integration profile than RV and LV
Main advantages	Longest human data and experience SIN RV vector design may address safety concerns	Better safety profile than RV vectors Can stably carry larger cargo Efficiently transduce nondividing HSC	Nonpathogenic, can carry a large cargo and may be safer than RV and LV
Main disadvantage	Clinically significant risk of insertion oncogenesis Lower capacity Does not transduce non-dividing cells	Might induce dysregulation/ disruption of cellular genes, albeit at low frequency	Still not in human trials

3. LV vectors can stably carry larger and more complex transgene cassettes with introns and regulatory elements, necessary for high globin gene expression.
4. In experimental systems, they have a safer integration profile: unlike RV vectors, which have an insertion bias for promoters and 5′ regulator regions of cellular

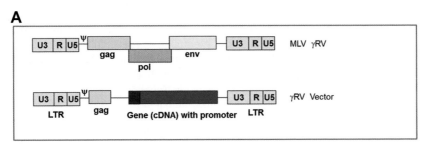

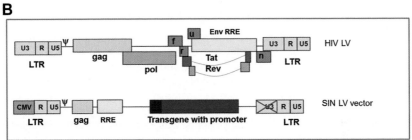

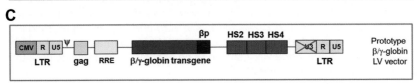

Fig. 4. Gene therapy viruses and vectors. The genome of both wild-type (*A*) murine MLV and (*B*) the HIV-1 virus and the gene therapy vectors derived from them. The initial RVs had full-length LTRs with intact U3 region (which carries the viral enhancer and promoter). With the current generation of LVs, the U3 region of the 3′ LTR is deleted, and in the 5′LTR, it is replaced by a cytomegalovirus (CMV) promoter in the 5′ LTR. The CMV promoter is only used in packaging the vector, and is not transmitted to host cells. The HIV envelope is replaced by VSV-G envelope. (*C*) A prototypic globin LV vector is shown.

genes, LV vectors usually insert within the introns of cellular genes, avoiding the regulatory elements near the transcription start site. Insertional dysregulation caused by abnormal splicing of endogenous cellular genes was noted with LV-based gene therapy experiments.[32,33] LCR-containing LV vectors had approximately 200-fold lower transforming potential compared with the conventional RV vectors.[33] Addition of insulator elements resulted in a further reduction in transforming activity of LCR-containing LV.[33] Thus, based on SIN LV design and supportive data, gene therapy with LV vectors is currently considered to have a lesser risk of insertional oncogenesis than RV vectors and higher efficacy at transferring genes into HSC.

INITIAL VECTOR DEVELOPMENT FOR β-THALASSEMIA

A decade long investigation with β-globin RV vectors resulted in: a) variable and low level expression of the β-globin transgene,[20,34] b) unstable vectors with multiple rearrangements,[35] and c) vectors with low titers.[36,37] In addition, it was found that only HS2 and HS3 elements of β-globin LCR were most important for expression and 3′ HS could be removed without affecting expression.[23,24] Vectors were made containing only core elements of HS2, HS3, and HS4 of the LCR to accommodate the transgene cassette into RV.[38,39] Another important observation was wide variation in gene expression, dependent on the site of integration.[39] These chromatin position effects led to the discovery and use of chromatin insulator elements, such as chicken hypersensitive site 4 (cHS4), into RV vectors.[40,41] Insulators are boundary elements flanking the gene cluster of interest and protect the transgene from silencing, resulting in position-independent expression, and have enhancer blocking activity.[41] The prototypic cHS4 insulator has 2 cores: a proximal 250-bp core element[42] and distal 400-bp element in which all the insulator activity of cHS4 resides.[43]

INITIAL DEVELOPMENT OF LV-BASED VECTORS FOR β-THALASSEMIA

Long-term correction of thalassemia with an LV vector in a murine thalassemia intermedia model was first reported by May and colleagues,[44] with an average increase in hemoglobin by 3 to 4 g/dL per LV vector copy and correction of red cell indices. LV vector–mediated correction of the thalassemia phenotype was also reported in other thalassemia mouse models.[45,46] However, in these studies multiple vector copies were needed for phenotypic correction because of variable transgene expression.[45,46] Further optimization of the LCR components was done by different investigators, which included larger HS2 to HS4 elements of LCR, incorporation of cHS4 insulator elements,[47] or the inclusion of HS I.[48] Later, correction of human β⁰-thalassemia cells was shown in human erythropoiesis models in vitro and in a xenograft model.[49] LV vectors carrying a mutated β-globin gene [that confers it with antisickling properties (βT87Q[50]] or a γ-globin gene were shown to be effective in corrections of both thalassemia and SCD in murine models.[51]

HUMAN GENE THERAPY FOR THALASSEMIA

The basic steps of gene therapy for hemoglobinopathies are shown in **Fig. 5**. In June 2007, the first successful gene therapy for a transfusion-dependent hemoglobin (Hb) $\beta^E\beta^0$-thalassemia was done using an SIN LV-based β^{T87Q} vector.[52] A transduction

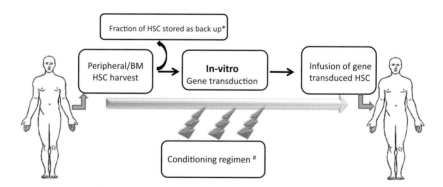

*- To be used if the gene transduced cells fails to engraft
#- High dose chemotherapy such as Busulfan

Fig. 5. Steps of gene transfer into humans. Autologous G-CSF mobilized peripheral blood HSC or bone marrow HSC are harvested and isolated to a pure population. The HSC are transduced for 24 to 48 hours with the gene therapy vector. Conditioning chemotherapy is given concurrently to open up HSC niche. The gene-transduced HSC are infused intravenously.

efficiency of about 30% was reported. The patient received myeloablative busulfan conditioning followed by infusion of 3.9×10^6 CD34+ cells/kg of gene-transduced HSC. After engraftment he had a gradual increase in gene-marked cells to 10% to 20%, and became transfusion independent with a stable hemoglobin of 8.5 to 9 g/dL by 2 years after gene transfer. Although the thalassemia phenotype was partially corrected with gene therapy there was an initial safety concern. Insertional site analysis showed clonal expansion at the high-mobility-group AT-hook 2 (HMGA2) locus in erythroid cells to 10% to 12%. However, the clone stabilized and, at 5 years after gene therapy, it contributed only 2% to 3% of the circulating nucleated cells, and the patient is still transfusion independent.[53] In addition, instability of tandem cHS4 core elements was noted in some cells. To date, 1 more patient has been enrolled in this protocol, but the outcome is not known.

In the United States, a group led by Sadelain and colleagues[54] started a phase 1 to 2 β-thalassemia gene therapy trial in 2011; so far 2 patients have been reported to have received gene-corrected CD34+ cells, and their outcome is awaited.

GENE THERAPY FOR SCD

Successes in β-thalassemia gene therapy led to similar studies in SCD. Both γ-globin–based and modified β-globin–based vectors have been developed for SCD gene therapy. Synthetic β-globin (β^{T87Q} and β^{AS3}) with antisickling properties has been developed by 2 different groups.[50,55] By making 3 amino acid substitutions to the normal human β-globin gene (T87Q, E22A, and G16D), Townes and colleagues[55] bioengineered a recombinant β-globin that prevents axial and lateral contacts in the sickle polymer. The recombinant β-globin designated β^{AS3} inhibits sickle hemoglobin polymerization in the deoxygenated state, and also provides a competitive advantage compared with sickle β-globin for interaction with the alpha globin.[55]

Pawliuk and colleagues[50] were the first to show correction of the SCD phenotype in a murine model by expressing β^{T87Q} with an LV vector. Later, Levasseur and colleagues[56] used a SIN LV vector carrying antisickling globin β^{AS3} to correct the phenotype in sickle mice with human α and β^s globin. The study also showed the feasibility of high gene transfer efficiency in HSC with long-term persistent expression without cytokine prestimulation. Romero and colleagues[57] recently used LV-based vector encoding β^{AS3} to show consistent expression of modified β-globin and reversal of RBC physiologic changes in red cells differentiated for CD34+ bone marrow stem cells derived from a patient with SCD.

Because γ-globin is known to have antisickling properties, gene therapy using γ-globin was considered. However, in adult life, the γ-globin transcripts are highly silenced; to circumvent this, γ-globin driven by β-globin promoters and enhancers were developed.[58,59] Pestina and colleagues[58] showed that the γ-globin gene driven by 3.1 kb of β-globin LCR and a 130-bp β-globin promoter resulted in increase in Hb by 2.6 g/dL/vector copy (VC) and amelioration of disease symptoms. In addition, replacement of γ-globin 3'-untranslated region (3'-UTR) with the β-globin 3'-UTR resulted in a higher Hb increment of 4.1 g/dL/VC.[58] Our group substituted the exons of γ-globin gene for β-globin in the β-globin vector and showed phenotypic correction in the humanized sickle mouse model.[59] In addition, by using reduced intensity conditioning and variable cell dose, we showed that HbF exceeding 10% and a stable chimerism of 20% gene-modified HSCs in the marrow results in phenotypic correction.[59] To date, no patient with SCD has been reported to be enrolled in clinical gene therapy trials, although our group has just opened a gene therapy trial for SCD in Cincinnati.

RECENT ADVANCES

Role of Mobilizing Agents to Achieve Adequate Stem Cell Dose

To achieve transfusion independence, an adequate number of gene-transduced HSCs have to be given. At present, G-CSF mobilized CD34+ and also bone marrow–derived HSCs have been used in gene therapy trials. Specific concerns with G-CSF mobilization in patients with thalassemia include marked leukocytosis and thrombocytosis, and risk for potential thrombotic events in splenectomized patients.[60] In addition, in patients with SCD, the use of G-CSF is contraindicated because there was a high incidence of mortality associated with its use.[61] Plerixafor (AMD3100) has been found to safely mobilize an adequate amount of CD 34+ cells in patients with thalassemia.[62] In addition, when plerixafor was used in combination with G-CSF, it resulted in a more primitive HSC phenotype with a high reconstitution potential and enrichment of CD34+ cell concentration in the BM.[63]

In Vivo Selection: Giving Survival Advantage to Transduced Stem Cells

One of the limitations of β-thalassemia gene therapy in human is to achieve good gene-marked HSC engraftment. Efforts have been made to identify ways to give selective survival advantage to gene-transduced HSCs. Zhao and colleagues[64] developed an LV vector encoding both human γ-globin and an enzyme, methylguanine methyltransferase (MGMT). The addition of MGMT rendered transduced cells resistant to cytotoxic effects of alkylating agents. Thus, when exposed to alkylating agents either before or after transplantation, survival advantage was shown in transduced HSCs compared with the untransduced HSCs.[64] By this approach they were able to achieve a higher number of γ-globin–expressing red cells and HbF, leading to resolution of anemia.[64] Although this approach has translational potential, exposure to additional alkylating agents is less likely to be tolerated in patients with SCD and thalassemia.

Newer Vectors

Although the safety of gene therapy has potentially increased by the use of SIN LV vectors, on integration site analysis they still insert in transcriptionally active sites. Newer vectors with potentially better safety profiles have been developed, of which FV-based vectors have shown promising preclinical results.

FV-based vectors have several unique advantages compared with existing RV-based and LV-based vectors (see **Table 2**). (1) FV is nonpathogenic; (2) FV tends to integrate into nongenic regions predominantly; and (3) it has the largest retrovirus genome compared with RV and LV, hence can be used to package a larger transgene cassette. However, the disadvantage is that, like RV, they require cell division before integration. Morianos and colleagues[65] recently showed that FV vectors with the α-globin HS40 regulatory element resulted in stable expression of human β-globin gene in erythroid cell lines, murine model of thalassemia, and erythroid cells derived from gene-transduced human CD34+ cells from patients with thalassemia.

Transcriptional Manipulation to Increase HbF

Hydroxyurea and other agents have been used to induce HbF in patients with SCD and thalassemia. The exact mechanism of how these medications cause an increase in HbF is still unclear. In recent years novel manipulation approaches have been used to activate the endogenously silent γ-globin expression to increase HbF levels. Recent reports have highlighted the role of KLF1 and BCL11A in repression of γ-globin expression in adult life.[66,67] Several proof-of-concept studies to suppress the level of expression of KLF1 and BCL11A by using short-hairpin RNA in erythroid progenitors and conditional knock-down in murine models have shown increase in γ-globin expression resulting in increased HbF without significantly affecting the erythropoiesis.[66–68] Apart from repression of transcription factors, another approach used for increasing the production of endogenous γ-globin is by activation of its promoter.[69] By using artificial zinc finger transcriptional activation factor, Wilber and colleagues[69] showed an increase in HbF in erythroblasts derived from human CD34+ cells.

At present, the dual approach of combining activation of endogenous γ-globin with either gene therapy using γ-globin vector or inducers of HbF such as 5-azacytidine have been tried.[68] Initial results are promising: if successful, this could result in high levels of HbF leading to potential therapeutic benefit in patients with SCD and β-thalassemia.

INDUCED PLURIPOTENT STEM CELL AND GENE EDITING APPROACH

Advances in induced pluripotent stem cells (iPSC) and gene editing technologies has offered a promising opportunity to correct genetic defects using autologous somatic cells. iPSC offer the potential for an endless supply of stem cells for gene manipulation and correction strategies.[70,71] iPSC are generated from mature somatic cells by forced reprogramming of genes to induce the repressed multilineage differentiation potential. The major advantage of iPSC in a setting of gene therapy is that it offers the possibility to screen and choose the ideal clone with safe integration and high transgene expression profile. Feasibility of this approach was recently shown by using an LV-mediated β-globin gene transfer in iPSC from patients with β-thalassemia.[72] The principles of gene editing and the use of iPSC are discussed below.

The ability to make targeted double-stranded DNA breaks (DSB) by using different site-directed endonuclease approaches have been exploited by researchers to correct the defects in the target genes. ZFNs,[73] transcription activator–like effector nucleases (TALENS),[74] and clustered regulatory interspaced short palindromic repeat (CRISPR/Cas) endonucleases[75] systems have been used to make site-specific DSBs. Following DSBs, the breaks in DNA are repaired by 2 mechanisms: nonhomologous end joining (NHEJ) and homology-directed repair (HDR)/homologous recombination. NHEJ mediates direct joining of the DNA ends in a DSB, which leads to a high incidence of insertion or deletion at the break site. However, in HDR, a homologous sequence is used as a template for generation of the missing DNA sequence at the break point. Despite the high fidelity of the HDR, the frequency of its occurrence is low. When site-directed DSB is combined with facilitated homologous recombination using a donor repair DNA element, the frequency of HDR could be significantly improved (**Fig. 6**). The ZFN system was the first of these systems to be established, and feasibility studies done in a human iPSC line has shown promising initial results.

ZFN-mediated correction of α-thalassemia has been shown in human iPSC.[76] Proof-of-concept studies have been reported using ZFN and TALEN for correction of SCD. Sebastiano and colleagues[77] reported in situ correction of SCD mutation in 2 iPSC cell lines derived from patients with sickle cell anemia; by this approach they reported mean target efficacy of correction to be 9.8%. However, the frequency of successful recombination is still low enough to warrant drug selection approaches, making it more complex and difficult to work with in somatic stem cells.[77]

Due to limited modularity of ZFN and low specificity leading to off-target effects, research has shifted to a more open platform with high specificity and modularity such as TALENs.[78] Sun and colleagues[79] recently showed correction of SCD mutation in iPSC cells with highly specific TALEN in combination with *piggyBack* transposon. At

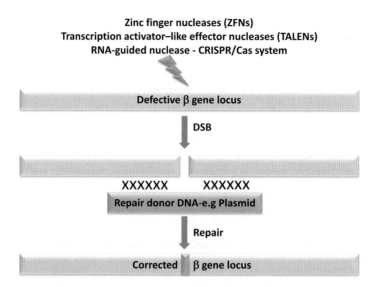

Fig. 6. Gene editing approach. Targeted DSB are made at the site of genetic defect using different customized site-specific endonucleases (ZFN/TALEN/CRISPR/Cas). Following DSB, a donor template strand with correct genome sequence is introduced, which facilitates homologous repair leading to correction of the underlying genetic defect. If the donor template is not provided, the DSB is repaired by NHEJ.

present, there are limited tools available to measure the off-target effects of the endonuclease-induced DSBs. Although the gene editing approach is promising, a lot of work is still needed in improving the specificity and efficiency of gene editing. Simultaneous advances in iPSC to generate long-term HSC could help realize the potential of gene editing approaches in correcting genetic defects in these disorders.

REFERENCES

1. Modell B. Global epidemiology of haemoglobin disorders and derived service indicators. London, UK: World Health Organization; 2008. p. 417–96.
2. Weatherall DJ. The thalassemias: disorders of globin synthesis. In: Kaushansky K, Lichtman M, Beutler E, et al, editors. Williams hematology. 8th edition. United States: McGraw-Hill; 2010.
3. Musallam KM, Cappellini MD, Taher AT. Iron overload in beta-thalassemia intermedia: an emerging concern. Curr Opin Hematol 2013;20:187–92.
4. Olivieri NF, Nathan DG, MacMillan JH, et al. Survival in medically treated patients with homozygous beta-thalassemia. N Engl J Med 1994;331:574–8.
5. Platt OS, Brambilla DJ, Rosse WF, et al. Mortality in sickle cell disease. Life expectancy and risk factors for early death. N Engl J Med 1994;330:1639–44.
6. Shenoy S. Hematopoietic stem-cell transplantation for sickle cell disease: current evidence and opinions. Ther Adv Hematol 2013;4:335–44.
7. Angelucci E. Hematopoietic stem cell transplantation in thalassemia. Hematology Am Soc Hematol Educ Program 2010;2010:456–62.
8. Walters MC, Patience M, Leisenring W, et al. Stable mixed hematopoietic chimerism after bone marrow transplantation for sickle cell anemia. Biol Blood Marrow Transplant 2001;7:665–73.

9. Mentzer WC, Heller S, Pearle PR, et al. Availability of related donors for bone marrow transplantation in sickle cell anemia. Am J Pediatr Hematol Oncol 1994;16:27–9.

10. La Nasa G, Argiolu F, Giardini C, et al. Unrelated bone marrow transplantation for beta-thalassemia patients: the experience of the Italian Bone Marrow Transplant Group. Ann N Y Acad Sci 2005;1054:186–95.

11. Goussetis E, Peristeri I, Kitra V, et al. HLA-matched sibling stem cell transplantation in children with beta-thalassemia with anti-thymocyte globulin as part of the preparative regimen: the Greek experience. Bone Marrow Transplant 2012;47:1061–6.

12. Fleischhauer K, Locatelli F, Zecca M, et al. Graft rejection after unrelated donor hematopoietic stem cell transplantation for thalassemia is associated with nonpermissive HLA-DPB1 disparity in host-versus-graft direction. Blood 2006; 107:2984–92.

13. La Nasa G, Giardini C, Argiolu F, et al. Unrelated donor bone marrow transplantation for thalassemia: the effect of extended haplotypes. Blood 2002;99:4350–6.

14. Thompson AL, Bridley A, Twohy E, et al. An educational symposium for patients with sickle cell disease and their families: results from surveys of knowledge and factors influencing decisions about hematopoietic stem cell transplant. Pediatr Blood Cancer 2013;60:1946–51.

15. Walters MC, Patience M, Leisenring W, et al. Barriers to bone marrow transplantation for sickle cell anemia. Biol Blood Marrow Transplant 1996;2:100–4.

16. Sankaran VG, Orkin SH. The switch from fetal to adult hemoglobin. Cold Spring Harb Perspect Med 2013;3:a011643.

17. Sankaran VG. Targeted therapeutic strategies for fetal hemoglobin induction. Hematology Am Soc Hematol Educ Program 2011;2011:459–65.

18. Musallam KM, Taher AT, Cappellini MD, et al. Clinical experience with fetal hemoglobin induction therapy in patients with beta-thalassemia. Blood 2013; 121:2199–212 [quiz: 372].

19. Voskaridou E, Christoulas D, Bilalis A, et al. The effect of prolonged administration of hydroxyurea on morbidity and mortality in adult patients with sickle cell syndromes: results of a 17-year, single-center trial (LaSHS). Blood 2010;115: 2354–63.

20. Cone RD, Weber-Benarous A, Baorto D, et al. Regulated expression of a complete human beta-globin gene encoded by a transmissible retrovirus vector. Mol Cell Biol 1987;7:887–97.

21. Karlsson S, Papayannopoulou T, Schweiger SG, et al. Retroviral-mediated transfer of genomic globin genes leads to regulated production of RNA and protein. Proc Natl Acad Sci U S A 1987;84:2411–5.

22. Grosveld F, van Assendelft GB, Greaves DR, et al. Position-independent, high-level expression of the human beta-globin gene in transgenic mice. Cell 1987; 51:975–85.

23. Collis P, Antoniou M, Grosveld F. Definition of the minimal requirements within the human beta-globin gene and the dominant control region for high level expression. EMBO J 1990;9:233–40.

24. Ellis J, Tan-Un KC, Harper A, et al. A dominant chromatin-opening activity in 5' hypersensitive site 3 of the human beta-globin locus control region. EMBO J 1996;15:562–8.

25. Jarman AP, Wood WG, Sharpe JA, et al. Characterization of the major regulatory element upstream of the human alpha-globin gene cluster. Mol Cell Biol 1991; 11:4679–89.

26. Cavazzana-Calvo M, Fischer A, Hacein-Bey-Abina S, et al. Gene therapy for primary immunodeficiencies: part 1. Curr Opin Immunol 2012;24:580–4.

27. Hacein-Bey-Abina S, Garrigue A, Wang GP, et al. Insertional oncogenesis in 4 patients after retrovirus-mediated gene therapy of SCID-X1. J Clin Invest 2008;118:3132–42.

28. Boztug K, Schmidt M, Schwarzer A, et al. Stem-cell gene therapy for the Wiskott-Aldrich syndrome. N Engl J Med 2010;363:1918–27.

29. Stein S, Ott MG, Schultze-Strasser S, et al. Genomic instability and myelodysplasia with monosomy 7 consequent to EVI1 activation after gene therapy for chronic granulomatous disease. Nat Med 2010;16:198–204.

30. Miyoshi H, Blomer U, Takahashi M, et al. Development of a self-inactivating lentivirus vector. J Virol 1998;72:8150–7.

31. Naldini L, Blomer U, Gage FH, et al. Efficient transfer, integration, and sustained long-term expression of the transgene in adult rat brains injected with a lentiviral vector. Proc Natl Acad Sci U S A 1996;93:11382–8.

32. Hargrove PW, Kepes S, Hanawa H, et al. Globin lentiviral vector insertions can perturb the expression of endogenous genes in beta-thalassemic hematopoietic cells. Mol Ther 2008;16:525–33.

33. Arumugam PI, Higashimoto T, Urbinati F, et al. Genotoxic potential of lineage-specific lentivirus vectors carrying the beta-globin locus control region. Mol Ther 2009;17:1929–37.

34. Dzierzak EA, Papayannopoulou T, Mulligan RC. Lineage-specific expression of a human beta-globin gene in murine bone marrow transplant recipients reconstituted with retrovirus-transduced stem cells. Nature 1988;331:35–41.

35. Novak U, Harris EA, Forrester W, et al. High-level beta-globin expression after retroviral transfer of locus activation region-containing human beta-globin gene derivatives into murine erythroleukemia cells. Proc Natl Acad Sci U S A 1990;87: 3386–90.

36. Plavec I, Papayannopoulou T, Maury C, et al. A human beta-globin gene fused to the human beta-globin locus control region is expressed at high levels in erythroid cells of mice engrafted with retrovirus-transduced hematopoietic stem cells. Blood 1993;81:1384–92.

37. Chang JC, Liu D, Kan YW. A 36-base-pair core sequence of locus control region enhances retrovirally transferred human beta-globin gene expression. Proc Natl Acad Sci U S A 1992;89:3107–10.

38. Leboulch P, Huang GM, Humphries RK, et al. Mutagenesis of retroviral vectors transducing human beta-globin gene and beta-globin locus control region derivatives results in stable transmission of an active transcriptional structure. EMBO J 1994;13:3065–76.

39. Sadelain M, Wang CH, Antoniou M, et al. Generation of a high-titer retroviral vector capable of expressing high levels of the human beta-globin gene. Proc Natl Acad Sci U S A 1995;92:6728–32.

40. Sun FL, Elgin SC. Putting boundaries on silence. Cell 1999;99:459–62.

41. Chung JH, Bell AC, Felsenfeld G. Characterization of the chicken beta-globin insulator. Proc Natl Acad Sci U S A 1997;94:575–80.

42. Recillas-Targa F, Pikaart MJ, Burgess-Beusse B, et al. Position-effect protection and enhancer blocking by the chicken beta-globin insulator are separable activities. Proc Natl Acad Sci U S A 2002;99:6883–8.

43. Arumugam PI, Urbinati F, Velu CS, et al. The 3' region of the chicken hypersensitive site-4 insulator has properties similar to its core and is required for full insulator activity. PloS one 2009;4:e6995.

44. May C, Rivella S, Callegari J, et al. Therapeutic haemoglobin synthesis in beta-thalassaemic mice expressing lentivirus-encoded human beta-globin. Nature 2000;406:82–6.
45. Rivella S, May C, Chadburn A, et al. A novel murine model of Cooley anemia and its rescue by lentiviral-mediated human beta-globin gene transfer. Blood 2003; 101:2932–9.
46. Persons DA, Hargrove PW, Allay ER, et al. The degree of phenotypic correction of murine beta -thalassemia intermedia following lentiviral-mediated transfer of a human gamma-globin gene is influenced by chromosomal position effects and vector copy number. Blood 2003;101:2175–83.
47. Arumugam PI, Scholes J, Perelman N, et al. Improved human beta-globin expression from self-inactivating lentiviral vectors carrying the chicken hypersensitive site-4 (cHS4) insulator element. Mol Ther 2007;15:1863–71.
48. Lisowski L, Sadelain M. Locus control region elements HS1 and HS4 enhance the therapeutic efficacy of globin gene transfer in beta-thalassemic mice. Blood 2007;110:4175–8.
49. Puthenveetil G, Scholes J, Carbonell D, et al. Successful correction of the human beta-thalassemia major phenotype using a lentiviral vector. Blood 2004; 104:3445–53.
50. Pawliuk R, Westerman KA, Fabry ME, et al. Correction of sickle cell disease in transgenic mouse models by gene therapy. Science 2001;294:2368–71.
51. Persons DA, Allay ER, Sabatino DE, et al. Functional requirements for phenotypic correction of murine beta-thalassemia: implications for human gene therapy. Blood 2001;97:3275–82.
52. Cavazzana-Calvo M, Payen E, Negre O, et al. Transfusion independence and HMGA2 activation after gene therapy of human beta-thalassaemia. Nature 2010;467:318–22.
53. Payen E, Leboulch P. Advances in stem cell transplantation and gene therapy in the beta-hemoglobinopathies. Hematology Am Soc Hematol Educ Program 2012;2012:276–83.
54. Boulad F. Gene therapy for hemoglobinopathies BMT tandem meeting. Salt Lake City, February 13–17, 2013.
55. Levasseur DN, Ryan TM, Reilly MP, et al. A recombinant human hemoglobin with anti-sickling properties greater than fetal hemoglobin. J Biol Chem 2004;279: 27518–24.
56. Levasseur DN, Ryan TM, Pawlik KM, et al. Correction of a mouse model of sickle cell disease: lentiviral/antisickling beta-globin gene transduction of unmobilized, purified hematopoietic stem cells. Blood 2003;102:4312–9.
57. Romero Z, Urbinati F, Geiger S, et al. Beta-globin gene transfer to human bone marrow for sickle cell disease. J Clin Invest 2013;123(8):3317–30.
58. Pestina TI, Hargrove PW, Jay D, et al. Correction of murine sickle cell disease using gamma-globin lentiviral vectors to mediate high-level expression of fetal hemoglobin. Mol Ther 2009;17:245–52.
59. Perumbeti A, Higashimoto T, Urbinati F, et al. A novel human gamma-globin gene vector for genetic correction of sickle cell anemia in a humanized sickle mouse model: critical determinants for successful correction. Blood 2009;114: 1174–85.
60. Taher AT, Otrock ZK, Uthman I, et al. Thalassemia and hypercoagulability. Blood Rev 2008;22:283–92.
61. Adler BK, Salzman DE, Carabasi MH, et al. Fatal sickle cell crisis after granulocyte colony-stimulating factor administration. Blood 2001;97:3313–4.

62. Yannaki E, Papayannopoulou T, Jonlin E, et al. Hematopoietic stem cell mobilization for gene therapy of adult patients with severe beta-thalassemia: results of clinical trials using G-CSF or plerixafor in splenectomized and nonsplenectomized subjects. Mol Ther 2012;20:230–8.

63. Yannaki E, Karponi G, Zervou F, et al. Hematopoietic stem cell mobilization for gene therapy: superior mobilization by the combination of plerixafor plus GCSF in patients with thalassemia major. Hum Gene Ther 2013;24(10):852–60.

64. Zhao H, Pestina TI, Nasimuzzaman M, et al. Amelioration of murine beta-thalassemia through drug selection of hematopoietic stem cells transduced with a lentiviral vector encoding both gamma-globin and the MGMT drug-resistance gene. Blood 2009;113:5747–56.

65. Morianos I, Siapati EK, Pongas G, et al. Comparative analysis of FV vectors with human alpha- or beta-globin gene regulatory elements for the correction of beta-thalassemia. Gene Ther 2012;19:303–11.

66. Zhou D, Liu K, Sun CW, et al. KLF1 regulates BCL11A expression and gamma-to beta-globin gene switching. Nat Genet 2010;42:742–4.

67. Sankaran VG, Menne TF, Xu J, et al. Human fetal hemoglobin expression is regulated by the developmental stage-specific repressor BCL11A. Science 2008;322:1839–42.

68. Xu J, Peng C, Sankaran VG, et al. Correction of sickle cell disease in adult mice by interference with fetal hemoglobin silencing. Science 2011;334:993–6.

69. Wilber A, Tschulena U, Hargrove PW, et al. A zinc-finger transcriptional activator designed to interact with the gamma-globin gene promoters enhances fetal hemoglobin production in primary human adult erythroblasts. Blood 2010;115:3033–41.

70. Takahashi K, Tanabe K, Ohnuki M, et al. Induction of pluripotent stem cells from adult human fibroblasts by defined factors. Cell 2007;131:861–72.

71. Park IH, Zhao R, West JA, et al. Reprogramming of human somatic cells to pluripotency with defined factors. Nature 2008;451:141–6.

72. Papapetrou EP, Lee G, Malani N, et al. Genomic safe harbors permit high beta-globin transgene expression in thalassemia induced pluripotent stem cells. Nat Biotechnol 2011;29:73–8.

73. Urnov FD, Miller JC, Lee YL, et al. Highly efficient endogenous human gene correction using designed zinc-finger nucleases. Nature 2005;435:646–51.

74. Bedell VM, Wang Y, Campbell JM, et al. In vivo genome editing using a high-efficiency TALEN system. Nature 2012;491:114–8.

75. Cho SW, Kim S, Kim JM, et al. Targeted genome engineering in human cells with the Cas9 RNA-guided endonuclease. Nat Biotechnol 2013;31:230–2.

76. Chang CJ, Bouhassira EE. Zinc-finger nuclease-mediated correction of alpha-thalassemia in iPS cells. Blood 2012;120:3906–14.

77. Sebastiano V, Maeder ML, Angstman JF, et al. In situ genetic correction of the sickle cell anemia mutation in human induced pluripotent stem cells using engineered zinc finger nucleases. Stem Cells 2011;29:1717–26.

78. Joung JK, Sander JD. TALENs: a widely applicable technology for targeted genome editing. Nat Rev Mol Cell Biol 2013;14:49–55.

79. Sun N, Zhao H. Seamless correction of the sickle cell disease mutation of the HBB gene in human induced pluripotent stem cells using TALENS. Biotechnol Bioeng 2013. [Epub ahead of print].

Therapeutic Strategies to Alter the Oxygen Affinity of Sickle Hemoglobin

Martin K. Safo, PhD[a], Gregory J. Kato, MD[b],*

KEYWORDS

- Sickle cell • 5-HMF • Antisickling • R state • Hemoglobin allosteric effectors

KEY POINTS

- The T state of sickle hemoglobin (HbS) is prone to polymerize, promoting red cell sickling.
- Stabilizers of the R state of HbS have the potential to directly inhibit sickling.
- R-state stabilizers also increase the affinity of HbS for oxygen.
- An R-state stabilizer, 5-hydoxymethyl-2-furfural (also known as Aes-103) is currently in clinical trials.

OXYGEN AFFINITY OF SICKLE ERYTHROCYTES

The erythrocytes in sickle cell disease have long been known to show decreased oxygen affinity compared with those from healthy volunteers.[1–4] This property is measured as an increase in the partial pressure of oxygen required to produce 50% oxygen saturation (P_{50}), discussed in further detail later. This decreased oxygen affinity is caused at least in part by increased intracellular concentration of 2,3-diphosphoglycerate (2,3-DPG) in erythrocytes, observed generally in all forms of anemia and considered a compensatory adaption that facilitates oxygen release from red cells to the tissues. 2,3-DPG is a product of anaerobic glycolysis, which has been found in recent years to be regulated in erythrocytes by oxygen-regulated sequestration and inactivation of glycolytic enzymes by the cytoskeletal protein band 3.[5–7] Among patients with sickle cell disease, P_{50} and 2,3-DPG levels vary widely, and more increased levels seem to decrease solubility of sickle hemoglobin (HbS),[8–10] and to

Disclosure: See last page of article.
[a] Department of Medicinal Chemistry, Institute for Structural Biology and Drug Discovery, School of Pharmacy, Virginia Commonwealth University, 800 E. Leigh Street, P.O. Box 980540, Richmond, VA 23219-1540, USA; [b] Division of Hematology-Oncology, Department of Medicine, Heart, Lung, Blood and Vascular Medicine Institute, University of Pittsburgh, 200 Lothrop Street, BST E1240, Pittsburgh, PA 15261, USA
* Corresponding author.
E-mail address: katogj@upmc.edu

increase red cell sickling under hypoxia,[7,11] although this has not been confirmed by all investigators.[12,13] In vitro manipulation of human sickle blood to reduce 2,3-DPG content in red cells also reduces hypoxia-induced sickling in vitro.[14] Preliminary investigation suggests that decreased oxygen affinity of HbS may be associated with greater clinical symptoms,[8,15] but more investigation is needed to confirm this association. Although decreased oxygen affinity may be adaptive in other anemias, it may be counteradaptive in sickle cell disease because of its promotion of the T state of HbS, which promotes sickling. These effects relate to alterations in the conformation of hemoglobin (Hb).

THE ALLOSTERIC STATES OF HB AND SICKLE CELL DISEASE

Hb has been shown to function in equilibrium between 2 classic states: the tense (T) state, which has low affinity for ligand, and the relaxed (R) state, which has high affinity for ligand.[16–19] The crystal structure of the T-state (unliganded or deoxygenated) or the R-state (liganded or oxygenated) Hb is each made up of 2 alpha-beta heterodimers ($\alpha1\beta1$ and $\alpha2\beta2$) arranged around a 2-fold axis of symmetry to form a central water cavity with the alpha cleft and beta cleft defining entries into the cavity (**Fig. 1**). The T→R allosteric transition is characterized by rotation of the $\alpha1\beta1$ dimer relative to the $\alpha2\beta2$ dimer, which significantly reshapes the central water cavity, resulting in several differences between the quaternary T and R structures. Most notable is the formation of a larger central water cavity; including the alpha and beta clefts in the quaternary T structure with respect to the quaternary R structure, as well as several different interdimer ($\alpha1\beta2$ or $\alpha2\beta1$, $\alpha1\alpha2$ and $\beta1\beta2$) hydrogen bond and/or salt-bridge interactions in the T or R structures that stabilize one state relative to the other. Despite the presence of βVal6 in HbS, normal and HbS molecules have identical quaternary structures.

The T and R structures were used to formulate the Monod-Wyman-Changeux[20] and the Koshland-Némethy-Filmer[21] allosteric models and later modified by Perutz[16–19] with his stereochemical construct. Since then, several R-like or T-like conformations within quaternary T and R states,[22–28] as well as distinct quaternary relaxed states (R2, R3, RR2, RR3, and so forth) that extend beyond the classic T→R transition[29,30] have been described and/or incorporated in modern allosteric models.[31,32] Like the

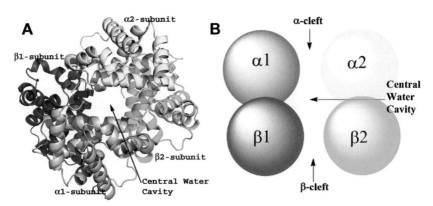

Fig. 1. Quaternary structure of human Hb. Alpha-1 subunit (*gray*), alpha-2 subunit (*yellow*), beta-1 subunit (*magenta*), and beta-2 subunit (*green*). (*A*) Ribbon diagram showing the 4 Hb subunits arranged around a central water cavity. (*B*) The Hb subunits showing access to the central water cavity via the alpha cleft and beta cleft.

R and T structures, the relaxed structures also show significant differences in the geometry of the central water cavities.[29,33–37] Unlike a quarter of a century ago, it is now widely accepted that Hb function involves an ensemble of relaxed Hb states in dynamic equilibrium.[29,33,36–40] One such recent evidence is that aromatic aldehydes that increase the oxygen affinity of HbS do so by binding to quaternary R2 structures and not the quaternary R structures to stabilize the relaxed state.[41,42] An ongoing study also suggests that thiols increase the oxygen affinity of Hb in part by forming a covalent adduct with βCys93 of both the quaternary R and R3 structures in a manner that should prevent formation of the characteristic T-state salt-bridge interaction between βAsp94 and βHis146 when the Hb transitions to the T state and in so doing shifts the allosteric equilibrium to the relaxed state (Martin K. Safo, unpublished data, 2013). Unless noted otherwise, the R state is used to represent the ensemble of relaxed states.

HB: A TARGET FOR DRUG DESIGN

The allosteric equilibrium of Hb is modulated by several endogenous heterotopic effectors, such as 2,3-DPG, and hydrogen ions (H^+); the former bind to the beta cleft and preferentially stabilizes the T state relative to the R state.[16,43,44] Stabilization of the R state shifts the oxygen binding curve or oxygen equilibrium curve (OEC) of Hb to the left, producing a high-affinity Hb that more readily binds and holds oxygen (**Fig. 2**). A shift toward the T state (right shift of the OEC) produces a low-affinity Hb that readily releases oxygen. The degree of shift in the OEC is reported as an increase or decrease in P_{50}, the oxygen tension at 50% Hb O_2 saturation, whereas the degree of allosteric character is indicated by the slope of the oxygen binding curve (n_{50}).

Several synthetic allosteric effectors of Hb (AEHs) also bind to the surface, alpha cleft or beta cleft, or the middle of the central water cavity to liganded Hb structure (in the R, R2, or R3 state) and/or unliganded Hb structure (in the T state) (see **Fig. 1**) to either shift the OEC to the left or to the right (see **Fig. 2**). The direction and magnitude of the shift depend on preferential stabilization of one state rather than the other through additional hydrogen bond and/or hydrophobic interactions that prevent the rotation associated with the allosteric transition and/or destabilization of a state by removing intersubunit interactions, which facilitates the allosteric movement.[37,42,45–49]

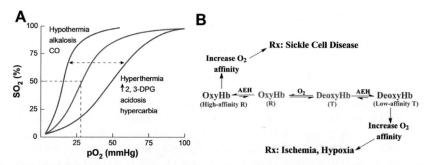

Fig. 2. The allosteric mechanism of Hb. (*A*) Oxygen equilibrium (or dissociation) curve of Hb. The normal P_{50} value is indicated by dashed lines. The left shift and right shift in the curves (*blue*) are associated with various conditions, including allosteric effectors of Hb (AEHs). (*B*) Modulation of Hb allosteric transition by synthetic AEHs. Stabilization of either the R state or T state (*blue*) has potential therapeutic applications. The R represents all identified relaxed states including R2, R3, RR2, RR3, and the classic R. deoxyHb, deoxygenated Hb; oxyHb, oxygenated Hb; Rx, reaction; So₂, oxygen saturation.

For example, RSR-13 (efaproxiral) and several other aromatic propionate analogues bind to the middle of the central water cavity of $Hb^{47,50-53}$; several angstroms away from the beta cleft where 2,3-DPG and other organic phosphates are known to bind.[31,43,44] The binding ties the two dimers together, preferentially stabilizing the T state relative to the R state to lower the affinity of Hb for O_2 and enhance its delivery to tissues in a manner physiologically similar to 2,3-DPG (see **Fig. 2**B). These AEHs have potential therapeutic applications in treating ischemia-related cardiovascular diseases, such as angina, myocardial ischemia, stroke, and trauma, for which more O_2 is needed to heal tissue or organs.[54-59] In contrast, a second class of AEHs, which includes several aromatic aldehydes, bind to Hb to increase its O_2 affinity by preferentially stabilizing the R state relative to the T state (see **Fig. 2**B). These compounds are potentially useful for the treatment of sickle cell disease.[41,42,46,60-64]

The availability of the crystal structures of T and the various relaxed states of Hb have contributed significantly to the design of quaternary state–specific AEHs. Because these compounds bind to locations separate from the substrate (heme pocket) or endogenous 2,3-DPG (beta cleft) binding sites, they are not restricted by the need to generate molecules with higher affinities than the natural ligands; moreover, these AEHs can elicit an effect regardless of the natural ligand concentration. Also, because the allosteric activity of Hb can be modulated to varying degrees, it allows the possibility of tailoring drug activity to the severity of the disease state. Some AEHs bind to the same allosteric sites of Hb, but produce different magnitudes of OEC shift and, in some instances, opposite shift.[41,42,45,47-49] Based on these observation, a general hypothesis was proposed that the effectors' ability to shift the allosteric equilibrium (ie, the effectors' potency and/or direction of shift) is caused not only by where the molecule binds but also by how it interacts with the Hb dimer-dimer interface to stabilize or destabilize that allosteric state.[48,49]

DEVELOPMENT OF ALLOSTERIC MODIFIERS OF HB TO TREAT SICKLE CELL DISEASE

As atomic-level understanding of Hb allosteric property and of the interactions between Hb molecules that contribute to Hb polymerization and formation of pathologic fibers became clear, several classes of compounds (eg, urea derivatives, amino acid derivatives, oligopeptides, carbohydrate derivatives, aromatic alcohols, and acids) were developed, most with the objective of disrupting HbS polymer formation.[65-71] However, most of these compounds had weak, if any, significant antisickling activity, probably because of weak binding to shallow cavities on the surface of the Hb protein, because such cavities do not exclude water and ions and do not provide the necessary environment for strong hydrophobic interactions.

The realization that the polymerization process is exacerbated by the low O_2 affinity of HbS as a result of unusually high concentration of 2,3-DPG in sickle red blood cells (RBCs) led to another rational approach to treat sickle cell disease by increasing the affinity of HbS for oxygen sufficiently to prevent premature release of oxygen, but not so extensively as to compromise tissue oxygenation. Sunshine and colleagues[72] were among the first to suggest that increasing the O_2 affinity of HbS by 4 mm Hg could lead to therapeutically significant inhibition of intracellular polymerization. This approach was also bolstered by the milder clinical severity observed in patients with sickle cell anemia in whom approximately 20% of the red cell Hb content is expressed as the high-O_2-affinity fetal Hb (HbF), which is now known to inhibit HbS polymerization.[73,74] The beginning of the 1970s saw the development of such AEHs, most notably aromatic aldehydes, aspirin derivatives, thiols, and isothiocyanates that form covalent adducts with Hb, modifying the protein's allosteric property to increase its oxygen affinity.[61,64,75–81] The Klotz group reported several benzaldehydes, including the food additive vanillin (**Fig. 3**), and showed that these compounds form a Schiff-base interaction with the amino terminus of alpha globin.[64] The interaction is sometimes described as transient covalent, lasting only for a short period of time, because the Schiff base exists in equilibrium between the bound and the free aldehyde. Several isothiocyanates (see **Fig. 3**) that form covalent adducts with Hb have also been reported for their antisickling activities, also by virtue of their ability to increase the oxygen affinity of Hb.[78] The aliphatic isothiocyanates (see **Fig. 3**) bind covalently to beta globin Cys93 to disrupt the native T-state salt-bridge interaction between βAsp94 and βHis146. This binding leads to T-state destabilization, explaining their left-shifting property.[78] Binding to the βCys93 was also suggested to explain the significant increase in the solubility of fully deoxygenated HbS by preventing direct polymer contacts.[78] In contrast, aromatic isothiocyanates (see **Fig. 3**) also react at the amino terminal amine on the alpha chain of Hb and show antisickling activities by increasing the oxygen affinity of HbS, which the investigators suggested to be caused by

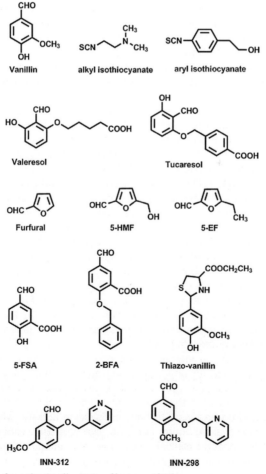

Fig. 3. Structures of synthetic allosteric effectors of Hb.

destabilization of the T state.[78] Although the isothiocyanates seem promising because they can be administered at low doses and less frequently, like other AEHs that form permanent covalent interactions with Hb their lack of specificity could lead to toxicity.

Peter Goodford's group was the first to use the classic R structure to design left-shifting aromatic aldehyde-acid AEHs that were postulated to cross-link the two symmetry-related alpha globin subunits via a Schiff-base interaction with the N-terminus of αVal1 of one alpha subunit and a hydrogen-bond interaction with the opposite αVal1 of the second alpha subunit, and stabilize the R state relative to the T state.[82,83] The study resulted in clinical-tested antisickling aromatic aldehydes that include valeresol (12C79; see **Fig. 3**) and tucaresol (589C80; see **Fig. 3**). A later study by Don Abraham suggested that the left-shifting properties of these agents were the result of 2 molecules (not 1 as proposed by Goodford), each forming a Schiff-base interaction with the N-terminus of the αVal1 nitrogen of the T structure (not the R structure as proposed by Goodford) in manner that destabilizes the T state and left shifts the OEC to the R state.[60] Valeresol underwent human testing, and although potent, was not orally bioavailable, and had a short duration of action of 3 to 4 hours following intravenousadministration.[84,85] Tucaresol was orally bioavailable with more favorable in vivo human pharmacokinetics than valeresol[84–88] but caused immune-mediated toxicity in longer-term phase-II studies.[89] Although shown not to bind as designed, the discovery of tucaresol and valeresol indicated proof of principle that the allosteric property of Hb could be altered pharmacologically.

Although Goodford and Abraham had proposed seemingly opposing views of the antisickling mechanism of left-shifting aromatic aldehydes, it was not until several years later that the exact mechanism underlying the antisickling effect of these compounds was identified.[42] Our group, working with aromatic aldehydes (eg, vanillin, furfural, 5-ethyl-2-furfural, and 5-hydoxymethyl-2-furfural [5-HMF]; see **Fig. 3**), showed that these compounds bind to the alpha cleft of both the quaternary R2 structure (and not the classic R structure) and quaternary T structure. Although binding adds to the stability of the R2 structure, it additionally destabilizes the T structure, which shifts the allosteric equilibrium to the R state and increases the oxygen affinity of Hb.[42] In contrast with the R2 structure, the alpha cleft of the R structure is sterically crowded because of the presence of the C-terminal residues αTyr140 and αArg141, thus precluding binding to these effectors.[42] When Peter Goodford proposed his design model, only the classic R and T structures were known. There are several aromatic aldehyde AEHs that also bind to the alpha cleft to form Schiff base with αVal1 nitrogen, but instead of left shifting the OEC, they decrease Hb affinity for oxygen.[37,48,49,90] An ortho-substituted or para-substituted carboxylate moiety (relative to the aldehyde functional group) in these right shifters, such as 5-formylsalicylic acid (see **Fig. 3**) and 2-(benzyloxy)-5-formylbenzoic acid (see **Fig. 3**), make intersubunit salt-bridge interactions with the guanidinium group of αArg141 on the opposite alpha subunit in the T structure that stabilizes the T state. The left-shifting aromatic aldehydes lack these carboxylate moieties.

With the important lesson learned about potential toxicity issues with covalent AEHs, it was realized that, for any antisickling agent to become a successful drug candidate, clinicians must start with a nontoxic or low-toxicity scaffold in designing new agents. Abraham revisited the food additive vanillin, which had previously been shown by Zaugg and colleagues[64] to have antisickling activity, which he translated into a phase-I clinical trial. Although nontoxic, like valeresol, vanillin was not orally bioavailable, and the phase-I clinical study was terminated. Aldehydes are subject to aldehyde dehydrogenase–mediated oxidative metabolism in human RBCs and liver, which may have been rapid for both vanillin and valeresol, explaining their non–oral bioavailability. A decade later, the prodrug of vanillin, in which the aldehyde group was protected by L-cysteine to form a thiazolidine complex (thiazovanillin; see **Fig. 3**), was shown to have significantly improved oral pharmacokinetic and pharmacodynamic properties compared with the corresponding free aldehyde vanillin, suggesting a viable strategy to improve oral bioavailability, as well as the efficacy of similar antisickling aldehydes.[91]

In a collaborative effort between Don Abraham, Martin Safo, Osheiza Abdulmalik, and Toshio Asakura, 5-HMF (see **Fig. 3**) was shown to have remarkable antisickling activity.[42,63] A single oral dose of 100 mg/kg of 5-HMF was sufficient to protect transgenic sickle mice from death from acute pulmonary sequestration of sickle cells after a hypoxic challenge,[63] whereas chronic administration of up to 375 mg/kg/d of 5-HMF for 2 years was nontoxic to rats or mice.[92] Acute oral median lethal dose for 50% of the test population (LD_{50}) values for rats were 2.5 to 5.0 g/kg for 5-HMF (US Environmental Protection Agency, 1992). 5-HMF also shows no in vitro cytotoxic effects on RBCs, and plasma proteins do not inhibit its binding to intracellular Hb.[42,63]

Crystal structures of 5-HMF and similar furfural analogues (**Fig. 4**) in complex with the quaternary T or R2 structure show that the compounds form Schiff-base interactions with the αVal1 nitrogen in a symmetry-related fashion. The binding of 5-HMF to the R2 structure adds additional intersubunit interaction through a series of direct and intricate water-mediated interactions that tie the two alpha subunits together and restrict the transition to the T state (see **Fig. 4**). The high specificity of 5-HMF for Hb is most likely caused by this intricate and strong hydrogen-bond network. Other less potent antisickling aldehydes, such as vanillin and furfural, lack this intricate sheath of water molecules, explaining their reduced allosteric activity.[42] In contrast with binding to the R2 structure, binding of 5-HMF, as well as other aldehydes, to the wider T structure alpha cleft always results in weak binding of the compounds, which does not seem to add additional intersubunit interaction across the dimer interface.[42] Binding, however, disrupts a T-state water-mediated bridge between

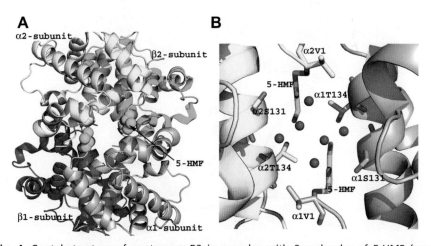

Fig. 4. Crystal structure of quaternary R2 in complex with 2 molecules of 5-HMF (*cyan spheres*). Hb subunits are in ribbons (alpha-1 subunit in gray, alpha-2 subunit in yellow, beta-1 subunit in magenta, and beta-2 subunit in green). (*A*) Two molecules of 5-HMF bound at the alpha cleft in a symmetry-related fashion to the N-terminal αVal1. (*B*) The bound 5-HMF molecules. Each molecule forms a Schiff-base interaction with the αVal1 nitrogen. The sheath of water molecules (*red spheres*) form intricate hydrogen-bond interactions with the bound compounds and the protein to tie the 2 alpha subunits together.

α1Val1 and the opposite subunit residue α1Arg141, effectively destabilizing the T structure and shifting the equilibrium to the R state.[42]

Based on the atomic interactions between Hb and 5-HMF or vanillin, several pyridyl derivatives of vanillin were developed by our group.[41,46] These compounds (INN) bind to the same Hb site as 5-HMF and have superior left-shifting ability and antisickling activities, some having as much as 90-fold and 2.5-fold more potency than vanillin and 5-HMF, respectively.[41,46] Similar to 5-HMF, the INN compounds also bind to the alpha cleft to form Schiff-base adducts with the N-terminal αVal1 nitrogen (**Fig. 5**), and through a series of direct and intricate water-mediated interactions (via the hydroxyl moiety) tie the two alpha subunits together to stabilize the relaxed state in the R2 form.[41] One of the studied compounds, INN-312, in addition to its left-shifting property, also stereospecifically inhibited polymer formation.[41] Binding of INN-312 at the alpha cleft disposes the methoxypyridine substituent (which is ortho to the alde-hyde group) toward the surface of the Hb tetramer to make contact with residues of the alpha-F helix (see **Fig. 5**), which was suggested to lead to destabilization of polymer contact.[41] Asn78α on the F helix has been implicated in stabilizing the HbS fiber; consistently, a variant Hb, Stanleyville (Asn78α ↔ Lsy78α) inhibits polymeriza-tion by destabilizing contacts between deoxy-HbS molecules.[93] This finding suggests a novel therapeutic approach involving the design of compounds that stereospecifi-cally inhibit deoxy-HbS polymer formation while increasing the oxygen affinity of Hb.

CLINICAL DEVELOPMENT

Aes-103 (5-HMF) has undergone preclinical testing for potential treatment of sickle cell disease, as described earlier, including results from the National Toxicology

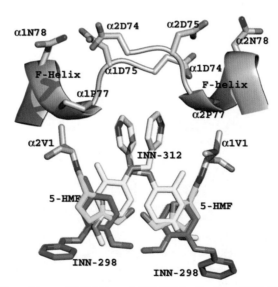

Fig. 5. Superposition of bound 5-HMF (*cyan*), INN-312 (*yellow*), and INN-298 (*magenta*) mol-ecules in the quaternary R2 structures. The Hb molecule (*gray*) is shown for the 5-HMF com-plex. All 3 AEHs form Schiff-base interactions with the αVal1 nitrogen. The meta-positioned methoxypyridine substituent (relative to the aldehyde moiety) in INN-298 is directed toward the center of the water cavity, whereas the ortho-positioned methoxypyridine substituent in INN-312 is directed toward the surface of the Hb to make contact with the F helix, which has been implicated in polymer formation.

Program.[92] It is an organic compound derived from decomposition of certain sugars, found commonly in small amounts in foods such as coffee and prunes. It increases the oxygen affinity of human sickle blood and inhibits hypoxia-induced sickling in vitro.[63,94,95] Short-term administration of high doses in healthy volunteers and patients having lung surgery has been well tolerated.[96,97] Aes-103 has progressed through phase-1, double-blind, placebo-controlled, dose-escalation safety and tolerability trials in healthy volunteers and adults with sickle cell disease (ClinicalTrials.gov identifier NCT01597401),[98] and is expected to enter phase 2 clinical trials.

Although the development of 5-HMF is encouraging, there are several challenges facing the use of covalent Hb modifiers as antisickling agents; some, enumerated earlier, include nonspecific binding, and, for aldehydes, rapid metabolism in vivo, which may compromise their effectiveness. However, a large body of data on vanillin and 5-HMF suggests that these aldehydes have little toxicity at high doses, and that they also provide a structural scaffold to design additional nontoxic AEHs. In addition, some antisickling aldehydes, such as 5-HMF and tucaresol, are less susceptible to rapid metabolism, and moreover there are proven ways to derivatize aldehydes into prodrugs that would protect the aldehydes if needed. Another challenging problem for the use of AEHs pertains to efficacy; namely, the difficulty with designing pharmaceutically useful agents capable of sustained modification of the large amounts of intracellular Hb (approximately 5 millimoles). Although this may seem pharmacologically challenging, therapeutic efficacy might require modification of only a fraction of HbS, as suggested by the mild clinical course of patients with about 20% HbF.[74,99,100] Modification of 10% to 24% of HbS was obtained in an early phase trial with tucaresol, showing the feasibility of modifying this percentage of Hb in vivo.[86] As discussed earlier, a decrease of as little as a 4 mm Hg in the P_{50} has been predicted to provide clinical benefit,[72] and this magnitude of change may be achievable in vivo.

SUMMARY

Pharmacologic stabilization of the R state of HbS offers a therapeutic strategy that directly inhibits the fundamental pathologic mechanism of sickle cell disease, the polymerization of HbS. Although challenges remain in the implementation of this strategy, one agent, 5-HMF (Aes-103), is currently in an active clinical trial to pursue the goal of directly inhibiting erythrocyte sickling in vivo. This is one of the first pharmaceutical agents designed expressly for sickle cell disease to enter clinical trials. Additional investigation of the potential usefulness of sickle erythrocyte P_{50} as a potential biomarker of clinical subphenotype is warranted now that such subphenotypes of sickle cell disease are becoming better defined.

DISCLOSURE AND FUNDING

Disclosure: Dr M.K. Safo is a co-owner of a patent for the use of 5-HMF in sickle cell disease, and he receives research funding from AesRx, LLC, a licensee for Aes-103 (5-HMF). Dr G.J. Kato has collaborated with AesRx, LLC, through a Clinical Trials Agreement between AesRx, LLC and the National Heart, Lung and Blood Institute.

Funding: M.K. Safo gratefully acknowledges research support from the Virginia Commonwealth University Presidential Research Initiative Program Award. The structural biology resources were provided in part by the National Cancer Institute to the VCU Massey Cancer Center (CA 16059-28). During the phase-1 clinical trials of Aes-103, G.J. Kato received research support from the National Heart, Lung and

Blood Institute Division of Intramural Research (1-ZIA-HL006149-01) with additional project support from the National Center for Advancing Translational Sciences Therapeutics for Rare and Neglected Diseases Program (1-ZIB-TR000002-01).

REFERENCES

1. Riggs SA, Wells M. The oxygen equilibrium of sickle-cell hemoglobin. Biochim Biophys Acta 1961;50:243–8.
2. Charache S, Grisolia S, Fiedler AJ, et al. Effect of 2,3-diphosphoglycerate on oxygen affinity of blood in sickle cell anemia. J Clin Invest 1970;49:806–12.
3. Seakins M, Gibbs WN, Milner PF, et al. Erythrocyte Hb-S concentration. An important factor in the low oxygen affinity of blood in sickle cell anemia. J Clin Invest 1973;52:422–32.
4. Milner PF. Oxygen transport in sickle cell anemia. Arch Intern Med 1974;133: 565–72.
5. Chu H, Breite A, Ciraolo P, et al. Characterization of the deoxyhemoglobin binding site on human erythrocyte band 3: implications for O_2 regulation of erythrocyte properties. Blood 2008;111:932–8.
6. Weber RE, Voelter W, Fago A, et al. Modulation of red cell glycolysis: interactions between vertebrate hemoglobins and cytoplasmic domains of band 3 red cell membrane proteins. Am J Physiol Regul Integr Comp Physiol 2004; 287:R454–64.
7. Rogers SC, Ross JG, d'Avignon A, et al. Sickle hemoglobin disturbs normal coupling among erythrocyte O_2 content, glycolysis, and antioxidant capacity. Blood 2013;121:1651–62.
8. Poillon WN, Kim BC, Welty EV, et al. The effect of 2,3-diphosphoglycerate on the solubility of deoxyhemoglobin S. Arch Biochem Biophys 1986;249:301–5.
9. Poillon WN, Kim BC. 2,3-Diphosphoglycerate and intracellular pH as interdependent determinants of the physiologic solubility of deoxyhemoglobin S. Blood 1990;76:1028–36.
10. Poillon WN, Robinson MD, Kim BC. Deoxygenated sickle hemoglobin. Modulation of its solubility by 2,3-diphosphoglycerate and other allosteric polyanions. J Biol Chem 1985;260:13897–900.
11. Jensen FB. The dual roles of red blood cells in tissue oxygen delivery: oxygen carriers and regulators of local blood flow. J Exp Biol 2009;212:3387–93.
12. Beutler E, Paniker NV, West C. The effect of 2,3-DPG on the sickling phenomenon. Blood 1971;37:184–6.
13. Swerdlow PH, Bryan RA, Bertles JF, et al. Effect of 2, 3-diphosphoglycerate on the solubility of deoxy-sickle hemoglobin. Hemoglobin 1977;1:527–37.
14. Poillon WN, Kim BC, Labotka RJ, et al. Antisickling effects of 2,3-diphosphoglycerate depletion. Blood 1995;85:3289–96.
15. Adhikary PK, Hara S, Dwivedi C, et al. Vaso-occlusive crisis episodes in sickle cell disease. J Med 1986;17:227–40.
16. Perutz MF, Wilkinson AJ, Paoli M, et al. The stereochemical mechanism of the cooperative effects in hemoglobin revisited. Annu Rev Biophys Biomol Struct 1998;27:1–34.
17. Perutz MF, Fermi G, Luisi B, et al. Stereochemistry of cooperative mechanisms in hemoglobin. Cold Spring Harb Symp Quant Biol 1987;52:555–65.
18. Perutz MF. Nature of haem-haem interaction. Nature 1972;237:495–9.
19. Perutz MF. Stereochemical mechanism of cooperative effects in haemoglobin. Biochimie 1972;54:587–8.

20. Monod J, Wyman J, Changeux JP. On the nature of allosteric transitions: a plausible model. J Mol Biol 1965;12:88–118.
21. Koshland DE Jr, Nemethy G, Filmer D. Comparison of experimental binding data and theoretical models in proteins containing subunits. Biochemistry 1966;5: 365–85.
22. Sawicki CA, Gibson QH. Quaternary conformational changes in human hemoglobin studied by laser photolysis of carboxyhemoglobin. J Biol Chem 1976; 251:1533–42.
23. Samuni U, Dantsker D, Juszczak LJ, et al. Spectroscopic and functional characterization of T state hemoglobin conformations encapsulated in silica gels. Biochemistry 2004;43:13674–82.
24. Song XJ, Simplaceanu V, Ho NT, et al. Effector-induced structural fluctuation regulates the ligand affinity of an allosteric protein: binding of inositol hexaphosphate has distinct dynamic consequences for the T and R states of hemoglobin. Biochemistry 2008;47:4907–15.
25. Wilson J, Phillips K, Luisi B. The crystal structure of horse deoxyhaemoglobin trapped in the high-affinity (R) state. J Mol Biol 1996;264:743–56.
26. Schumacher MA, Dixon MM, Kluger R, et al. Allosteric transition intermediates modelled by crosslinked haemoglobins. Nature 1995;375:84–7.
27. Abraham DJ, Peace RA, Randal RS, et al. X-ray diffraction study of did and tetra-ligated T-state hemoglobin from high salt crystals. J Mol Biol 1992;227: 480–92.
28. Cavanaugh JS, Rogers PH, Anyone A. Crystallographic evidence for a new ensemble of ligand-induced allosteric transitions in hemoglobin: the T-to-T(high) quaternary transitions. Biochemistry 2005;44:6101–21.
29. Jenkins JD, Moseyed FN, Danso-Danquah R, et al. Structure of relaxed-state human hemoglobin: insight into ligand uptake, transport and release. Acta Crystallogr D Biol Crystallogr 2009;65:41–8.
30. Janin J, Wodak SJ. The quaternary structure of carbonmonoxy hemoglobin ypsilanti. Proteins 1993;15:1–4.
31. Yonetani T, Tsuneshige A. The global allostery model of hemoglobin: an allosteric mechanism involving homotropic and heterotropic interactions. C R Biol 2003;326:523–32.
32. Henry ER, Bettati S, Hofrichter J, et al. A tertiary two-state allosteric model for hemoglobin. Biophys Chem 2002;98:149–64.
33. Safo MK, Abraham DJ. The enigma of the liganded hemoglobin end state: a novel quaternary structure of human carbonmonoxy hemoglobin. Biochemistry 2005;44:8347–59.
34. Safo MK, Burnett JC, Moseyed FN, et al. Structure of human carbonmonoxyhemoglobin at 2.16 A: a snapshot of the allosteric transition. Acta Crystallogr D Biol Crystallogr 2002;58:2031–7.
35. Mueser TC, Rogers PH, Anyone A. Interface sliding as illustrated by the multiple quaternary structures of liganded hemoglobin. Biochemistry 2000;39:15353–64.
36. Silva MM, Rogers PH, Anyone A. A third quaternary structure of human hemoglobin A at 1.7-A resolution. J Biol Chem 1992;267:17248–56.
37. Safo MK, Ahmed MH, Ghatge MS, et al. Hemoglobin-ligand binding: understanding Hb function and allostery on atomic level. Biochim Biophys Acta 2011;1814:797–809.
38. Gong Q, Simplaceanu V, Lukin JA, et al. Quaternary structure of carbonmonoxyhemoglobins in solution: structural changes induced by the allosteric effector inositol hexaphosphate. Biochemistry 2006;45:5140–8.

39. Lukin JA, Kontaxis G, Simplaceanu V, et al. Quaternary structure of hemoglobin in solution. Proc Natl Acad Sci U S A 2003;100:517–20.

40. Schumacher MA, Zheleznova EE, Poundstone KS, et al. Allosteric intermediates indicate R2 is the liganded hemoglobin end state. Proc Natl Acad Sci U S A 1997;94:7841–4.

41. Abdulmalik O, Ghatge MS, Moseyed FN, et al. Crystallographic analysis of human hemoglobin elucidates the structural basis of the potent and dual anti-sickling activity of pyridyl derivatives of vanillin. Acta Crystallogr D Biol Crystallogr 2011;67:920–8.

42. Safo MK, Abdulmalik O, Danso-Danquah R, et al. Structural basis for the potent antisickling effect of a novel class of five-membered heterocyclic aldehydic compounds. J Med Chem 2004;47:4665–76.

43. Anyone A. X-ray diffraction study of binding of 2,3-diphosphoglycerate to human deoxyhaemoglobin. Nature 1972;237:146–9.

44. Richard V, Dodson GG, Mauguen Y. Human deoxyhaemoglobin-2,3-diphosphoglycerate complex low-salt structure at 2.5 A resolution. J Mol Biol 1993;233:270–4.

45. Safo MK, Bruno S. Allosteric effectors of hemoglobin: past, present and future. In: Mozzarelli A, Bettati S, editors. Chemistry and biochemistry of oxygen therapeutics: from transfusion to artificial blood. Hoboken, NJ: John Wiley; 2011. p. 285–300.

46. Nnamani IN, Joshi GS, Danso-Danquah R, et al. Pyridyl derivatives of benzaldehyde as potential antisickling agents. Chem Biodivers 2008;5:1762–9.

47. Safo MK, Moure CM, Burnett JC, et al. High-resolution crystal structure of deoxy hemoglobin complexed with a potent allosteric effector. Protein Sci 2001;10:951–7.

48. Abraham DJ, Safo MK, Boyiri T, et al. How allosteric effectors can bind to the same protein residue and produce opposite shifts in the allosteric equilibrium. Biochemistry 1995;34:15006–20.

49. Boyiri T, Safo MK, Danso-Danquah RE, et al. Bisaldehyde allosteric effectors as molecular ratchets and probes. Biochemistry 1995;34:15021–36.

50. Abraham DJ, Wireko FC, Randal RS, et al. Allosteric modifiers of hemoglobin: 2-[4-[[(3,5-disubstituted anilino)carbonyl]methyl]phenoxy]-2-methylpropionic acid derivatives that lower the oxygen affinity of hemoglobin in red cell suspensions, in whole blood, and in vivo in rats. Biochemistry 1992;31:9141–9.

51. Randal RS, Mahran MA, Mehanna AS, et al. Allosteric modifiers of hemoglobin. 1. Design, synthesis, testing, and structure-allosteric activity relationship of novel hemoglobin oxygen affinity decreasing agents. J Med Chem 1991;34:752–7.

52. Chen Q, Lalezari I, Nagel RL, et al. Liganded hemoglobin structural perturbations by the allosteric effector L35. Biophys J 2005;88:2057–67.

53. Lalezari I, Lalezari P, Poyart C, et al. New effectors of human hemoglobin: structure and function. Biochemistry 1990;29:1515–23.

54. Hou H, Khan N, Grinberg OY, et al. The effects of Efaproxyn (efaproxiral) on subcutaneous RIF-1 tumor oxygenation and enhancement of radiotherapy-mediated inhibition of tumor growth in mice. Radiat Res 2007;168:218–25.

55. Grinberg OY, Miyake M, Hou H, et al. The dose-dependent effect of RSR13, a synthetic allosteric modifier of hemoglobin, on physiological parameters and brain tissue oxygenation in rats. Adv Exp Med Biol 2003;530:287–96.

56. Khandelwal SR, Randal RS, Lin PS, et al. Enhanced oxygenation in vivo by allosteric inhibitors of hemoglobin saturation. Am J Physiol 1993;265:H1450–3.

57. Kunert MP, Liard JF, Abraham DJ. RSR-13, an allosteric effector of hemoglobin, increases systemic and iliac vascular resistance in rats. Am J Physiol 1996;271: H602–13.
58. Suh JH, Stea B, Nabid A, et al. Phase III study of efaproxiral as an adjunct to whole-brain radiation therapy for brain metastases. J Clin Oncol 2006;24:106–14.
59. Scott C, Suh J, Stea B, et al. Improved survival, quality of life, and quality-adjusted survival in breast cancer patients treated with efaproxiral (efaproxyn) plus whole-brain radiation therapy for brain metastases. Am J Clin Oncol 2007;30:580–7.
60. Wireko FC, Abraham DJ. X-ray diffraction study of the binding of the antisickling agent 12C79 to human hemoglobin. Proc Natl Acad Sci U S A 1991;88: 2209–11.
61. Abraham DJ, Mehanna AS, Wireko FC, et al. Vanillin, a potential agent for the treatment of sickle cell anemia. Blood 1991;77:1334–41.
62. Swerdlow PS, Orringer EP, Abraham DJ. Dietary management of sickle cell anaemia with vanillin. Free Radic Res Commun 1992;17:351–2.
63. Abdulmalik O, Safo MK, Chen Q, et al. 5-Hydroxymethyl-2-furfural modifies intracellular sickle haemoglobin and inhibits sickling of red blood cells. Br J Haematol 2005;128:552–61.
64. Zaugg RH, Walder JA, Klotz IM. Schiff base adducts of hemoglobin. Modifications that inhibit erythrocyte sickling. J Biol Chem 1977;252:8542–8.
65. Mehanna AS. Sickle cell anemia and antisickling agents then and now. Curr Med Chem 2001;8:79–88.
66. Sheh L, Mokotoff M, Abraham DJ. Design, synthesis, and testing of potential antisickling agents. 9. Cyclic tetrapeptide homologs as mimics of the mutation site of hemoglobin S. Int J Pept Protein Res 1987;29:509–20.
67. Patwa DC, Abraham DJ, Hung TC. Design, synthesis, and testing of potential antisickling agents. 6. Rheologic studies with active phenoxy and benzyloxy acids. Blood Cells 1987;12:589–601.
68. Abraham DJ, Perutz MF, Phillips SE. Physiological and x-ray studies of potential antisickling agents. Proc Natl Acad Sci U S A 1983;80:324–8.
69. Perutz MF, Fermi G, Abraham DJ, et al. Hemoglobin as a receptor of drugs and peptides: X-ray studies of the stereochemistry of binding. J Am Chem Soc 1986; 108:1064–78.
70. Abraham DJ, Gazze DM, Kennedy PE, et al. Design, synthesis, and testing of potential antisickling agents. 5. Disubstituted benzoic acids designed for the donor site and proline salicylates designed for the acceptor site. J Med Chem 1984;27:1549–59.
71. Abraham DJ, Mokotoff M, Sheh L, et al. Design, synthesis, and testing of antisickling agents. 2. Proline derivatives designed for the donor site. J Med Chem 1983;26:549–54.
72. Sunshine HR, Hofrichter J, Eaton WA. Requirement for therapeutic inhibition of sickle haemoglobin gelation. Nature 1978;275:238–40.
73. Wood WG, Pembrey ME, Serjeant GR, et al. Hb F synthesis in sickle cell anaemia: a comparison of Saudi Arab cases with those of African origin. Br J Haematol 1980;45:431–45.
74. Pembrey ME, Wood WG, Weatherall DJ, et al. Fetal haemoglobin production and the sickle gene in the oases of eastern Saudi Arabia. Br J Haematol 1978;40:415–29.
75. Garel MC, Domenget C, Caburi-Martin J, et al. Covalent binding of glutathione to hemoglobin. I. Inhibition of hemoglobin S polymerization. J Biol Chem 1986; 261:14704–9.

76. Caburi-Martin J, Garel MC, Domenget C, et al. Contact inhibition within hemoglobin S polymer by thiol reagents. Biochim Biophys Acta 1986;874:82–9.

77. Garel MC, Domenget C, Galacteros F, et al. Inhibition of erythrocyte sickling by thiol reagents. Mol Pharmacol 1984;26:559–65.

78. Park S, Hayes BL, Marankan F, et al. Regioselective covalent modification of hemoglobin in search of antisickling agents. J Med Chem 2003;46:936–53.

79. Zaugg RH, Walder JA, Walder RY, et al. Modification of hemoglobin with analogs of aspirin. J Biol Chem 1980;255:2816–21.

80. Walder JA, Zaugg RH, Iwaoka RS, et al. Alternative aspirins as antisickling agents: Acetyl-3,5-dibromosalicylic acid. Proc Natl Acad Sci U S A 1977;74:5499–503.

81. Walder JA, Zaugg RH, Walder RY, et al. Diaspirins that cross-link beta chains of hemoglobin: Bis(3,5-dibromosalicyl) succinate and bis(3,5-dibromosalicyl) fumarate. Biochemistry 1979;18:4265–70.

82. Beddell CR, Goodford PJ, Kneen G, et al. Substituted benzaldehydes designed to increase the oxygen affinity of human haemoglobin and inhibit the sickling of sickle erythrocytes. Br J Pharmacol 1984;82:397–407.

83. Merrett M, Stammers DK, White RD, et al. Characterization of the binding of the anti-sickling compound, BW12C, to haemoglobin. Biochem J 1986;239: 387–92.

84. Keidan AJ, Franklin IM, White RD, et al. Effect of BW12C on oxygen affinity of haemoglobin in sickle-cell disease. Lancet 1986;1:831–4.

85. Fitzharris P, McLean AE, Sparks RG, et al. The effects in volunteers of BW12C, a compound designed to left-shift the blood-oxygen saturation curve. Br J Clin Pharmacol 1985;19:471–81.

86. Arya R, Rolan PE, Wootton R, et al. Tucaresol increases oxygen affinity and reduces haemolysis in subjects with sickle cell anaemia. Br J Haematol 1996; 93:817–21.

87. Rolan PE, Mercer AJ, Wootton R, et al. Pharmacokinetics and pharmacodynamics of tucaresol, an antisickling agent, in healthy volunteers. Br J Clin Pharmacol 1995;39:375–80.

88. Rolan PE, Parker JE, Gray SJ, et al. The pharmacokinetics, tolerability and pharmacodynamics of tucaresol (589C80; 4[2-formyl-3-hydroxyphenoxymethyl] benzoic acid), a potential anti-sickling agent, following oral administration to healthy subjects. Br J Clin Pharmacol 1993;35:419–25.

89. Rhodes J. Discovery of immunopotentiatory drugs: current and future strategies. Clin Exp Immunol 2002;130:363–9.

90. Safo MK, Boyiri T, Burnett JC, et al. X-ray crystallographic analyses of symmetrical allosteric effectors of hemoglobin: compounds designed to link primary and secondary binding sites. Acta Crystallogr D Biol Crystallogr 2002;58:634–44.

91. Zhang C, Li X, Lian L, et al. Anti-sickling effect of MX-1520, a prodrug of vanillin: an in vivo study using rodents. Br J Haematol 2004;125:788–95.

92. Available at: http://ntp.niehs.nih.gov/go/TS-M950006. Accessed January 1, 2014.

93. Rhoda MD, Martin J, Blouquit Y, et al. Sickle cell hemoglobin fiber formation strongly inhibited by the Stanleyville II mutation (alpha 78 Asn leads to Lys). Biochem Biophys Res Commun 1983;111:8–13.

94. Mendelsohn LG, Pedoeim L, van Beers EJ, et al. Effect of Aes-103 anti-sickling agent on oxygen affinity and stability of red blood cells from patients with sickle cell anemia. ASH Annual Meeting Abstracts. Blood 2012;120(21):85.

95. van Beers EJ, Samsel L, Mendelsohn LG, et al. Imaging flow cytometry for fully automated quantification of percentage of sickled cells in sickle cell anemia. ASH Annual Meeting Abstracts. Blood 2012;120(21):2105.

96. Gatterer H, Greilberger J, Philippe M, et al. Short-term supplementation with alpha-ketoglutaric acid and 5-hydroxymethylfurfural does not prevent the hypoxia induced decrease of exercise performance despite attenuation of oxidative stress. Int J Sports Med 2013;34:1–7.
97. Matzi V, Lindenmann J, Muench A, et al. The impact of preoperative micronutrient supplementation in lung surgery. A prospective randomized trial of oral supplementation of combined alpha-ketoglutaric acid and 5-hydroxymethylfurfural. Eur J Cardiothorac Surg 2007;32:776–82.
98. Stern W, Mathews D, McKew J, et al. A phase 1, first-in-man, dose-response study of Aes-103 (5-HMF), an anti-sickling, allosteric modifier of hemoglobin oxygen affinity in healthy Norman volunteers. ASH Annual Meeting Abstracts. Blood 2012;120(21):3210.
99. Padmos MA, Roberts GT, Sackey K, et al. Two different forms of homozygous sickle cell disease occur in Saudi Arabia. Br J Haematol 1991;79:93–8.
100. el-Hazmi MA. Heterogeneity and variation of clinical and haematological expression of haemoglobin S in Saudi Arabs. Acta Haematol 1992;88:67–71.

Targeted Fetal Hemoglobin Induction for Treatment of Beta Hemoglobinopathies

Susan P. Perrine, MD[a],*, Betty S. Pace, MD[b],
Douglas V. Faller, MD, PhD[c]

KEYWORDS

- Fetal hemoglobin • Genetic modifiers • Sickle cell disease • Beta-thalassemia
- Stress signaling

KEY POINTS

- Fetal globin reduces clinical events initiated by sickle hemoglobin polymerization, because it cannot participate in the process.
- Fetal globin chains reduce excess alpha globin and globin chain imbalance in β-thalassemia, improving total hemoglobin levels.
- Target levels of fetal globin that reduce clinical severity in sickle cell disease and β-thalassemia are established from natural mutations, modifiers, and from treatment trials.
- Genetic modifiers related to the beta globin locus and/or to erythroid cell stress signaling and survival influence responses to different therapeutics.
- Combinations of therapeutics with differing molecular mechanisms and that promote erythroid survival offer new opportunities for personalized, highly active treatment.

INTRODUCTION

β-Thalassemia syndromes are common monogenic disorders worldwide, characterized by molecular mutations that cause deficiency of the beta globin chain of adult hemoglobin (HbA; $\alpha_2\beta_2$), and an excess of unmatched alpha globin chains.[1-8] Excess

This work was supported by grants from the National Institutes of Health, R01 DK-52962, R41 HL-108516, and R41 HL-110727 (S.P. Perrine) and HL-69234 (B.S. Pace).
Conflict of Interest Statement: S.P. Perrine and D.V. Faller are inventors on patents owned by Boston University and licensed to HemaQuest Pharmaceuticals, which is conducting clinical trials of sodium 2,2-dimethylbutyrate.
[a] Hemoglobinopathy-Thalassemia Research Unit, Cancer Center, Department of Medicine, Pediatrics, Pharmacology and Experimental Therapeutics, Boston University School of Medicine, 72 East Concord Street, L-909, Boston, MA 02118, USA; [b] Department of Pediatrics and Biochemistry and Molecular Biology, Georgia Regents University, Augusta, GA 30912, USA; [c] Cancer Center, Boston University School of Medicine, Boston, MA 02118, USA
* Corresponding author.
E-mail address: sperrine@bu.edu

Hematol Oncol Clin N Am 28 (2014) 233–248
http://dx.doi.org/10.1016/j.hoc.2013.11.009
0889-8588/14/$ – see front matter © 2014 Elsevier Inc. All rights reserved.

alpha globin damages the red blood cell membrane and causes apoptosis of developing erythroblasts and intramedullary hemolysis.[1–8] Clinical observations and previous trials of fetal globin inducers have shown that patients with β-thalassemia benefit from natural persistence of, or pharmacologic induction of, another type of globin that is normally suppressed before birth and in infancy: fetal hemoglobin (HbF; HBG, gamma globin).[1–20] Patients with higher gamma globin levels than their counterparts with the same mutations often do not require transfusions as regularly or as early in life as patients with lower levels of gamma globin. Inheritance of a single modifying trait that increases HbF, such as a single nucleotide polymorphism (SNP) in BCL11A, without any other genetic difference, can produce higher total hemoglobin up to 1 g/dL.[21] The impact of HbF is particularly notable in infants with sickle cell disease (SCD), who survive in utero in a highly hypoxic environment that would produce completely sickled cells with no oxygen delivery without the presence of HbF in every red blood cell. Other natural models of the benefit of increased HbF include sickle cell populations with milder disease and greater than or equal to 20% HbF in Saudi Arabia and in India (the Arabian Indian haplotype), whereas 30% HbF in S-HPFH produces a benign condition. The National Institutes of Health Natural History Study and multiple studies of hydroxyurea (HU) showed the highly significant ameliorating effects of HbF at levels greater than 8.6% or 0.5 g/dL.[22–26] In addition, treatment trials, such as those conducted with arginine butyrate, have increased HbF from a mean of 7% to 21% and reduced hospital days by 3-fold.[15] Inducing gamma globin expression by even small increments is recognized as a therapeutic avenue that should be amenable to broad application, because the gamma globin genes are universally present and normally integrated in hematopoietic stem cells.[1,2,27] Although a single chemotherapeutic drug, hydroxyurea, is commercially available and has had variable effects, several important principles for this approach have been defined in trials of prior generations of therapeutics.[22–27] The recent discovery of new therapeutic candidates now offers a renaissance for this approach.

EXPERIENCE IN TRIALS OF PRIOR GENERATION HBF INDUCERS

Table 1 lists several therapeutics that induce HbF and are being clinically investigated. Proof of principle of HbF induction was shown in previous clinical trials of several drugs in which pharmacologic reactivation of gamma globin expression reduced anemia and even eliminated transfusion requirements in patients with β-thalassemia.[27] HbF induction has been accomplished with chemotherapeutic agents, particularly 5-azacytidine, and 5-aza-2-deoxycytidine (decitabine),[14–20] and with short-chain fatty acids (SCFAs), such as arginine butyrate (AB) and sodium phenylbutyrate.[2,9,10,12,13,15,28] 5-Azacytidine and decitabine have shown high potency with responses in 12 of 13 patients in one study, including adult patients with SCD who do not respond to hydroxyurea.[17] Cellular abnormalities were all reduced after HbF levels were increased.[17]

A therapeutic that is not cytotoxic is preferable for a long-term therapy in β-thalassemia, because with cumulative dosing with hydroxyurea total hemoglobin (Hgb) levels increase, usually by less than 1 g/dL but also tend to decline over time.[16,17] The first-generation SCFAs had limitations of rapid metabolism and high dose requirements; AB and phenylbutyrate are also global histone deacetylase (HDAC) inhibitors that inhibit erythropoiesis through cell cycle arrest.[2] Erythropoiesis-stimulating agents are beneficial, but require parenteral administration and are too costly for lifelong therapy.[19,29–32] Nevertheless, these three classes of therapeutics reduced anemia and rendered some patients with thalassemia transfusion independent.[2,9,10,27] Therapeutics that require lower doses and oral administration would allow broader application,

Table 1
HbF-inducing therapeutics with clinical experience

Therapeutic Class	Therapeutic Name	Current Development Status/Activity
Demethylating agents	5-Azacytadine, decitabine	Potent HbF inducer; IV use only; myelosupressive, mutagenic
	Decitabine + THU	Low-dose metronomic regimen promotes erythroid differentiation, active in phase 2 trials
		THU inhibits metabolizing enzyme, allows oral use
		Active in baboons; in phase I–II SCD dosing trial in progress
Ribonucleotide reductase inhibitor	Hydroxyurea (Droxia)	Activity through transient cytostasis; sole drug approved for SCD, oral
		High activity in young children; beneficial in 50% of adults; increases mean HbF by 2%–3%, reduces clinical events in SCD; improves erythropoiesis, increases mean total Hgb in HbE β-thalassemia by 0.6 g/dL. Clinical benefit, improved SCD survival with HbF >0.5 g/dL
HDAC inhibitors	Vorinostat	Oral; in phase1/2 trial in SCD
	Panobinostat	Oral, active in transgenic sickle mice
	HDAC1/2 inhibitors MS-275	In vitro activity, in preclinical development. Active in vitro and in vivo in baboons, in phase 3 cancer trial; suppresses BCL11A
Short-chain fatty acid derivatives	Arginine butyrate	Intermittent dosing increased HbF 3-fold in SCD, and total Hgb >3 g/dL in β-thalassemia; low bioavailability (IV injection) HDAC inhibitor, suppresses BCL11A, displaces HDAC3 from gamma promoter
	Sodium phenylbutyrate	Oral, low bioavailability, requires large doses, increases HbF in SCD and total Hgb in 50% of patients with thalassemia
	Sodium 2,2-dimethylbutyrate	Oral derivative, displaces HDAC2 from promoter; promotes erythroid survival through Bcl-xL survival protein; long half-life, active in patients with SCD and β-thalassemia, in phase 2 trials
Thalidomide derivatives	Pomalidomide	In vitro and in vivo transgenic mice activity, activity observed in phase 1–2 trials in SCD
LSD-1 inhibitors	Tranylcypromine	Inhibits corepressor LSD-1, which binds TR2/TR4 nuclear receptors in the gamma globin promoter to silence expression; active in β-YAC mice; use in psychiatric disorders
	Benserazide	Displaces HDAC3, LSD-1 from promoter, active in SCD/thalassemia progenitors, baboons, transgenic mice; long-term clinical use as PK enhancer for amino acids
Stress signaling enhancer	Salubrinal	Inhibits dephosphorylation of, and increases eIF2αP, with enhanced stress signaling and thalassemic erythroid survival, promotes translation of HbF

Abbreviations: HDAC, histone deacetylase; IV, intravenous; PK, pharmacokinetic; THU, tetrahydrouridine.

particularly in regions where thalassemia is common globally and transfusions carry particularly high risks of infection.[2]

Several observations in the earlier trials were informative regarding magnitude of responses, and patterns of response, in patients with differing β-thalassemia mutations. Several inducers (5-azacytidine, phenylbutyrate, AB, and erythropoietin [EPO]) produced significant hematologic responses with increases in total hemoglobin of 2 to 5 g/dL or more greater than baseline. Although the clinical trials have been small, patients with diverse thalassemia syndromes had significant responses, including transfusion independence.[2,10–19] Collins and colleagues[9] found that sodium phenylbutyrate increased total Hgb by 2 g/dL greater than baseline, and that responses occurred more frequently in patients with EPO levels greater than 160 mU/mL. Increases in total Hgb levels of 1 to 5 g/dL greater than baseline were achieved when these agents were administered for at least 3 to 6 months.[9,10,33] This finding is remarkable, because thalassemic cells survive for only a few days,[4–8] compared with the normal red cell survival of 120 days.

Of the chemotherapeutic agents, hydroxyurea (HU) treatment has increased total Hgb by 0.6 to 1.0 g/dL in patients with HbE/β-thalassemia, and, although the effect was not as great in magnitude, it significantly reduced hemolysis, which is a cause of many complications.[2,16,17] Hajjar and Pearson[13] reported that gamma globin increased rapidly with HU treatment, with a 6-week treatment time frame required for a peak response, but that it was followed by a decline in total Hgb, suggesting cellular growth inhibition.[15] 5-Azacytidine increased total Hgb levels by an average of 2.5 g/dL (range 1–4 g/dL), even in end-stage patients with life-threatening severe anemia.[1,2,18,19]

Of the SCFAs and HDAC inhibitors, AB, administered first frequently, 4 to 5 days/wk, and then intermittently, twice per month, increased total Hgb levels by 1 to 5 g/dL (mean 2.9 g/dL) when administered for 3 to 6 months.[10] AB treatment rendered patients transfusion independent for several years with home therapy, given 4 nights every other week to avoid the (reversible) antiproliferative effects common to HDAC inhibitors. In a trial using pulse, or intermittent, AB, HbF increased by a mean of 3-fold in 9 of 11 patients, increasing from 7% to 21%, and hospital days were reduced from 80/y to 20/y.[15] AB has been safe in long-term use, with no significant butyrate-related adverse events in more than 16 patient-years of home administration provided by parents.[12,13] EPO preparations increased Hgb levels by 1 to 3 g/dL more than baseline in patients with thalassemia intermedia, and decreased transfusion requirements in thalassemia major.[34] HbF did not increase with EPO or darbopoietin therapy, so that only thalassemic red blood cell production increased, rather than red cells corrected for globin chain imbalance as occurs with the HbF inducers. However, EPO trials highlight the importance of maintenance of healthy erythroid cells for fetal globin to be induced by any pharmacologic or biologic treatment. These trials all show proof of principle of the usefulness of therapeutic induction of gamma globin with or without enhancement of erythropoiesis in patients with β-thalassemia and SCD.

MOLECULAR TARGETS: HBG GLOBIN TRANSCRIPTION AND THE FETAL GLOBIN PROGRAM

The temporal and tissue-specific expression of the betalike globin genes, including ζ, $^A\gamma$, $^G\gamma$, δ, and β, are controlled at multiple levels. Within the beta globin cluster, there are cis-acting promoter elements for each gene and a distal trans-acting element designated the locus control region (LCR). Looping of the LCR in close proximity to the individual cis-promoter elements and competition between the globin genes for interaction with the LCR regulates their developmentally regulated expression. Mice transgenic for constructs containing the beta and gamma globin genes and their cis-acting elements, together with the LCR, show appropriate stage-specific and tissue-specific expression of fetal and adult globin.[5]

There is a broad range of basal HbF globin levels among individuals, defined by their inherited fetal globin program. SNPs and mutations/deletions within the beta globin cluster account for a portion of this variation. Genetic loci beyond the beta globin cluster, which regulate the fetal globin program, have recently been identified by genome-wide association studies (GWAS) and subsequently validated. Two of these elements, the *HBS1L-MYB* intergenic interval on chromosome 6 and *BCL11A* on chromosome 2, seem to be responsible for an estimated 15% to 20% respectively of individual variation in HbF globin levels.[35,36] Since their discovery, correlative studies have shown that SNPs within these loci that result in increased levels of HbF ameliorate the severity of SCD and β-thalassemia.[29,37] Certain mutations within the *KLF1* transcription factor also result in persistent high-level expression of gamma globin after birth.[38]

HBS1L-MYB Intergenic Interval

c-Myb is a transcription factor, initially identified as a proto-oncogene in leukemogenic retroviruses, which is required for definitive hematopoiesis. The activity/level of Myb is reciprocally related to the basal level of fetal globin expression.

KLF-1 (EKLF)

KLF-1 is a transcription factor that binds to a CACCC element in the beta promoter (and a similar element in the gamma A and gamma G promoters, albeit with lesser affinity) and drives high-level adult-stage beta globin expression.[38] Repression of KLF-1 activity reduces beta globin transcription and reciprocally enhances gamma globin expression, reversing its developmental silencing.[39]

BCL11A

BCL11A was identified as a major regulator of basal fetal expression patterns in GWAS[36] and was later shown to be a transcriptional repressor that is required for the maintenance of silencing of fetal or embryonic globin expression in human and murine erythroid cells, respectively.[40] BCL11A interacts with multiple erythroid transcription factors and with the NuRD nucleosome remodeling a deacetylase complex, promoting physical interactions between the LCR and the beta globin promoter, enhancing beta globin transcription, and reciprocally suppressing gamma globin. These genetic modifiers of the fetal globin program also show interactive regulation of each other. c-Myb influences KLF-1 expression.[39] The KLF-1 protein, in addition to directly activating beta globin transcription, also activates BCL11A expression, which also directly induces beta globin expression.[41,42]

TARGETED GAMMA GLOBIN ACTIVATION THROUGH THE CACCC ELEMENT

Understanding fetal globin gene regulation by identifying various cis-acting elements and their interacting trans-acting factors has been a goal for many years to develop therapeutic targets. A key element regulating the betalike globin genes is the CACCC box, located in the proximal promoter (**Fig. 1**). Naturally occurring mutations in the beta-CACCC box cause β-thalassemia[43–45] and deletion of the gamma-CACCC box significantly attenuates gamma globin promoter activity.[46,47] Transcription factors belonging to the Sp1/Krüppel-like factor (KLF) family recognize CACCC/GC boxes to regulate gene transcription. The founding member KLF-1 (EKLF) is an

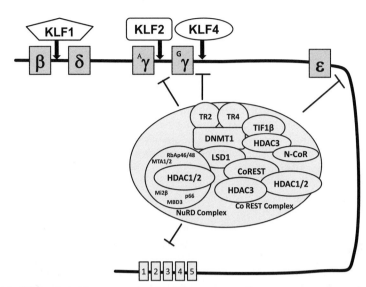

Fig. 1. Modifiers of globin gene expression. Components of repressor complexes that inhibit the HBG promoter and transcription, shown by the bars. Small-molecule therapeutics inhibit specific repressor components. Sites at which 2 activators (KLF-2 and KLF-4) act on the HBG, and 1 activator (KLF-1) binds the HBB promoter and is displaced to the HBG promoter by selected drugs, are shown by *arrows*.

erythroid-specific factor and positive regulator of the beta globin gene.[48] KLF-1 is critical for hemoglobin switching, and targeting this factor has not been achieved for effective therapy for the hemoglobinopathies. Recent insights into repressive factors such as KLF-1 that silence gamma globin expression during development offer new approaches to reactivate HbF expression. Knockdown of the repressor factor *BCL11A*, known to be activated by KLF-1, increases HbF in cultured erythroblasts and ameliorates the SCD phenotype in transgenic mice.[49–52] Transcription factors involved in gamma globin activation earlier in development remain to be discovered.

Other KLF family members have been investigated for their roles as gamma globin regulators. Previous reports showed that KLF-13 (FKLF-2), associates with creb binding protein (CBP)/p300 to activate gamma globin transcription,[53] although FKLF-2 did not enhance the endogenous gene.[51] A subsequent study in K562 cells showed that KLF-2, KLF-5, and KLF-13 positively regulate and KLF-8 negatively regulates the gamma globin gene through the CACCC element.[54] Furthermore, an essential role for KLF-4 in primitive erythropoiesis was shown in zebrafish.[55] Pace and colleagues recently defined KLF-4 as a positive regulator of gamma globin expression in human primary erythroid cells through KLF-4 binding to the CACCC box; moreover, CBP inhibits the ability of KLF-4 to activate the gamma globin promoter.[56] These studies define novel molecular mechanisms by which the Sp1/KLF family of factors might be targeted for therapeutic gamma globin gene activation.

THERAPEUTIC APPROACHES DIRECTED TO INCREASING GAMMA GLOBIN TRANSCRIPTION

The identification of transcription factors and other genetic modifiers that influence the fetal globin program in a cell suggests the possibility of targeting these components directly as a method to enhance HbF expression in the beta hemoglobinopathies.

These modifiers were validated as targets using genetic methodology, including knock-outs and small hairpin RNA, but these approaches do not yet have clinical application. Instead, less direct approaches, using small molecules that affect more readily drugable components of transcriptional activator or repressor complexes, including epigenetic modifiers, have been the first to be tested clinically. **Table 1** shows several drug classes that are, or have been, clinically studied.

Demethylation of the Silenced Gamma Globin Genes

The first such approach used 5-azacytadine, a DNA demethylating agent. It had been observed that the silenced gamma globin genes in the adult were heavily cytosine methylated, as were other genes known to be silenced after embryonic or fetal life (although it was later shown that the methylation occurred long after the gamma globin genes were transcriptionally silenced).[57] 5-Azacytidine is a potent inhibitor of the enzyme responsible for maintaining this methylation, DNA N-methyl transferase (DNMT1). The hypothesis that the gamma globin genes could be reactivated by this DNA demethylating agent was validated in primate studies[58] and small clinical studies in which demethylation of the fetal globin genes and their coincident reactivation were shown.[15,16] Because the demethylating activity of 5-azacytidine could not be separated from its potent cytotoxicity, interpretation of these studies was confounded as to whether the mechanism of reinduction was via direct demethylation or indirectly via stress erythropoiesis.[16] More recently, support for this approach has been generated using decitabine, a metabolite of 5-azacytidine that retains its potent DNMT1 inhibitory activity, but is far less cytotoxic, and more effective when used in a low dose on a regular, but intermittent (metronomic) regimen. Decitabine has been shown in clinical studies of SCD and β-thalassemia to be a potent inducer of HbF, with activity even in severely affected adult patients who do not respond to hydroxyurea.[17] Transcriptional repression of the fetal globin gene is accomplished in large part by site-specific binding of a DNA-binding protein and subsequent recruitment of several different types of corepressor proteins that contribute to gene silencing. For example, the nuclear receptors TR2 and TR4 (TR2/TR4) bind to direct repeat elements in human embryonic and fetal globin gene promoters and play a critical role in the silencing of these genes by recruiting DNMT1, and the NuRD and LSD-1/CoREST repressor complexes and histone deacetylase 3 (HDAC3), which then effect coordinated epigenetic chromatin modifications.[59] Deacetylation of histones and the consequent formation of nucleosomes and resulting compaction of chromatin is a primary epigenetic mechanism of gene silencing. HDAC2 and HDAC3 have also been identified at the silenced gamma globin promoter by chromatin immunoprecipitation.[60] Knockdown of HDAC3 by small interfering RNA is sufficient to induce transcription of the silenced gamma globin gene promoter in primary erythroid progenitors.[60] In a similar way, knockdown of HDAC1 or HDAC2 has been shown to be sufficient to induce gamma globin gene expression in some in vitro systems[34] and is now being studied in progenitors cultured from patients with hemoglobinopathies.

The first HDAC inhibitory agent tested clinically in the beta hemoglobinopathies was the short-chain fatty acid arginine butyrate (AB), which, when used in frequent and then intermittent dosing regimens, produced significant hematologic and clinical responses in 9 of 11 patients with SCD and long-term elimination of transfusion dependency in patients with β-thalassemia.[15] Its activity partly led to current evaluation of several oral HDAC inhibitors. Pulse administration overcame the reversible growth inhibitory activity of AB and phenylbutyrate (SCFAs).[15,27] Irreversible cytotoxicity of other HDAC inhibitors, including benzamides, cyclic tetrapeptides, and hydroxamates, may be more challenging for effective dosing, but are worthwhile to investigate. New generations of short-chain (aliphatic) fatty acids have been developed through pharmacophore modeling that lack HDAC inhibitory activity and do not inhibit erythroid progenitor cell proliferation. At least one such derivative, sodium 2,2-dimethylbutyrate (SDMB), has been studied in dose-ranging trials in both SCD and β-thalassemia, has induced HbF in both conditions to different degrees in various conditions (**Fig. 2**), and is now in late phase II clinical trials in SCD.[61,62]

The molecular mechanisms through which these drug candidates act are still being elucidated. One class of short-chain fatty acid derivatives (SCFAD) identified through computational modeling, typified by RB7 (3-2ox-2H chromen-3yl benzoic acid), mediated high-level fetal globin induction through dissociation of HDAC3 (but not HDAC1 or 2) and its adaptor protein NCoR, specifically from the gamma globin gene promoter.[60,63] KLF-1 was simultaneously actively recruited to endogenous gamma globin gene promoters and away from the beta globin promoter, as was the core ATPase BRG1 subunit of the human SWI/WNF complex, a ubiquitous multimeric complex that regulates gene expression by remodeling nucleosomal structure.[64] Both KLF-1 and BRG1 were required for induction of gamma globin transcription by these short-chain fatty acid derivatives.

SCFAs and their derivatives have been shown to modify the expression or binding of other established genetic modifiers of basal gamma globin gene expression. For example, exposure to butyrate decreases the levels of BCL11A in cultured hematopoietic cells[65] and induces dissociation of the HDAC3/NCoR repressor complex from the gamma globin promoter.[60,64] SDMB is not an inhibitor of HDACs but induces dissociation of HDAC2 from the gamma globin promoter.

A NOVEL MECHANISM OF HDAC3 DISPLACEMENT AND RECRUITMENT OF EKLF

Combinations of therapeutic agents are necessary to control most medical conditions. Gamma globin inducers with higher potency than the original therapies have been

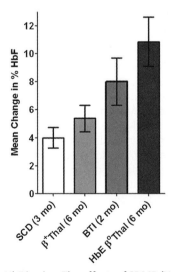

Fig. 2. Novel SCFAD induces HbF in vivo. The effects of SDMB (HQK-1001) at doses from 20 to 50 mg/kg/dose in inducing HbF (mean response) at greater than baseline levels in 4 hemoglobinopathy trials. The duration of treatment and the patient population are shown. β-Thalassemia intermedia (BTI) included patients with HbE-β⁰-thalassemia and β⁰/β⁺-thalassemia.

discovered recently in screening programs using high-throughput screening or molecular modeling, and drug candidates with complimentary mechanisms of action can now be applied.[44,66,67] Cytotoxic agents are not suitable for simultaneously dosed combinations, because this would likely result in greater degrees of erythroid cell apoptosis, but such agents can be used sequentially. A precedent for combination therapy with butyrate and 5-azacytidine was first noted in laboratory models by Stamatoyannopoulos[5]; the two drugs produced a synergistic, 3-fold increase in gamma globin expression compared with the significant levels induced by each drug alone.[2] We have found greater responses, with both additive and synergistic effects, with combinations of therapeutics in erythroid cell culture studies and in animal models with hydroxyurea, decitabine, or an oral HDAC inhibitor, MS-275, plus an SCFAD that is not a global HDAC inhibitor, SDMB.[34,66] In clinical trials of AB and EPO, patients with β^+-thalassemia tended to have lower HbF levels (<30%) and lower baseline EPO levels (<130 mU/mL) than patients with at least one β^0-thalassemia mutation.[34] The β^+-thalassemia group responded to a combination of butyrate plus EPO with larger increases in total hemoglobin than with either agent administered alone, whereas patients with a single β^0-thalassemia mutation, who had higher baseline EPO levels (>130 mU/mL), responded well to butyrate, increasing total Hgb levels by 2 to 4 g/dL. Added EPO conferred no additional benefit in this group.[2,27,34] In contrast, patients with baseline EPO levels less than 80 mU/mL required the combination of AB and EPO to elicit an equally high hematologic response (with an increase in total hemoglobin of 3 g/dL more than baseline).[27] These clinical and laboratory findings indicate that combinations of therapeutics with complimentary, but distinct, molecular mechanisms of actions can produce significantly greater responses than single agents.[34]

DUAL-ACTION INDUCERS, INCLUDING TRANSLATION AND ENHANCED ERYTHROID CELL SURVIVAL

The beneficial therapeutic effects of sodium phenylbutyrate, AB, and isobutyramide all suggested that an oral SCFAD that does not cause cell cycle arrest could offer benefit for long-term treatment in β-thalassemia. An oral butyrate derivative, SDMB, stimulated gamma globin production in erythroid cell cultures, anemic baboons, and transgenic mice and enhances thalassemic erythroid cell survival through Bcl-family prosurvival proteins.[27,68] In toxicology testing, SDMB has had an excellent safety profile in long-term animal studies in 2 species, tested negative in mutagenicity testing, and has favorable pharmacokinetics in normal humans, with a half-life of 9 to 11 hours at 2 to 20 mg/kg/dose, allowing once per day dosing.[69] SDMB is therefore a good candidate for single-use therapy in some patients and for combined modality therapy, because it can be used with cytotoxic therapeutics that suppress erythropoiesis, such as the global HDAC inhibitors, decitabine, or hydroxyurea. SDMB has undergone initial evaluation in short-term (2 month) studies in patients with β-thalassemia intermedia (BTI) with dose escalation from 10 to 40 mg/kg/dose, as shown in **Fig. 2**. HbF increased by a mean of 9% more than baseline, particularly at 20 mg/kg, as shown in **Fig. 2**.[69] With dual actions on fetal globin induction and enhancing erythroid cell survival, SDMB may provide a safe maintenance therapeutic, to which the cytotoxic agents might be intermittently added or pulsed.[27,68,70] Small, 2-month and 6-month trials in BTI and HbE β^0-thalassemia also produced HbF responses, to differing degrees, with induction as high as 22% more than baseline (see **Fig. 2**). Because hematologic effects of hydroxyurea require at least 6 months of treatment,[16,17] a longer trial is in progress with SDMB in SCD. Other agents with dual molecular actions include butyrate, which has epigenetic HDAC inhibitory actions, displaces HDAC3 and recruits remodeling complexes and KLF-1 to the HBG promoter, suppresses BCL11A, and enhances CREB1 binding in the HBG promoter.[61] Benserazide is an oral agent that induces the gamma globin gene promoter in association with reduction in HDAC3 and LSD-1 binding. Decitabine-tetrahydrouridine, which inhibits DNMT1, promotes erythroid differentiation at low (noncytotoxic) concentrations. The monoamine oxidase inhibitor tranylcypromine was recently shown to activate HbF in the β-YAC transgenic mice by the inhibition of LSD-1 in vivo.[71,72] Novel mechanisms reported recently that should greatly enhance therapeutic activity are enhancement of erythroid stress signaling through the HR1-eIF2αP, and translational effects, reported by Hahn and Lowrey[73] and Chen and Perrine.[74]

THE INFLUENCE OF QUANTITATIVE TRAIT LOCI

HbF and proportions of F cells can vary by 10-fold in different normal people and in patients with the same molecular mutations, making it difficult to predict whether thalassemia intermedia or major result from the same globin mutations within individual patients.[35] The influence of specific genetic modifiers, including SNPs and quantitative trait loci (QTL), which alter basal HbF levels in both normal people and people with hemoglobinopathy and ameliorate clinical severity, is now recognized to be influenced primarily by the presence of 3 genetic modifiers.[21,36–38,57–59] These modifiers include the T allele present at promoter nucleotide (nt) –158 5' upstream of the HbG (^{G}γ-globin gene) on chromosome 11p15 (rs7482144), which is associated with increased HbF levels during stress erythropoiesis (as in SCD and β-thalassemia).[65,75] This SNP and 2 other QTLs account for nearly 50% of the variation in basal HbF/F-cell levels.[21,36,38,58,60,63–65,75–77] Genome-wide SNP association studies by Thein and colleagues[20] found that BCL11A is a major QTL for HbF and F-cell production in normal individuals and in patients with β-thalassemia, and this was subsequently confirmed in SCD.[21,36,38,41,58] BCL11A has profound effects in preventing the fetal-to-adult globin switch when absent.[60,63–65,75–77] Thein and colleagues[20] also showed that the HBS1L-MYB intergenic polymorphism (HMIP) on chromosome 6q23 exerts significant negative effects.[38,58,65,76,77] Other groups have confirmed that BCL11A on chromosome 2p16 is a major HbF QTL in populations with or without beta hemoglobinopathies. Further, Chui and colleagues showed that BCL11A is a transcriptional repressor of HbG (^{G}γ-globin) proximal promoter activity, which is abolished by butyrate.[36,65] Galenello and colleagues showed that an SNP in this gamma globin repressor is associated with higher HbF levels and an increase in total hemoglobin in patients with thalassemia.[21,33,41,60] Our group previously identified alterations in protein binding in nucleated erythroid cells of patients who responded to butyrate therapy.[27] Recent findings showed that treatment of erythroid progenitor cells with butyrate or the higher potency agent RB7, causes displacement of a repressor complex containing HDAC3 from the gamma globin promoter, leading to histone acetylation, new binding of EKLF, and a remodeling complex Brg-Brm, followed by gamma globin transcription.[27,28,33,35,68,70,78] HbF inducers that suppress BCL11A, such as MS-275 and resveratrol, were identified in high-throughput screening of diverse chemical libraries, including a library already approved by the US Food and Drug Administration.[44,66]

Differences in QTLs occur commonly, and differing QTL profiles may have contributed to the variability in patient responses to differing therapeutic candidates, making definitive correction of globin imbalance in thalassemia unpredictable. In recent analyses of patients with SCD and thalassemia enrolled in clinical trials of SDMB, more than 50% of the randomly enrolled subjects had at least one high-basal-HbF genotype at the *BCL11A* or *Xmn-I* locus, and 70% of Thai patients with HbE β-thalassemia had a high HbF QTL genotype.[63] As in the Sardinian population, QTLs in the Thai thalassemia population that alter HbF profoundly affected the severity of thalassemia, with SNPs in BCL11A (which should functionally diminish the repression of fetal globin) producing an average 1 g/dL higher total hemoglobin levels in patients who otherwise had the same thalassemia globin mutations.[29,36,63] Sheehan and colleagues[66,79] performed genome screening in infants receiving hydroxyurea therapy and found a panel of polymorphisms unrelated to the globin locus but influencing cell survival, senescence, iron transport, and pharmacokinetics that are associated with either greater or lesser responses to hydroxyurea. It is similarly likely that the presence or absence of polymorphisms in influential genetic modifiers linked to the globin locus and to genes affecting cell survival or stress signaling (QTL) affects the ability of different therapeutics to induce HbF in diverse patients. Our group found that homozygosity for one SNP, in the gene AKAP12, which is associated with lower responses to hydroxyurea,[79] is associated with greater in vitro responses to SDMB and benserazide (**Fig. 3**). Such investigations are at an early stage but already suggest that evaluating the QTL profiles of patients may provide biomarkers to target trials of distinct HbF inducers in the subsets of patient who are most likely to respond well to an individual therapeutic.

In addition to tailoring by QTL profiles, administering a therapeutic combination consisting of an epigenetic modifier (eg, an HDAC inhibitor such as butyrate or MS-275, or a demethylating agent such as decitabine)[43] with a promoter-targeted

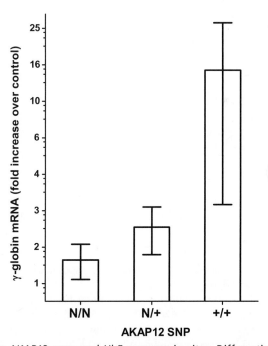

Fig. 3. SNPs in the AKAP12 gene and HbF response in vitro. Differential responses to an inducer in sickle cell erythroid progenitors ± SNPs in AKAP12, a gene affecting erythroid cell senescence. Homozygosity for an SNP in AKAP12 is associated with a 7-fold greater gamma globin mRNA responses greater than baseline in erythroid progenitors treated with benserazide, shown in the far right bar, compared with the magnitude of induction in wild-type progenitors.

agent that is not a global HDAC inhibitor, such as benserazide, or SDMB, and agents that enhance erythroid stress signaling and survival would provide complimentary therapeutic effects.[28,34,61,62,66,73,74] Clinical trials and, ultimately, definitive therapy can then be tailored to patient subsets predicted to have a greater response to individual agents.

SUMMARY

Reactivation of fetal globin, known as nature's remedy, has proved more challenging than was initially anticipated, and may be best achieved when treatment is initiated before the natural decline is complete in the young infant or child. Proof of concept has been shown with several individual small-molecule therapeutics with induction of fetal globin to partially or even fully correct globin chain balance, reducing the anemia in β-thalassemia with 3 different classes of therapeutics.[34] Patients with β^+-thalassemia mutations, without coinherited β^0-thalassemia mutations, typically have lower baseline EPO levels and require 2 different therapeutic agents for optimal hematologic responses in prior trials, whereas the presence of a single β^0 globin gene mutation was associated with rapid and greater responses to butyrate alone. Chemotherapeutic agents and HDAC inhibitors, which inhibit cellular proliferation, can be used intermittently, particularly in β-thalassemia, because the cellular growth arrest they induce may accelerate erythroid cell apoptosis. Clinical trials can now target specific therapies to patients characterized for globin-related and other cellular QTL profiles. New generations of oral noncytotoxic HbF inducers, such as SDMB, low-dose decitabine-tetrahydrouridine, or benserazide can be used in combinations with epigenetic modifiers and with agents that increase translation. Combining therapeutics with epigenetic and promoter-targeted mechanisms with agents that reduce disordered erythropoiesis should particularly benefit the many patients with thalassemia who live chronically with low hemoglobin levels (<7 g/dL) and patients with SCD who do not respond well to hydroxyurea. A challenge to adapting this approach to its full potential is that therapeutics must first be tested individually, before being combined, as in other conditions such as oncology. With a growing number of candidates, reactivating the fetal gamma globin gene to compensate for the mutated globin genes should be possible for many patients.

ACKNOWLEDGMENTS

The authors greatly appreciate the assistance of Richard Ghalie in providing data summaries of SDMB and Michael Boosalis for technical illustrations.

REFERENCES

1. Steinberg MH, Rodgers GP. Pharmacologic modulation of fetal hemoglobin. Medicine 2001;80:328–44.
2. Perrine SP. Fetal globin stimulant therapies in the beta-hemoglobinopathies: principles and current potential. Pediatr Ann 2008;37:339–46.
3. Gallo E, Massaro P, Miniero R, et al. The importance of the genetic picture and globin synthesis in determining the clinical and haematological features of thalassaemia intermedia. Br J Haematol 1979;41:211–21.
4. Schrier SL. Pathobiology of thalassemic erythrocytes. Curr Opin Hematol 1997; 4:75–8.
5. Stamatoyannopoulos G. Control of globin gene expression during development and erythroid differentiation. Exp Hematol 2005;33:259–71.

6. Centis F, Tabellini L, Lucarelli G, et al. The importance of erythroid expansion in determining the extent of apoptosis in erythroid precursors in patients with beta-thalassemia major. Blood 2000;96:3624–9.
7. Mathias LA, Fisher TC, Zeng L, et al. Ineffective erythropoiesis in beta-thalassemia major is due to apoptosis at the polychromatophilic normoblast stage. Exp Hematol 2000;28:1343–53.
8. Pootrakul P, Sirankapracha P, Hemsorach S, et al. A correlation of erythrokinetics, ineffective erythropoiesis, and erythroid precursor apoptosis in Thai patients with thalassemia. Blood 2000;96:2606–12.
9. Collins AF, Pearson HA, Giardina P, et al. Oral sodium phenylbutyrate therapy in homozygous beta thalassemia: a clinical trial. Blood 1995;85:43–9.
10. Perrine SP, Ginder GD, Faller DV, et al. A short-term trial of butyrate to stimulate fetal-globin-gene expression in the beta-globin disorders. N Engl J Med 1993; 328:81–6.
11. Cao H, Stamatoyannopoulos G, Jung M. Induction of human gamma globin gene expression by histone deacetylase inhibitors. Blood 2004;103:701–9.
12. Cappellini D, Graziadei MG, Ciceri L, et al. Oral isobutyramide therapy in patients with thalassemia intermedia: results of a phase II open study. Blood Cells Mol Dis 2000;26:105–11.
13. Hajjar FM, Pearson HA. Pharmacologic treatment of thalassemia intermedia with hydroxyurea. J Pediatr 1994;125:490–2.
14. Singer ST, Kuypers FA, Olivieri NF, et al. Fetal haemoglobin augmentation in E/beta(0) thalassaemia: clinical and haematological outcome. Br J Haematol 2005;131:378–88.
15. Atweh GF, Sutton M, Nassif I, et al. Sustained induction of fetal hemoglobin by pulse butyrate therapy in sickle cell disease. Blood 1999;93:790–7.
16. Ley TJ, DeSimone J, Anagnou NP, et al. 5-Azacytidine selectively increases gamma-globin synthesis in a patient with beta+ thalassemia. N Engl J Med 1982;307:1469–75.
17. Saunthararajah Y, Hillery CA, Lavelle D, et al. Effects of 5-aza-2'-deoxycytidine on fetal hemoglobin levels, red cell adhesion, and hematopoietic differentiation in patients with sickle cell disease. Blood 2003;102:3865–70.
18. Bourantas K, Economou G, Georgiou J. Administration of high doses of recombinant human erythropoietin to patients with beta-thalassemia intermedia: a preliminary trial. Eur J Haematol 1997;58:22–5.
19. Galanello R, Barella S, Turco MP, et al. Serum erythropoietin and erythropoiesis in high- and low-fetal hemoglobin beta-thalassemia intermedia patients. Blood 1994;83:561–5.
20. Thein SL, Menzel S, Lathrop M, et al. Control of fetal hemoglobin: new insights emerging from genomics and clinical implications. Hum Mol Genet 2009;18: R216–23.
21. Sankaran VG, Xu J, Byron R, et al. A functional element necessary for fetal hemoglobin silencing. N Engl J Med 2011;365(9):807–14.
22. Wang WC, Ware RE, Miller ST, et al. Hydroxycarbamide in very young children with sickle- cell anaemia: a multicentre, randomized, controlled trial (BABY HUG). Lancet 2011;377:1663–72.
23. Charache S, Terrin ML, Moore RD, et al. Effect of hydroxyurea on frequency of painful crises in sickle cell anemia. Investigators of the Multicenter Study of Hydroxyurea in Sickle Cell Anemia. N Engl J Med 1995;332(2):1317–22.
24. Platt OS, Brambilla DJ, Rosse WF, et al. Mortality in sickle cell disease. Life expectancy and risk factors for early death. N Engl J Med 1994;330:1639–44.

25. Steinberg MH, Barton F, Castro O, et al. Effect of hydroxyurea on mortality and morbidity in adult sickle cell anemia: risks and benefits up to 9 years of treatment. JAMA 2003;289:1645–51.
26. Steinberg MH, McCarthy WF, Castro O, et al. The risks and benefits of long-term use of hydroxyurea in sickle cell anemia: a 17.5 year follow-up. Am J Hematol 2010;85:403–8.
27. Perrine SP, Castaneda SA, Chui DH, et al. Fetal globin gene inducers: novel agents and new potential. Ann N Y Acad Sci 2010;1202:158–64.
28. Fucharoen S, Siritanaratkul N, Winichagoon P, et al. Hydroxyurea increases hemoglobin F levels and improves the effectiveness of erythropoiesis in beta-thalassemia/hemoglobin E disease. Blood 1996;87:887–92.
29. Nuinoon M, Makarasara W, Mushiroda T, et al. A genome-wide association identified the common genetic variants influence disease severity in beta0-thalassemia/hemoglobin E. Hum Genet 2010;127:303–14.
30. Jiang J, Best S, Menzel S, et al. cMYB is involved in the regulation of fetal hemoglobin production in adults. Blood 2006;108:1077–83.
31. Garner C, Mitchell J, Hatzis T, et al. Haplotype mapping of a major quantitative-trait locus for fetal hemoglobin production, on chromosome 6q23. Am J Hum Genet 1998;62:1468–74.
32. Labie D, Pagnier J, Lapoumeroulie C, et al. Common haplotype dependency of high G gamma-globin gene expression and high Hb F levels in beta-thalassemia and sickle cell anemia patients. Proc Natl Acad Sci U S A 1985; 82:2111–4.
33. Uda M, Galanello R, Sanna S, et al. Genome-wide association study shows BCL11A associated with persistent fetal hemoglobin and amelioration of the phenotype of beta-thalassemia. Proc Natl Acad Sci U S A 2008;105:1620–5.
34. Bradner JE, Mak R, Tanguturi SK, et al. Chemical genetic strategy identifies histone deacetylase 1 (HDAC1) and HDAC2 as therapeutic targets in sickle cell disease. Proc Natl Acad Sci U S A 2010;107(28):12617–22.
35. Thein SL, Menzel S. Discovering the genetics underlying foetal haemoglobin production in adults. Br J Haematol 2009;145:455–67.
36. Sedgewick AE, Timofeev N, Sebastiani P, et al. BCL11A is a major HbF quantitative trait locus in three different populations with beta-hemoglobinopathies. Blood Cells Mol Dis 2008;41(3):255–8.
37. Lettre G, Sankaran VG, Bezerra MA, et al. DNA polymorphisms at the BCL11A, HBS1L-MYB, and beta-globin loci associate with fetal hemoglobin levels and pain crises in sickle cell disease. Proc Natl Acad Sci U S A 2008;105(33): 11869–74.
38. Guy LG, Mei Q, Perkins AC, et al. Erythroid Kruppel-like factor is essential for beta-globin gene expression even in absence of gene competition, but is not sufficient to induce the switch from gamma-globin to beta-globin gene expression. Blood 1998;91(7):2259–63.
39. Bianchi E, Zini R, Salati S, et al. c-myb supports erythropoiesis through the transactivation of KLF1 and LMO2 expression. Blood 2010;116(22):e99–110.
40. Bauer DE, Kamran SC, Orkin SH. Reawakening fetal hemoglobin: prospects for new therapies for the beta-globin disorders. Blood 2012;120(15):2945–53.
41. Borg J, Papadopoulos P, Georgitsi M, et al. Haploinsufficiency for the erythroid transcription factor KLF1 causes hereditary persistence of fetal hemoglobin. Nat Genet 2010;42(9):801–5.
42. Zhou D, Liu K, Sun CW, et al. KLF1 regulates BCL11A expression and gamma-to beta-globin gene switching. Nat Genet 2010;42(9):742–4.

43. Kulozik AE, Bellan-Koch A, Bail S, et al. Thalassemia intermedia: moderate reduction of beta globin gene transcriptional activity by a novel mutation of the proximal CACCC promoter element. Blood 1991;77:2054–8.
44. Orkin SH, Antonarakis SE, Kazazian HH Jr. Base substitution at position -88 in a beta- thalassemic globin gene. Further evidence for the role of distal promoter element ACACCC. J Biol Chem 1984;259:8679–81.
45. Orkin SH, Kazazian HH Jr, Antonarakis SE, et al. Linkage of beta-thalassaemia mutations and beta-globin gene polymorphisms with DNA polymorphisms in human beta-globin gene cluster. Nature 1982;296:627–31.
46. Lin HJ, Han CY, Nienhuis AW. Functional profile of the human fetal gamma-globin gene upstream promoter region. Am J Hum Genet 1992;51:363–70.
47. Ulrich MJ, Ley TJ. Function of normal and mutated gamma-globin gene promoters in electroporated K562 erythroleukemia cells. Blood 1990;75:990–9.
48. Miller IJ, Bieker JJ. A novel, erythroid cell-specific murine transcription factor that binds to the CACCC element and is related to the Kruppel family of nuclear proteins. Mol Cell Biol 1993;13:2776–86.
49. Sankaran VG, Xu J, Ragoczy T, et al. Developmental and species-divergent globin switching are driven by BCL11A. Nature 2009;60:1093–7.
50. Sankaran VG, Menne TF, Xu J, et al. Human fetal hemoglobin expression is regulated by the developmental stage-specific repressor BCL11A. Science 2008;322:1839–42.
51. Xu J, Sankaran VG, Ni M, et al. Transcriptional silencing of gamma-globin by BCL11A involves long-range interactions and cooperation with SOX6. Genes Dev 2010;24:783–98.
52. Yi Z, Cohen-Barak O, Hagiwara N, et al. Sox6 directly silences epsilon globin expression in definitive erythropoiesis. PLoS Genet 2006;2:e14.
53. Song CZ, Keller K, Murata K, et al. Functional interaction between coactivators CBP/p300, PCAF, and transcription factor FKLF2. J Biol Chem 2002;277: 7029–36.
54. Zhang P, Basu P, Redmond LC, et al. A functional screen for Kruppel-like factors that regulate the human gamma-globin gene through the CACCC promoter element. Blood Cells Mol Dis 2005;35:227–35.
55. Gardiner MR, Gongora MM, Grimmond SM, et al. A global role for zebrafish klf4 in embryonic erythropoiesis. Mech Dev 2007;124:762–74.
56. Kalra I, Alam M, Choudhary P, et al. KLF4 activates HBG gene expression in primary erythroid cells. Br J Haematol 2011;154:248–59.
57. Perrine SP, Greene MF, Cohen RA, et al. Delayed fetal globin switching in infants of diabetic mothers is associated with specific DNA hypomethylation. FEBS Lett 1988;228:139–43.
58. DeSimone J, Heller P, Hall L, et al. 5-Azacytidine stimulates fetal hemoglobin synthesis in anemic baboons. Proc Natl Acad Sci U S A 1982;79(14):4428–31.
59. Cui S, Kolodziej KE, Obara N, et al. Nuclear receptors TR2 and TR4 recruit multiple epigenetic transcriptional corepressors that associate specifically with the embryonic beta-type globin promoters in differentiated adult erythroid cells. Mol Cell Biol 2011;31(16):3298–311.
60. Mankidy R, Faller DV, Mabaera R, et al. Short-chain fatty acids induce gamma-globin gene expression by displacement of a HDAC3-NCoR repressor complex. Blood 2006;108:3179–86.
61. Kutlar A, Ataga K, Reid M, et al. A phase I/II trial of HQK-1001, a fetal globin gene inducer, in sickle cell disease. Am J Hematol 2012;87(11):1017–21. http://dx.doi.org/10.1002/ajh.23306.

62. Fuchareon S, Inati A, Siritanaraku N, et al. A randomized phase I/II trial of HQK-1001, an oral foetal globin gene inducer, in beta thalassemia intermedia and HbE beta thalassemia. Br J Haematol 2013;161(4):587–93. http://dx.doi.org/10.1111/bjh.12304.

63. Bohacek R, Boosalis MS, McMartin C, et al. Identification of novel small-molecule inducers of fetal hemoglobin using pharmacophore and 'PSEUDO' receptor models. Chem Biol Drug Des 2006;67:318–28.

64. Perrine SP, Mankidy R, Boosalis MS, et al. Erythroid Kruppel-like factor (EKLF) is recruited to the gamma-globin gene promoter as a co-activator and is required for gamma-globin gene induction by short-chain fatty acid derivatives. Eur J Haematol 2009;82:466–76.

65. Chen Z, Luo HY, Steinberg MH, et al. BCL11A represses HBG transcription in K562 cells. Blood Cells Mol Dis 2009;42:144–9.

66. Sheehan VA, Luo Z, Flanagan JM, et al. Genetic modifiers of sickle cell anemia in the Baby HUG cohort: influence on laboratory and clinical phenotypes. Am J Hematol 2013. [Epub ahead of print]. http://dx.doi.org/10.1002/ajh.23457.

67. Lavelle D, Vaikus K, Ling Y, et al. Effects of tetrahydrouridine on pharmacokinetics and pharmacodynamics of oral decitabine. Blood 2012;119:1240–7. http://dx.doi.org/10.1182/blood-2011-08-371690.

68. Perrine SP, Welch WC, Keefer J, et al. Evaluation of safety and pharmacokinetics of sodium 2, 2 dimethylbutyrate, a novel short chain fatty acid derivative, in a phase 1, double-blind, placebo-controlled, single- and repeat-dose studies in healthy volunteers. J Clin Pharmacol 2011;51:1186–94. http://dx.doi.org/10.1177/0091270010379810.

69. Sangerman JI, Boosalis MS, Shen L, et al. Identification of new and diverse inducers of fetal hemoglobin with high throughput screening (HTS) [abstract]. Blood 2010;116:4277.

70. Perrine S, Faller DV, Shen L, et al. HQK-1001 has additive HbF-inducing activity in combination with hydroxyurea and decitabine [abstract]. Blood 2009;114:977.

71. Shi L, Cui S, Engel JD, et al. Lysine-specific demethylase 1 is a therapeutic target for fetal hemoglobin induction. Nat Med 2013;19:291–4.

72. Sangerman J, Lee MS, Yao X, et al. Mechanisms for fetal hemoglobin induction by histone deacetylase inhibitors involves gamma globin activation by CREB1 and ATF-2. Blood 2006;108(10):3590–9.

73. Hahn CK, Lowrey CH. Eukaryotic initiation factor 2alpha phosphorylation mediates fetal hemoglobin induction through a post-transcriptional mechanism. Blood 2013;122(4):477–85. http://dx.doi.org/10.1182/blood-2013-03-491043.

74. Chen JJ, Perrine S. Stressing HbF synthesis: role of translation? Blood 2013; 122:467–8. http://dx.doi.org/10.1182/blood-2013-06-506139.

75. Castaneda S, Boosalis MS, Emery D, et al. Enhancement of growth and survival and alterations in Bcl-family proteins in beta-thalassemic erythroid progenitors by novel short-chain fatty acid derivatives. Blood Cells Mol Dis 2005;35:217–26.

76. Boosalis MS, Bandyopadhyay R, Bresnick EH, et al. Short-chain fatty acid derivatives stimulate cell proliferation and induce STAT-5 activation. Blood 2001;97:3259–67.

77. Pace BS, White GL, Dover GJ, et al. Short-chain fatty acid derivatives induce fetal globin expression and erythropoiesis in vivo. Blood 2002;100:4640–8.

78. Ikuta T, Kan YW, Swerdlow PS, et al. Alterations in protein-DNA interactions in the gamma globin gene promoter in response to butyrate therapy. Blood 1998;92:2924–33.

79. Sheehan VA, Howard TA, Sabo A, et al. Genetic predictors of hemoglobin F response to hydroxyurea in sickle cell anemia. Blood 2012;120. Abstract 241.

Does Erythropoietin Have a Role in the Treatment of β-Hemoglobinopathies?

Eitan Fibach, PhD[a],*, Eliezer A. Rachmilewitz, MD[b]

KEYWORDS

- Erythropoietin • Thalassemia • Sickle cell anemia • Erythrocytes • Oxidative stress
- Antioxidants

KEY POINTS

- The clinical experience with erythropoietin (Epo) treatment in β-hemoglobinopathies is limited, and well-controlled clinical trials have not been performed.
- Its high cost and route of administration (by injection) are obvious obstacles, especially in underdeveloped countries, where these diseases are prevalent.
- We believe that patients with non–transfusion-dependent thalassemia, with low hemoglobin (Hb) levels (<7.0 g/dL) or patients with thalassemia minor, in whom precipitating factors such as infections, operations, pregnancy, and so forth can significantly decrease their Hb levels, might benefit from Epo treatment, at least temporarily.
- We suggest that from the data summarized in this review, the time has come to define, by studying in vitro and in vivo models, as well as by controlled clinical trials, the rationale for treating patients with various forms of thalassemia and sickle cell anemia with Epo alone or in combination with other medications.

Erythropoietin (Epo), a hormone released in response to hypoxia mainly in the kidneys, is the major regulator of red blood cell (RBC) production (erythropoiesis). By binding to a surface receptor, it stimulates proliferation and inhibits apoptosis of erythroid progenitors and precursors in the bone marrow.[1,2] The clinically approved, commercially available, recombinant human Epo preparations include epoetin-α, epoetin-β, and the long-acting darbepoetin-α, all effective stimulators of erythropoiesis. They are widely used for the treatment of chronic anemia of different causes (eg, in patients treated by chemotherapy[3] or hemodialysis[4–6] as well as in patients with myelodysplastic syndrome).[7]

The β-hemoglobinopathies, β-thalassemia and sickle cell anemia (SCA), are hereditary hemolytic anemias caused by mutations in the β-globin cluster. In β-thalassemia,

[a] Department of Hematology, Hadassah–Hebrew University Medical Center, Ein-Kerem, Jerusalem 91120, Israel; [b] Department of Hematology, Wolfson Medical Center, Holon 58100, Israel
* Corresponding author.
E-mail address: Fibach@yahoo.com

Hematol Oncol Clin N Am 28 (2014) 249–263
http://dx.doi.org/10.1016/j.hoc.2013.11.002
0889-8588/14/$ – see front matter © 2014 Elsevier Inc. All rights reserved.

the mutations reduce (β^+) or abolish (β^0) the synthesis of β-globin chain and consequently the production of hemoglobin (Hb) A ($\alpha_2\beta_2$).[8] In SCA, the mutation causes a structural change in the β-globin (β^S), leading to production of an abnormal Hb (HbS). Despite the state of chronic anemia, the level of serum Epo in thalassemia, and to some extent in SCA, is low relative to the degree of anemia,[9–11] probably because of its increased use and consumption. Several studies reported improvement of the anemia in these patients after treatment with Epo.[12–17] For example, darbepoetin-α was shown to substantially increase Hb levels in patients with HbE–β-thalassemia.[18]

Although the therapeutic effect of Epo is mainly related to stimulation of erythropoiesis, since Epo is a pleiotropic cytokine, its administration into patients with β-hemoglobinopathies can be associated with a variety of beneficial and deleterious effects. This review presents the indications and contraindications (pros and cons) for the potential role of Epo as a treatment in such patients.

EPO AND ERYTHROPOIESIS

The main effect of Epo is on erythropoiesis. Epo is a 30.4-kDa glycoprotein produced primarily in the adult kidney under the control of an oxygen-sensing mechanism.[1,2] Low tissue oxygen tension induces EPO gene expression through both transcriptional activation and messenger RNA stabilization.[19] The mechanism involves activation of hypoxia inducible factor 1, a transcription factor that binds to a hypoxia responsive element in the 3′ flanking region of the EPO gene. The erythropoietic effect of Epo is mediated by a surface homodimeric Epo receptor (EpoR), a class 1 cytokine receptor,[20] which is present on erythroid progenitors and precursors.[21] After binding to the receptor, a signal transduction cascade is initiated, which involves the activation of a cytoplasmic, nonreceptor protein tyrosine kinase, Jak2, and the downstream signaling molecule Stat5, a cryptic cytoplasmic transcription factor.[22]

In the β-hemoglobinopathies, erythropoiesis is increased in the bone marrow and often in extramedullary sites. However, it is mostly ineffective; it does not result in mature RBC because of increased apoptosis.[23] Because Epo affects erythropoiesis by stimulating proliferation and by preventing apoptosis,[24] it can be speculated that Epo treatment would reduce ineffective erythropoiesis. Although all erythroid precursors in the β-hemoglobinopathies carry the mutated genotype, their abnormal phenotypic expression varies: in SCA, most precursors produce β^S-globin, and in β-thalassemia, low or no β-globin chains (depending on the genotype) and, therefore, have an excess of α-globin chains, the main cause for membrane damage and, consequently, short survival. In both diseases, some cells produce β-like δ-globin and γ-globin chains. By binding to α-chains, these β-like chains form HbA$_2$ ($\alpha_2\delta_2$) and fetal Hb (HbF) ($\alpha_2\gamma_2$) and thereby reduce the α-chain excess in β-thalassemia and the HbS in SCA. Consequently, these cells are less damaged and survive longer. Epo stimulates both types of precursors, thereby increasing the total erythroid mass of both the pathologic and the less pathologic RBCs.

EPO AND HBF

HbF plays an important role in the pathophysiology of thalassemia and SCA (**Fig. 1**). Epidemiologic studies have indicated that increased HbF ameliorates the clinical symptoms of the underlying disease.[25] HbF production can be specifically stimulated by a variety of pharmacologic agents,[26] including hydroxyurea which is the only clinically approved drug, mainly in SCA.[27] The mechanism of hydroxyurea

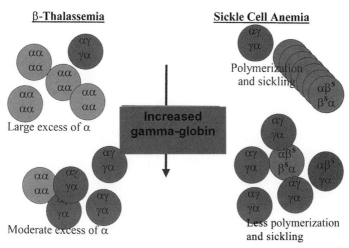

Fig. 1. The effect of increased γ-globin production on the cytopathology of RBC in β-hemo-globinopathies. In β-thalassemia, erythroid cells contain low or no β-globin chains (depending on the genotype) and, therefore, have an excess of α-globin chains. These free chains form insoluble and unstable α_4 tetrameres, which damage erythroid precursors and mature RBC. In SCA, β^S-globin chains bind α-globin chains to form HbS, which on deoxygenating conditions undergo polymerization, leading to RBC sickling. Increased γ-globin chains bind α-chains to form HbF. In β-thalassemia, this factor reduces the α-chain excess, and the α_4 formation. In SCA, this factor reduces HbS concentration, polymerization and, consequently, RBC sickling. In both cases, cells are less damaged and survive longer, ameliorating the state of anemia.

stimulation of γ-globin synthesis and HbF production is still unclear; it has been suggested that it involves nitric oxide generation.[28]

In addition to its effect on total Hb by increasing the production of RBC, Epo treatment can specifically stimulate HbF, by stimulating γ-globin gene expression. However, the effect of Epo is not straightforward. Using a culture system for growing human erythroid precursors,[29] we found that a constant high level of Epo significantly increased the yield of erythroid cells and total Hb, but it had no effect on the proportion of HbF. However, when Epo concentration was reduced during the culture period, the proportion of HbF increased compared with cultures treated with a fixed, high or low, Epo concentration. The possible mechanism of this effect involves changes in the intensity of the stimulus that Epo exerts on Hb-producing precursors (**Fig. 2**). This stimulus is influenced by the availability of surface EpoR and by the concentration of Epo. EpoR is decreased during cell maturation,[21] resulting in a decrease in HbF production content from high in early precursors to low, when HbA takes over in mature RBC.[30] Epo concentration decreases after Epo treatment of anemic patients, in whom serum Epo level fluctuates from high (after administration) to low (because of its short survival in vivo).[31] When high HbF-containing erythroid precursors are shifted from high to low Epo, their maturation is synchronized and accelerated, shortening the period of HbA production, leaving a relatively high proportion of HbF.[29] Changes in Epo levels, and thereby in Epo stimulus, also occur in stress erythropoiesis, which is associated with increased HbF.[32] Attempts to increase HbF in vivo, either by Epo alone or in combination with hydroxyurea, produced contradictory results.[12,17,33–37] This situation could be because of the different timing, dose, and frequency of Epo administration similar to the results in cultured cells mentioned earlier.

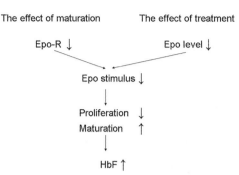

Fig. 2. The effect of the Epo stimulus on HbF. The proportion of HbF changes during maturation (from high in early precursors to low, as HbA takes over, in mature cells[30]) and after Epo treatment of anemic patients. We hypothesize that these changes are mediated by a decrease in the intensity of the stimulus that Epo exerts on Hb-producing precursors. During maturation, the Epo signal is diminished because of a decrease in surface EpoR, whereas after Epo treatment, Epo levels decrease precipitately after administration because of its short survival in vivo.[31] A shift from high to low Epo signaling decreases the rate of proliferation and accelerates the rate of maturation, thus, shortening the period of HbA production, leaving a relatively high proportion of HbF.[29]

EPO AND IRON OVERLOAD

Iron overload (IO) is a major problem in patients with thalassemia and to some extent, also in SCA, affecting both morbidity and mortality, mainly in older patients. The major cause of IO in thalassemia is repeated blood transfusions, the main therapeutic modality in the severe forms of the disease, which introduce iron (in the form of Hb in the transfused RBC) beyond the capacity of the body to dispose of it. Another cause of IO, which exists even in nontransfused patients,[38] is increased iron uptake from the gastrointestinal tract, which is mediated by reduced production of hepcidin, the master regulator of iron homeostasis. Hepcidin inhibits iron transport across the gut mucosa, thereby preventing excess iron absorption and inhibits transport of iron out of macrophages (where iron is stored), thus lowering its mobilization. Hepcidin functions by binding to the iron export channel ferroportin, which is located on the basolateral surface of the enterocytes and the plasma membrane of reticuloendothelial macrophages. Binding to ferroportin leads to its intracellular degradation and consequently reduces iron uptake and mobilization. Hepcidin is produced in the liver, and its production is regulated by multiple factors, including iron and cytokines such as interleukin 6. In thalassemia, hepcidin production is reduced, leading to increased iron absorption. The main cause for the low levels of hepcidin in thalassemia is believed to be augmented erythropoiesis, in which the body attempts, ineffectively, to overcome the anemia. The mechanism in not clear, but it was suggested to involve an increase in the synthesis of the growth differentiation factor 15 (GDF-15).[39]

Iron is transported in the circulation bound to transferrin and is taken up by cells through a transferrin receptor.[40] Inside the cells, most of the iron is bound, in a redox-inactive form, to various components such as Hb, heme, and cytochrome C, and the excess is stored in ferritin.[41] When serum iron exceeds the binding capacity of transferrin, it is present in the form of non–transferrin-bound iron.[42] This form of iron enters cells through transferrin-independent pathways to form labile iron pool (LIP),[43] which was suggested as a transitory intermediate between the cellular iron pools.[44] LIP is redox active and participates, through the Fenton and Haber-Weiss reactions, in the generation of reactive oxygen species (ROS), which, when present in excess, are cytotoxic. It is postulated that this is the main reason of morbidity and mortality caused by IO in major organs of patients with thalassemia. The administration of Epo can affect IO in 2 different indirect ways through its effect on erythropoiesis: on the one hand, it increases the use of iron, with a decrease in iron levels, but on the other hand, it may increase iron uptake by reducing hepcidin production, via GDF-15, with an increase in iron levels (**Fig. 3**).

Administration of Epo is usually supplemented by iron. This factor may be crucial for anemia associated with iron deficiency, when iron supply is a limiting factor of erythropoiesis, but it may not be required when iron supply is abundant. We studied the effect of iron supplementation in patients with chronic renal failure on dialysis,[45] in whom the kidneys fail to produce Epo, and consequently, the patients suffer from anemia. These patients are treated by weekly injections of Epo, which is usually supplemented with intravenous iron. By using T2-weighted magnetic resonance imaging, we have shown iron deposition in the liver, spleen, and pancreas. Stopping iron supplementation for up to 1 year reduced IO (monitored by decrease in serum ferritin and transferrin saturation levels), without interfering with the Hb-stimulating effect of Epo, indicating that under these conditions, the stored iron could be mobilized for erythropoiesis. These results raise the question of the minimal iron supplementation required in order to support erythropoiesis during Epo treatment and suggest that in patients with IO, such as in thalassemia, Epo may be given to increase the Hb level without iron supplementation. It is possible that such iron-free Epo treatment may reduce the consequences of IO by mobilizing iron not only from macrophages but also from parenchymal cells of vital organs (heart, liver), which are the main target of IO damage.

EPO AND OXIDATIVE STRESS

In β-thalassemia, as well as in SCA, although the primary lesion is mutations in the β-globin gene, the damage to the RBC and other cells is mediated in part by oxidative

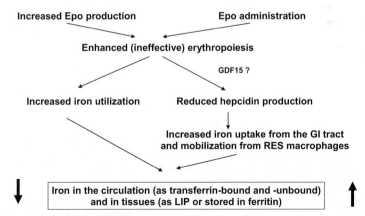

Fig. 3. The effects of Epo on IO. Increased Epo levels, either by augmented endogenous production because of a state of anemia-induced hypoxia or after Epo treatment, enhance erythropoiesis by stimulating the proliferation of erythroid precursors. This process may have opposing effects on IO: on one hand, it increases iron use, thus reducing its levels, but on the other hand, it reduces hepcidin production (probably mediated by increased production of GDF-15), thus increasing iron uptake and mobilization. In thalassemia, the latter effect prevails.

stress.[46,47] The homeostasis of the cellular oxidative status is maintained by the balance between oxidants, such as the ROS and antioxidants, such as reduced glutathione (GSH). When the balance is tilted by an increase in oxidants or a decrease in antioxidants, oxidative stress ensues. It has been shown that in thalassemia and SCA, RBC are under oxidative stress, caused mainly by IO, as discussed earlier.[48,49]

Another contributor to oxidative stress in thalassemic RBC is Hb instability. Excess α-globin chains form unstable tetramers that dissociate into monomers, which, after a change in their tertiary structure, are oxidized first to methemoglobin and then to hemichromes.[50] The following steps of the subunit disintegration are release of heme and iron while the protein precipitates both in the cytosol and the plasma membrane. The outcome of this chain of events is increased formation of ROS, which is catalyzed by free iron, with deleterious effects on the membrane lipids and proteins, including oxidation of membrane protein band 4.1 and a decrease in spectrin/band 3 ratio.[51]

Using flow cytometry, we showed increased generation of ROS with a concurrent decreased content of GSH, in thalassemic RBC compared with normal RBC at basal level, as well as after an oxidative insult, such as treatment of the cells with H_2O_2.[52,53] These effects were associated with RBC membrane changes, including lipid peroxidation and externalization of phosphatidylserine, a marker of cell senescence.[54] The changes in the RBC membranes resulted in increased susceptibility to hemolysis and to phagocytosis by macrophages.[55] Oxidative stress was also found in the polymorphonuclears[56] and platelets[52] of these patients, explaining, in part, their propensity for recurrent infections and thromboembolic complications.[57]

Several studies suggested that Epo reduces oxidative stress: starvation of rats, which reduces endogenous Epo production, was found to increase lipid peroxidation of the RBC membrane, whereas administration of Epo reversed the effect.[58] Improved antioxidant status was also found after Epo treatment of newborn rabbits. This situation could be caused by use of excess iron for developing erythroid precursors, as discussed earlier, thus making it unavailable for ROS generation.[59]

The antioxidant effect of Epo treatment was first suggested for patients with chronic renal failure on dialysis. RBC in these patients are under oxidative stress, which results in externalization of phosphatidylserine, a marker of senescence, which tags RBC for elimination by phagocytosis.[60,61] Epo treatment of these patients resulted in reduced lipid peroxidation concomitant with an increase in superoxide dismutase, catalase, and other antioxidant activities.[62–67] It also caused, within 4 hours, a decrease in the number of RBC showing surface phosphatidylserine.[54,68,69] Thus, although the main effect of Epo is related to stimulation of erythropoiesis and improvement in the anemia, as discussed earlier, it was suggested that in these patients, the Epo effect may also be associated with prolonging the life span of mature RBC.[70]

These reports raise the question: can Epo reduce oxidative stress in thalassemia and SCA? In an attempt to answer this question, we investigated the effect of Epo on the oxidative status on normal and β-thalassemic RBC and platelets.[71] When diluted human blood samples were incubated with Epo, ROS levels were decreased and GSH levels were concurrently increased in RBC and platelets from both normal and thalassemic donors compared with untreated cells. These effects were time dependent, starting within 10 to 15 minutes after exposure to Epo. The effect was noted in both unstimulated and H_2O_2-stimulated cells, indicating that Epo decreased the basal ROS of the cells as well as their ability to generate ROS in response to oxidative stress. We further correlated the effects of Epo on oxidative stress, senescence markers, and susceptibility to undergo hemolysis and phagocytosis in thalassemic RBC incubated in their autologous plasma for 3 days with or without Epo. The results showed that concomitant with the decrease in ROS and the increase in GSH, Epo treatment increased their staining with calcein and decreased their exposure of PS, markers of cell senescence, as well as hemolysis and phagocytosis.

The in vivo effects of Epo were shown 2 hours after its intraperitoneal injection (5000 U/kg) to heterozygous (Hbb$^{th3/+}$) β-thalassemic mice. The ROS and lipid peroxides of their RBC were significantly reduced with a concomitant increase in GSH levels compared with control mice.[71]

Although in these studies, the effects on oxidative stress required Epo concentrations Epo (1–2 U/mL) higher than normal serum levels, continuous, accumulative subthreshold effects, which could not be detected by the methodology used, at physiologic Epo concentrations are possible. Epo is obviously not a practical antioxidant drug, because it is less potent and more expensive than other antioxidants, and, in addition, has to be administrated by injection. Nevertheless, under conditions at which Epo levels are very high, such as during severe anemia (eg, after massive bleeding or in aplastic anemia), or after its administration to patients on hemodialysis or after chemotherapy, its protective effect as an antioxidant on RBC and platelet survival should also be considered.

The mechanism underlying the short-term effect of Epo on the oxidative stress of mature RBC is not clear. Epo affects erythroid cells through their surface EpoR, but mature RBC (and reticulocytes) seem to lack EpoR.[21,72] However, Myssina and colleagues[69] reported binding of radiolabeled Epo to a low, albeit detectable, number of high-affinity EpoR on mature RBC. Mihov and colleagues[73] reported that not only can recombinant human Epo bind specifically to mouse peripheral blood RBC but it can also upregulate their nitric oxide production. Interaction of Epo with the mature RBC membrane was also reported by Baciu and Ivanof.[74] To probe the possibility that EpoR is involved in mediating the effect of Epo on mature RBC, we inhibited Jak-2, a crucial step in the signal transduction pathway by EpoR, by Jak inhibitor I.[75] Treatment of thalassemic RBC with this inhibitor did not inhibit the antioxidant effect of Epo.[71]

Alternatively, the protective effect of Epo may be mediated through scavenging activity in the extracellular milieu; Epo contains more basic than acidic amino acids and many charged residues[76] that may act as a "sink" for ROS (eg, hydroxyl radicals).[77] Moreover, Epo is a highly sialidated glycoprotein.[78] It has been reported that mucin, a typical sialic acid containing high-molecular-weight glycoprotein, is an antioxidant and that sialic acid is crucial for this activity.[79] Mucin was also shown to enhance the antioxidant activity of polyphenols, probably by increasing their solubility.[80] Sialic acid may also function intracellularly; Oetke and colleagues,[81] using human hematopoietic cell lines, which are hyposialylated because of a deficiency in de novo sialic acid biosynthesis, reported efficient uptake and incorporation of free sialic acid. Other studies reported that thalassemic RBC have a lower content of sialic acid than normal RBC,[82,83] and that sialic acid can be taken up by human RBC.[84,85] In our experiments, using several methodologies, Epo, at the concentrations tested, did not show any ROS scavenging activity in a cell-free system.[71]

EPO AND NONHEMATOPOIETIC CELLS

Distinct from its essential role in the regulation of RBC production, Epo is involved in diverse nonhematopoietic biological functions.[86] In addition to its production in the kidney (and in the liver in fetal life), localized Epo production has been shown in various sites (eg, the neural tissue, the female genital tract, the placenta, and the testis). Functional EpoR expression has been documented in many nonhematopoietic cell types, suggesting their ability to respond to Epo (for review, see Ref.[87]).

Epo is known to have a protective effect in nonerythroid cells, such as neuronal cells and cardiomyocytes.[88] For example, significant improvement was reported in patients with stroke, who were treated with Epo within 8 hours after the onset of neurologic symptoms.[89] The mechanism of Epo-induced protection in nonerythroid cells was reported to involve several signaling pathways, including the Jak-2/STAT,[90] a crucial pathway of its erythropoietic effect.[91] However, the effect of Epo in nonerythroid cells is probably unrelated to its effect on erythropoiesis; the effect on erythropoiesis requires the continuous presence of Epo, whereas a brief exposure is sufficient for neuroprotection.[92] Consequently, desialylated Epo, which has high affinity for EpoR but a short life span (and therefore reduced erythropoietic effect), is neuroprotective.[93] Carbamylated Epo, another Epo analogue, which does not bind to EpoR and lacks erythropoietic activity, confers neuroprotection and cardioprotection.[94–96]

The receptor complex mediating the Epo protective effects in nonerythroid cells differs from EpoR with respect to the affinity for Epo, molecular weight, and associated proteins (reviewed in Ref.[97]). It was suggested that the protective effect of carbamylated Epo is mediated through a heteroreceptor complex comprising EpoR and a β-receptor subunit (CD131), a signal-transducing subunit shared by receptors to several cytokines.[97]

The protective effect of Epo on nonerythroid cells may have a significant beneficial effect also in thalassemia. The main causes of morbidity and mortality in older patients with thalassemia are associated with damage to cells of vital organs caused by IO-mediated oxidative stress. If Epo can directly alleviate the stress of these cells, in addition to improving the chronic anemia, it may contribute significantly to amelioration of a variety of symptoms of the disease.

EPO AND MALIGNANCY

As the life expectancy of thalassemic patients increases, the likelihood of developing malignancies increases as well.[98] In recent years, several studies have reported the association of thalassemia with malignancies, in the liver and hematopoietic system (eg, Ref.[99]). A possible link between these 2 diseases could be IO, which has been reported to be associated with various malignancies, including in the liver and in the hematopoietic system.[100,101] In vitro studies related IO and malignant transformation, mainly through the generation of ROS,[102] which can initiate the generation of a neoplastic clone through genetic or epigenetic alterations.

Anemia is an independent prognostic factor in patients with cancer.[103] The pathophysiology of malignancy-related anemia can be related to the anemia of chronic disease, nutritional deficiencies, bleeding, hemolysis, bone marrow involvement with malignant cells, and chemoradiotherapy. A direct relationship has been reported between acute anemia and intratumoral hypoxia,[104] although the effect of chronic anemia is more difficult to interpret.[105] There is also evidence that anemia might be associated with a reduced response to radiotherapy,[106] chemotherapy,[107] and surgery.[108]

The use of Epo in malignancies focuses on its anemia-correcting effect. It reduces blood transfusion requirements, improves the quality of life,[109] and improves survival.[110] In addition, Epo has been shown in animal models to restore radiosensitivity[111] and chemosensitivity.[112] Nevertheless, 2 randomized trials of the effect of Epo on progression-free survival reported negative results.[113,114] The expression of EpoR on cancer cells[87] suggests that Epo treatment may exert direct effects on these cells, stimulating their proliferation, inhibiting their apoptosis, and modulating their sensitivity to chemoradiation therapy. Epo may also affect the tumor microenvironment; Epo or EpoR knockout embryos showed defects in angiogenesis. A recent study showed that Epo-EpoR signaling stimulates pathologic angiogenesis of diabetic retinopathy[37]; however, its role in tumor angiogenesis, a process that is essential for tumor progression and metastasis, has not been established.

Epo may also have a therapeutic effect in malignancy. Epo treatment was reported to be associated with prolonged survival of patients with multiple myeloma. This clinical observation, which was supported by studies on murine myeloma models,[115] is most probably not a direct one on the myeloma cells, but through stimulation of the immune system.[116]

In summary, the main effect of Epo in thalassemia, and to some extent also in SCA, is related to stimulation of erythropoiesis, by which the number of RBC and the Hb levels are increased. Both abnormal RBC and less abnormal RBC, containing HbA2 or HbF, are stimulated. However, Epo is a pleiotropic cytokine, and its administration into thalassemic patients can be associated with a variety of effects, both beneficial and deleterious: (1) specific stimulation of HbF production, thereby decreasing the α-globin chain excess (the main pathologic factor in RBC); (2) modulation of IO by increased iron use and increased iron uptake; and (3) amelioration of oxidative stress, by a direct effect or indirectly by its effect on iron. This factor should delay the senescence and removal of RBC, as well as reduce cytotoxicity to other cells in vital organs. Epo may also affect a variety of diseases in these patients, including malignancy, stroke, thrombosis, hypertension, and so forth.

The clinical experience with Epo treatment in β-hemoglobinopathies is limited, and well-controlled clinical trials have not been performed. Its high cost and route of administration (by injection) are obvious obstacles, especially in underdeveloped countries, where these diseases are prevalent. We believe that patients with non–transfusion-dependent thalassemia, with low Hb levels (<7.0 g/dL) or patients with thalassemia minor, in whom precipitating factors such as infections, operations, pregnancy, and so forth can significantly decrease their Hb levels, might benefit from Epo treatment, at least temporarily. We suggest that from the data summarized in this review, the time has come to define, by studying in vitro and in vivo models, as well as by controlled clinical trials, the rationale for treating patients with various forms of thalassemia and SCA with Epo alone or in combination with other medications.

REFERENCES

1. Krantz SB. Erythropoietin. Blood 1991;77(3):419–34.
2. Jelkmann W. Erythropoietin: structure, control of production, and function. Physiol Rev 1992;72(2):449–89.
3. Beutel G, Ganser A. Risks and benefits of erythropoiesis-stimulating agents in cancer management. Semin Hematol 2007;44(3):157–65.
4. Kaupke CJ, Kim S, Vaziri ND. Effect of erythrocyte mass on arterial blood pressure in dialysis patients receiving maintenance erythropoietin therapy. J Am Soc Nephrol 1994;4(11):1874–8.
5. Coladonato JA, Frankenfield DL, Reddan DN, et al. Trends in anemia management among US hemodialysis patients. J Am Soc Nephrol 2002;13(5):1288–95.
6. Eschbach JW. Anemia management in chronic kidney disease: role of factors affecting epoetin responsiveness. J Am Soc Nephrol 2002;13(5):1412–4.
7. Santini V. Clinical use of erythropoietic stimulating agents in myelodysplastic syndromes. Oncologist 2011;16(Suppl 3):35–42.
8. Rund D, Rachmilewitz E. Beta-thalassemia. N Engl J Med 2005;353(11):1135–46.
9. Manor D, Fibach E, Goldfarb A, et al. Erythropoietin activity in the serum of beta thalassemic patients. Scand J Haematol 1986;37(3):221–8.

10. Dore F, Bonfigli S, Gaviano E, et al. Serum erythropoietin levels in thalassemia intermedia. Ann Hematol 1993;67(4):183–6.
11. Pulte D, Nagalla S, Caro J. Erythropoietin levels in patients with sickle cell disease not in vaso-occlusive crisis. Blood 2012;120(21):A3242.
12. Goldberg MA, Brugnara C, Dover GJ, et al. Hydroxyurea and erythropoietin therapy in sickle cell anemia. Semin Oncol 1992;19(3 Suppl 9):74–81.
13. Olivieri NF, Freedman MH, Perrine SP, et al. Trial of recombinant human erythropoietin: three patients with thalassemia intermedia. Blood 1992;80(12):3258–60.
14. Rachmilewitz EA, Aker M, Perry D, et al. Sustained increase in haemoglobin and RBC following long-term administration of recombinant human erythropoietin to patients with homozygous beta-thalassaemia. Br J Haematol 1995;90(2):341–5.
15. Rachmilewitz EA, Aker M. The role of recombinant human erythropoietin in the treatment of thalassemia. Ann N Y Acad Sci 1998;850:129–38.
16. Kohli-Kumar M, Marandi H, Keller MA, et al. Use of hydroxyurea and recombinant erythropoietin in management of homozygous beta0 thalassemia. J Pediatr Hematol Oncol 2002;24(9):777–8.
17. Chaidos A, Makis A, Hatzimichael E, et al. Treatment of beta-thalassemia patients with recombinant human erythropoietin: effect on transfusion requirements and soluble adhesion molecules. Acta Haematol 2004;111(4):189–95.
18. Singer ST, Vichinsky EP, Sweeters N, et al. Darbepoetin alfa for the treatment of anaemia in alpha- or beta- thalassaemia intermedia syndromes. Br J Haematol 2011;154(2):281–4.
19. Ebert BL, Bunn HF. Regulation of the erythropoietin gene. Blood 1999;94(6): 1864–77.
20. Lodish HF, Hilton DJ, Klingmuller U, et al. The erythropoietin receptor: biogenesis, dimerization, and intracellular signal transduction. Cold Spring Harb Symp Quant Biol 1995;60:93–104.
21. Broudy VC, Lin N, Brice M, et al. Erythropoietin receptor characteristics on primary human erythroid cells. Blood 1991;77(12):2583–90.
22. Ihle JN, Stravapodis D, Parganas E, et al. The roles of Jaks and Stats in cytokine signaling. Cancer J Sci Am 1998;4(Suppl 1):S84–91.
23. Rivella S. Ineffective erythropoiesis and thalassemias. Curr Opin Hematol 2009; 16(3):187–94.
24. Sui X, Krantz SB, Zhao ZJ. Stem cell factor and erythropoietin inhibit apoptosis of human erythroid progenitor cells through different signalling pathways. Br J Haematol 2000;110(1):63–70.
25. Olivieri NF. Reactivation of fetal hemoglobin in patients with beta-thalassemia. Semin Hematol 1996;33(1):24–42.
26. Gambari R, Fibach E. Medicinal chemistry of fetal hemoglobin inducers for treatment of beta-thalassemia. Curr Med Chem 2007;14(2):199–212.
27. Ware RE, Aygun B. Advances in the use of hydroxyurea. Hematology Am Soc Hematol Educ Program 2009;62–9.
28. Cokic VP, Smith RD, Beleslin-Cokic BB, et al. Hydroxyurea induces fetal hemoglobin by the nitric oxide-dependent activation of soluble guanylyl cyclase. J Clin Invest 2003;111(2):231–9.
29. Fibach E, Schechter AN, Noguchi CT, et al. Reducing erythropoietin in cultures of human erythroid precursors elevates the proportion of fetal haemoglobin. Br J Haematol 1994;88(1):39–45.
30. Dalyot N, Fibach E, Rachmilewitz EA, et al. Adult and neonatal patterns of human globin gene expression are recapitulated in liquid cultures. Exp Hematol 1992;20(9):1141–5.

31. Cho SH, Lim HS, Ghim JL, et al. Pharmacokinetic, tolerability, and bioequivalence comparison of three different intravenous formulations of recombinant human erythropoietin in healthy Korean adult male volunteers: an open-label, randomized-sequence, three-treatment, three-way crossover study. Clin Ther 2009;31(5):1046–53.
32. Alter BP. Fetal erythropoiesis in stress hematopoiesis. Exp Hematol 1979; 7(Suppl 5):200–9.
33. Bourantas KL, Georgiou I, Seferiadis K. Fetal globin stimulation during a short-term trial of erythropoietin in HbS/beta-thalassemia patients. Acta Haematol 1994;92(2):79–82.
34. Breymann C, Fibach E, Visca E, et al. Induction of fetal hemoglobin synthesis with recombinant human erythropoietin in anemic patients with heterozygous beta-thalassemia during pregnancy. J Matern Fetal Med 1999;8(1):1–7.
35. Little JA, McGowan VR, Kato GJ, et al. Combination erythropoietin-hydroxyurea therapy in sickle cell disease: experience from the National Institutes of Health and a literature review. Haematologica 2006;91(8):1076–83.
36. Rodgers GP, Dover GJ, Uyesaka N, et al. Augmentation by erythropoietin of the fetal-hemoglobin response to hydroxyurea in sickle cell disease. N Engl J Med 1993;328(2):73–80.
37. Saraf S, Molokie R, Gowhari M, et al. Clinical efficacy and safety of erythroid stimulating agents in sickle cell disease. Blood 2012;120. Abstract 3218.
38. Musallam KM, Rivella S, Vichinsky E, et al. Non-transfusion-dependent thalassemias. Haematologica 2013;98(6):833–44.
39. Tanno T, Noel P, Miller JL. Growth differentiation factor 15 in erythroid health and disease. Curr Opin Hematol 2010;17(3):184–90.
40. Wang J, Pantopoulos K. Regulation of cellular iron metabolism. Biochem J 2011; 434(3):365–81.
41. Konijn AM, Meyron-Holtz EG, Fibach E, et al. Cellular ferritin uptake: a highly regulated pathway for iron assimilation in human erythroid precursor cells. Adv Exp Med Biol 1994;356:189–97.
42. Breuer W, Hershko C, Cabantchik ZI. The importance of non-transferrin bound iron in disorders of iron metabolism. Transfus Sci 2000;23(3):185–92.
43. Prus E, Fibach E. The labile iron pool in human erythroid cells. Br J Haematol 2008;142(2):301–7.
44. Jacobs A. Low molecular weight intracellular iron transport compounds. Blood 1977;50(3):433–9.
45. Ghoti H, Rachmilewitz EA, Simon-Lopez R, et al. Evidence for tissue iron overload in long-term hemodialysis patients and the impact of withdrawing parenteral iron. Eur J Haematol 2012;89(1):87–93.
46. Pavlova LE, Savov VM, Petkov HG, et al. Oxidative stress in patients with beta-thalassemia major. Prilozi 2007;28(1):145–54.
47. Wood KC, Granger DN. Sickle cell disease: role of reactive oxygen and nitrogen metabolites. Clin Exp Pharmacol Physiol 2007;34(9):926–32.
48. Chan AC, Chow CK, Chiu D. Interaction of antioxidants and their implication in genetic anemia. Proc Soc Exp Biol Med 1999;222(3):274–82.
49. Shinar E, Rachmilewitz EA. Oxidative denaturation of red blood cells in thalassemia. Semin Hematol 1990;27(1):70–82.
50. Rachmilewitz EA, Harari E. Intermediate hemichrome formation after oxidation of three unstable hemoglobins (Freiburg, Riverdale-Bronx and Koln). Hamatol Bluttransfus 1972;10:241–50.

51. Advani R, Sorenson S, Shinar E, et al. Characterization and comparison of the red blood cell membrane damage in severe human alpha- and beta-thalassemia. Blood 1992;79(4):1058–63.

52. Amer J, Goldfarb A, Fibach E. Flow cytometric analysis of the oxidative status of normal and thalassemic red blood cells. Cytometry A 2004;60(1):73–80.

53. Amer J, Etzion Z, Bookchin RM, et al. Oxidative status of valinomycin-resistant normal, beta-thalassemia and sickle red blood cells. Biochim Biophys Acta 2006;1760(5):793–9.

54. Lang F, Lang KS, Lang PA, et al. Mechanisms and significance of eryptosis. Antioxid Redox Signal 2006;8(7–8):1183–92.

55. Amer J, Atlas D, Fibach E. N-acetylcysteine amide (AD4) attenuates oxidative stress in beta-thalassemia blood cells. Biochim Biophys Acta 2008;1780(2):249–55.

56. Amer J, Fibach E. Chronic oxidative stress reduces the respiratory burst response of neutrophils from beta-thalassaemia patients. Br J Haematol 2005;129(3):435–41.

57. Eldor A, Rachmilewitz EA. The hypercoagulable state in thalassemia. Blood 2002;99(1):36–43.

58. Biswas T, Ghosal J, Ganguly C, et al. Effect of erythropoietin on the interchange of cholesterol and phospholipid between erythrocyte membrane and plasma. Biochem Med Metab Biol 1986;35(2):120–4.

59. Bany-Mohammed FM, Slivka S, Hallman M. Recombinant human erythropoietin: possible role as an antioxidant in premature rabbits. Pediatr Res 1996;40(3):381–7.

60. Lang KS, Lang PA, Bauer C, et al. Mechanisms of suicidal erythrocyte death. Cell Physiol Biochem 2005;15(5):195–202.

61. Freikman I, Ringel I, Fibach E. Oxidative stress-induced membrane shedding from RBCs is Ca flux-mediated and affects membrane lipid composition. J Membr Biol 2011;240(2):73–82.

62. Turi S, Nemeth I, Varga I, et al. The effect of erythropoietin on the cellular defence mechanism of red blood cells in children with chronic renal failure. Pediatr Nephrol 1992;6(6):536–41.

63. Rud'ko IA, Balashova TS, Pokrovskii IuA, et al. The effect of human recombinant erythropoietin on the lipid peroxidation processes and antioxidant protection of the erythrocytes in patients with chronic kidney failure on hemodialysis. Gematol Transfuziol 1993;38(3):24–6 [in Russian].

64. Delmas-Beauvieux MC, Combe C, Peuchant E, et al. Evaluation of red blood cell lipoperoxidation in hemodialysed patients during erythropoietin therapy supplemented or not with iron. Nephron 1995;69(4):404–10.

65. Cavdar C, Camsari T, Semin I, et al. Lipid peroxidation and antioxidant activity in chronic haemodialysis patients treated with recombinant human erythropoietin. Scand J Urol Nephrol 1997;31(4):371–5.

66. Sommerburg O, Grune T, Hampl H, et al. Does long-term treatment of renal anaemia with recombinant erythropoietin influence oxidative stress in haemodialysed patients? Nephrol Dial Transplant 1998;13(10):2583–7.

67. Boran M, Kucukaksu C, Balk M, et al. Red cell lipid peroxidation and antioxidant system in haemodialysed patients: influence of recombinant human erythropoietin (r-HuEPO) treatment. Int Urol Nephrol 1998;30(4):507–12.

68. Bonomini M, Sirolli V, Settefrati N, et al. Increased erythrocyte phosphatidylserine exposure in chronic renal failure. J Am Soc Nephrol 1999;10(9):1982–90.

69. Myssina S, Huber SM, Birka C, et al. Inhibition of erythrocyte cation channels by erythropoietin. J Am Soc Nephrol 2003;14(11):2750–7.

70. Polenakovic M, Sikole A. Is erythropoietin a survival factor for red blood cells? J Am Soc Nephrol 1996;7(8):1178–82.

71. Amer J, Dana M, Fibach E. The antioxidant effect of erythropoietin on thalassemic blood cells. Anemia 2010;2010:978710.

72. Sawada K, Krantz SB, Dai CH, et al. Purification of human blood burst-forming units-erythroid and demonstration of the evolution of erythropoietin receptors. J Cell Physiol 1990;142(2):219–30.

73. Mihov D, Vogel J, Gassmann M, et al. Erythropoietin activates nitric oxide synthase in murine erythrocytes. Am J Physiol Cell Physiol 2009;297(2):C378–88.

74. Baciu I, Ivanof L. Erythropoietin interaction with the mature red cell membrane. Ann N Y Acad Sci 1983;414:66–72.

75. Pedranzini L, Dechow T, Berishaj M, et al. Pyridone 6, a pan-Janus-activated kinase inhibitor, induces growth inhibition of multiple myeloma cells. Cancer Res 2006;66(19):9714–21.

76. Lai PH, Everett R, Wang FF, et al. Structural characterization of human erythropoietin. J Biol Chem 1986;261(7):3116–21.

77. Rowley DA, Halliwell B. Superoxide-dependent and ascorbate-dependent formation of hydroxyl radicals in the presence of copper salts: a physiologically significant reaction? Arch Biochem Biophys 1983;225(1):279–84.

78. Inoue N, Takeuchi M, Asano K, et al. Structures of mucin-type sugar chains on human erythropoietins purified from urine and the culture medium of recombinant Chinese hamster ovary cells. Arch Biochem Biophys 1993;301(2):375–8.

79. Ogasawara Y, Namai T, Yoshino F, et al. Sialic acid is an essential moiety of mucin as a hydroxyl radical scavenger. FEBS Lett 2007;581(13):2473–7.

80. Ginsburg I, Koren E, Shalish M, et al. Saliva increases the availability of lipophilic polyphenols as antioxidants and enhances their retention in the oral cavity. Arch Oral Biol 2012;57(10):1327–34.

81. Oetke C, Hinderlich S, Brossmer R, et al. Evidence for efficient uptake and incorporation of sialic acid by eukaryotic cells. Eur J Biochem 2001;268(16): 4553–61.

82. Calatroni A, Barberi I, Salpietro C. Altered sialic acid contents of red blood cell membrane preparations in homozygous beta-thalassemia. Ital J Biochem 1978; 27(2):94–103.

83. Kahane I, Ben-Chetrit E, Shifter A, et al. The erythrocyte membranes in beta-thalassemia. Lower sialic acid levels in glycophorin. Biochim Biophys Acta 1980;596(1):10–7.

84. Bulai T, Bratosin D, Artenie V, et al. Uptake of sialic acid by human erythrocyte. Characterization of a transport system. Biochimie 2003;85(1–2):241–4.

85. Yousef GM, Ordon MH, Foussias G, et al. Molecular characterization, tissue expression, and mapping of a novel Siglec-like gene (SLG2) with three splice variants. Biochem Biophys Res Commun 2001;284(4):900–10.

86. Ogunshola OO, Bogdanova AY. Epo and non-hematopoietic cells: what do we know? Methods Mol Biol 2013;982:13–41.

87. Hardee ME, Arcasoy MO, Blackwell KL, et al. Erythropoietin biology in cancer. Clin Cancer Res 2006;12(2):332–9.

88. Joyeux-Faure M. Cellular protection by erythropoietin: new therapeutic implications? J Pharmacol Exp Ther 2007;323(3):759–62.

89. Ehrenreich H, Hasselblatt M, Dembowski C, et al. Erythropoietin therapy for acute stroke is both safe and beneficial. Mol Med 2002;8(8):495–505.

90. Zhang F, Wang S, Cao G, et al. Signal transducers and activators of transcription 5 contributes to erythropoietin-mediated neuroprotection against

hippocampal neuronal death after transient global cerebral ischemia. Neurobiol Dis 2007;25(1):45–53.

91. Ofir R, Qing W, Krup M, et al. Identification of genes induced by interleukin-3 and erythropoietin via the Jak-Stat5 pathway using enhanced differential display-reverse southern. J Interferon Cytokine Res 1997;17(5): 279–86.

92. Morishita E, Masuda S, Nagao M, et al. Erythropoietin receptor is expressed in rat hippocampal and cerebral cortical neurons, and erythropoietin prevents in vitro glutamate-induced neuronal death. Neuroscience 1997;76(1): 105–16.

93. Erbayraktar S, Yilmaz O, Gokmen N, et al. Erythropoietin is a multifunctional tissue-protective cytokine. Curr Hematol Rep 2003;2(6):465–70.

94. Fiordaliso F, Chimenti S, Staszewsky L, et al. A nonerythropoietic derivative of erythropoietin protects the myocardium from ischemia-reperfusion injury. Proc Natl Acad Sci U S A 2005;102(6):2046–51.

95. Leist M, Ghezzi P, Grasso G, et al. Derivatives of erythropoietin that are tissue protective but not erythropoietic. Science 2004;305(5681):239–42.

96. Moon C, Krawczyk M, Paik D, et al. Erythropoietin, modified to not stimulate red blood cell production, retains its cardioprotective properties. J Pharmacol Exp Ther 2006;316(3):999–1005.

97. Brines M, Grasso G, Fiordaliso F, et al. Erythropoietin mediates tissue protection through an erythropoietin and common beta-subunit heteroreceptor. Proc Natl Acad Sci U S A 2004;101(41):14907–12.

98. Poggi M, Sorrentino F, Pascucci C, et al. Malignancies in beta-thalassemia patients: first description of two cases of thyroid cancer and review of the literature. Hemoglobin 2011;35(4):439–46.

99. Karimi M, Giti R, Haghpanah S, et al. Malignancies in patients with beta-thalassemia major and beta-thalassemia intermedia: a multicenter study in Iran. Pediatr Blood Cancer 2009;53(6):1064–7.

100. Borgna-Pignatti C, Vergine G, Lombardo T, et al. Hepatocellular carcinoma in the thalassaemia syndromes. Br J Haematol 2004;124(1):114–7.

101. Joosten E, Meeuwissen J, Vandewinckele H, et al. Iron status and colorectal cancer in symptomatic elderly patients. Am J Med 2008;121(12):1072–7.

102. Toyokuni S. Role of iron in carcinogenesis: cancer as a ferrotoxic disease. Cancer Sci 2009;100(1):9–16.

103. Caro JJ, Salas M, Ward A, et al. Anemia as an independent prognostic factor for survival in patients with cancer: a systemic, quantitative review. Cancer 2001; 91(12):2214–21.

104. Hirst DG. What is the importance of anaemia in radiotherapy? The value of animal studies. Radiother Oncol 1991;20(Suppl 1):29–33.

105. Harrison LB, Chadha M, Hill RJ, et al. Impact of tumor hypoxia and anemia on radiation therapy outcomes. Oncologist 2002;7(6):492–508.

106. Nordsmark M, Overgaard M, Overgaard J. Pretreatment oxygenation predicts radiation response in advanced squamous cell carcinoma of the head and neck. Radiother Oncol 1996;41(1):31–9.

107. Teicher BA, Holden SA, al-Achi A, et al. Classification of antineoplastic treatments by their differential toxicity toward putative oxygenated and hypoxic tumor subpopulations in vivo in the FSaIIC murine fibrosarcoma. Cancer Res 1990;50(11):3339–44.

108. Hockel M, Schlenger K, Hockel S, et al. Tumor hypoxia in pelvic recurrences of cervical cancer. Int J Cancer 1998;79(4):365–9.

109. Glaspy J. The impact of epoetin alfa on quality of life during cancer chemotherapy: a fresh look at an old problem. Semin Hematol 1997;34(3 Suppl 2): 20–6.
110. Bohlius J, Langensiepen S, Schwarzer G, et al. Recombinant human erythropoietin and overall survival in cancer patients: results of a comprehensive meta-analysis. J Natl Cancer Inst 2005;97(7):489–98.
111. Ning S, Hartley C, Molineux G, et al. Darbepoietin alfa potentiates the efficacy of radiation therapy in mice with corrected or uncorrected anemia. Cancer Res 2005;65(1):284–90.
112. Thews O, Kelleher DK, Vaupel P. Erythropoietin restores the anemia-induced reduction in cyclophosphamide cytotoxicity in rat tumors. Cancer Res 2001; 61(4):1358–61.
113. Henke M, Laszig R, Rube C, et al. Erythropoietin to treat head and neck cancer patients with anaemia undergoing radiotherapy: randomised, double-blind, placebo-controlled trial. Lancet 2003;362(9392):1255–60.
114. Leyland-Jones B, Semiglazov V, Pawlicki M, et al. Maintaining normal hemoglobin levels with epoetin alfa in mainly nonanemic patients with metastatic breast cancer receiving first-line chemotherapy: a survival study. J Clin Oncol 2005; 23(25):5960–72.
115. Mittelman M, Zeidman A, Kanter P, et al. Erythropoietin has an anti-myeloma effect–a hypothesis based on a clinical observation supported by animal studies. Eur J Haematol 2004;72(3):155–65.
116. Prutchi-Sagiv S, Golishevsky N, Oster HS, et al. Erythropoietin treatment in advanced multiple myeloma is associated with improved immunological functions: could it be beneficial in early disease? Br J Haematol 2006;135(5):660–72.

Inflammatory Mediators of Endothelial Injury in Sickle Cell Disease

Carolyn C. Hoppe, MD

KEYWORDS

- Inflammation • Mediators • Sickle cell

KEY POINTS

- Inflammation plays a critical role in the complex pathophysiology of sickle cell disease (SCD) and drives both the acute and chronic processes leading to vascular injury.
- Mediators of inflammation, such as cellular adhesion molecules, cytokines, leukotrienes (LTs), and nuclear factor (NF)-κB signaling factors, represent potential therapeutic targets in SCD.

INTRODUCTION

SCD is now recognized as a complex disease characterized by acute and chronic inflammation. The incidence of nearly every clinical manifestation of SCD correlates with white blood cell (WBC) count, indicating a role for leukocytes and inflammation in the pathophysiology of SCD. Leukocytosis is common in SCD patients and is manifested by elevation in monocyte and neutrophil counts,[1–3] accompanied by elevated levels of circulating inflammatory cytokines, including tumor necrosis factor α (TNF-α), interleukin (IL)-1, and IL-8. Elevated levels of these cytokines have been shown to exacerbate sickling in experimental models and correlate with clinical vasoocclusive severity. Leukocytosis is associated with a decreased life expectancy and, when observed in infancy, predicts future disease severity.[4,5] Clinically, elevated baseline WBC counts have been associated with acute chest syndrome (ACS), decline in lung function, and ischemic stroke in children with sickle cell anemia (SCA).[6–8] Reports of acute vasoocclusive pain events, ACS multiorgan failure, and death after administration of myeloid colony-stimulating factors (granulocyte colony-stimulating factor or granulocyte-macrophage colony-stimulating factor) suggest that the association of leukocytosis and poor outcome may be causal. The reduced incidence of vasoocclusive pain and ACS episodes in patients on hydroxyurea (HU) is thought due, in part, to the myelosuppressive effect of the drug.[9]

Financial Disclosure and Conflict of Interest: The author has nothing to disclose.
Department of Hematology-Oncology, Children's Hospital & Research Center Oakland, 747 52nd Street, Oakland, CA 94609, USA
E-mail address: choppe@mail.cho.org

Hematol Oncol Clin N Am 28 (2014) 265–286
http://dx.doi.org/10.1016/j.hoc.2013.11.006
0889-8588/14/$ – see front matter © 2014 Elsevier Inc. All rights reserved.

Genetic associations with inflammation also support the involvement of inflammatory pathways in the pathophysiology of SCD and may partly explain the phenotypic heterogeneity of the disease. Associations between variants in the transforming growth factor β1 (TGF-β)/bone morphogenetic protein 6 pathway and pulmonary hypertension, stroke, and osteonecrosis in SCD have been replicated in 4 independent studies.[10–14]

Studies showing an increased risk of severe disease in SCA patients with elevated levels of TNF-α receptor-1 (TNF-R1) and vascular cell adhesion molecule (VCAM)-1 are supported by findings from a genome-wide association study of a link between disease severity and polymorphisms in VCAM-1 and in ADP-ribosylation factor guanine nucleotide-exchange factor 2 (ARFGEF2), a gene involved in TNF-R1 release.[15]

Another recent gene-centric association identified an association between ACS and a variant (rs6141803) located in close proximity to a gene (COMMD7) that is highly expressed in pulmonary endothelial cells (ECs), interacts with NF-κB signaling, and is differentially expressed when exposed to oxidant heme species.[16]

Individuals with SCA who express the integral red blood cell (RBC) membrane glycoprotein, Duffy antigen receptor for chemokines (DARC), were found to have higher steady-state WBC counts and levels of DARC-binding chemokines; IL-8; and regulated on activation, normal T cell expressed and secreted (RANTES) compared with individuals who were negative for the allele, FY*B^{null}.[17] The DARC modulates the bioavailability of proinflammatory chemokines, including RANTES (CCL5) and IL-8 (CXCL8), which are inactivated once bound to RBCs.

Gene expression studies have shown that sickle RBCs, either directly or indirectly, promote endothelial up-regulation of TNF-α and IL-1 genes.[18–20] Jison and colleagues[21] demonstrated differential expression of 112 genes involved in inflammation, heme metabolism, cell cycle regulation, antioxidant responses, and angiogenesis in peripheral blood mononuclear cells from SCD patients at baseline.

The importance of the vascular endothelium and its participation in the inflammatory response in SCD has become increasingly appreciated and is convincingly related to its activation by inflammatory stimuli and abnormal expression of adhesion molecules. Circulating ECs from individuals with SCA exhibit an activated phenotype with abnormal expression of adhesion molecules, selectins, tissue factor (TF), and up-regulated heme oxygenase-1 (HO-1).[22–24] Biologic modifiers triggering endothelial activation during sickle vasoocclusive episodes include hypoxia; oxidant molecules; cytokines, in particular TNF-α and IL-1; and thrombin.[25,26]

Adhesive interactions between sickle RBCs, leukocytes, platelets, and the vascular endothelium cause vasoocclusion, ischemia, and reperfusion injury that result in acute vasoocclusive pain episodes, ACS and, over time, ischemic organ damage. The development of sickle cell mouse models that mimic sickle cell vasoocclusion and ischemia-reperfusion injury in humans has provided critical information about the pathobiology of SCD. Because inflammation plays a significant role in the development of acute clinical manifestations and chronic vascular injury in SCD, pharmacologic strategies aimed at pathways of inflammation may have both therapeutic and preventative value.

This review summarizes the accumulated evidence from clinical and experimental studies that implicate the inflammatory response in the development of vascular injury associated with SCD. Despite the broad impact of inflammation on acute complications and chronic vascular disease in SCD, no directed antiinflammatory therapies for the treatment or prevention of vasoocclusive events currently exist. An integrated approach using a combination of therapeutic agents directed at individual components of the inflammatory response may ultimately be necessary to make a clinical impact on this debilitating disease.

OVERVIEW OF SICKLE CELL DISEASE PATHOPHYSIOLOGY

Vasoocclusion and transient ischemia-reperfusion events underlie the chronic vascular damage that occurs in SCD.[22,27] Hemoglobin polymerization and depolymerization cause not only RBC sickling and hemolysis but also a cascade of cellular interactions mediated by a host of inflammatory proteins (**Table 1**).[28,29]

Repeated cycles of sickling cause premature destruction of RBCs with release of hemoglobin and reactive heme iron. These products of hemolysis are a major source of oxidant stress, depleting nitric oxide (NO) through hemoglobin-mediated scavenging, consumption by reactive oxygen species (ROS), and arginase-mediated substrate depletion.[30–35] Even under ambient conditions, sickle mice develop reperfusion injury with excessive ROS generation in response to hypoxic episodes.[36–38]

The abnormal adhesion of sickle cells to vascular endothelium involves multiple ligands and receptors and correlates strongly with clinical severity of vasoocclusive pain.[39] Membrane alterations in subpopulations of RBCs expose adhesive receptors and/or phophatidylserine (PS) that promote RBC-endothelial interaction and make them vulnerable to removal or breakdown by enzymes, such as secretory phospholipase A2 (sPLA2), which in turn generates active lipid mediators, such as lysophospholipids and fatty acids, and the release of cytosolic enzymes, including arginase. RBCs

Table 1
Mediators of inflammation in sickle cell disease

Type	Name	Cellular Source	Main Effects
Cytokines	TNF-α, IL-1	EC, monocytes, neutrophils, mast cells, platelets	EC activation Adhesion molecule expression Coagulation (induces thrombin, PAF) Vascular permeability
Acute-phase reactants	IL-6, CRP	EC	Vascular permeability
Chemokines	IL-8	EC, leukocytes, monocytes, mast cells	TNF, IL-1 regulation EC activation Leukocyte activation, chemotaxis
	PAF	Leukocytes, mast cells	Leukocyte adhesion, chemotaxis
Eicosanoids LTs	PGI2, PGE2	Leukocytes, mast cells	Vasodilation
	LTB4		SRBC adhesion to neutrophils/EC neutrophil chemotaxis, adhesion
	LTE4		Bronchoconstriction, airway edema
Phospholipases	sPLA2		Lipid breakdown (cell membranes), cytokine induction
Vasoactive amines	Histamine	Mast cells, basophils	Vasodilation, permeability
	Serotonin	Platelets	Platelet aggregation
	NO	EC	Vasodilation Antioxidant (–)Adhesion molecule expression (–)Platelet aggregation
	ET-1	EC	Vasoconstriction ROS production
Platelet factors	IL-1, CD40LG TNFSF14 PF-4	Platelets	EC activation, SRBC adhesion EC adhesion molecule expression Coagulation; binds heparins on EC surface

Abbreviations: PG, prostaglandin; SRBC, sickled RBC; (–), inhibitory effect.

show evidence of lipid peroxidation and oxidative damage to structural proteins,[40–42] and plasma levels of lipid peroxidation products are elevated in SCD patients, indicative of ongoing oxidative stress.[43–45]

The generation of ROS in sickle RBC is mediated by NADPH oxidase, an enzyme regulated by protein kinase C, Rac GTPase, and intracellular Ca++ signaling and further augmented by TGF-β1 and endothelin-1 (ET-1).[46] Cell-free hemoglobin released by PS-exposing RBC may contribute to NO depletion.[47] Abnormal PS expression on RBC activates the endothelium, permitting exposure of thrombospondin and consequent generation of procoagulants, TF, and thrombin.[48–50]

The capture of sickle RBCs by adherent leukocytes has been demonstrated both in vitro and in sickle mice and represents a critical step leading to formation of heterocellular aggregates and microvascular obstruction in the process of vasoocclusion.[51] These sickle RBC–leukocyte interactions are provoked by abnormal membrane exposure of PS, intercellular adhesion molecule (ICAM)-4, and autologous immunoglobulins, which can bind leukocyte β2 integrins.[38] Consistent with these results, sickle RBC–leukocyte interactions were abrogated with improvement in blood flow in E-selectin knockout mice, emphasizing the role of E-selectin as a mediator of neutrophil adhesion. Based on these findings, a multistep model for the pathogenesis of sickle cell vasoocclusion has been proposed, highlighting the interaction of adherent leukocytes with sickle RBC and the endothelium (**Fig. 1**).[52]

CYTOPROTECTIVE MEDIATORS
Nitric Oxide

NO, a potent vasodilator, also mediates inflammation in SCD by countering oxidative stress, down-regulating expression of endothelial adhesion molecules, and inhibiting platelet aggregation.

Patients with SCD exhibit a chronic state of NO deficiency, which is further exacerbated during vasoocclusive pain episodes and ACS as a result of consumption by plasma hemoglobin and ROS (superoxides and xanthine oxidase) generated during ischemia-reperfusion cycles.[53] Endogenously produced inhibitors of NO synthase (NOS), such as asymmetric dimethylarginine, are also increased in SCD patients and may further limit NO availability.

The inhibitory effect of NO on leukocyte adhesion is supported by studies showing that

1. NO donors (eg, nitroprusside) decrease leukocyte adherence induced by inflammation.
2. NOS inhibitors increase recruitment of adherent leukocytes.
3. Depletion of NO by ROS (superoxide) promotes leukocyte adherence.
4. Scavenging of ROS by superoxide dismutase increases NO bioavailability and prevents leukocyte adhesion.

Endothelin-1

ET-1, a potent long-acting vasoconstrictor, counteracts the effects of NO in response to inflammatory stimuli, hypoxia, and shear stress. ET-1 is induced by sickle RBCs in vitro and mediates ROS generation through RBC NADPH oxidase activity.[46] Treatment with an ET-1 receptor antagonist lowered RBC-associated protein disulfide isomerase oxidant activity in sickle mice.[54]

Levels of ET-1 are increased in SCD patients during acute vasoocclusive pain episodes and may remain elevated for weeks thereafter, suggesting that it may be partly responsible for prolongation of vasoocclusive pain symptoms.[18,55–57] As the

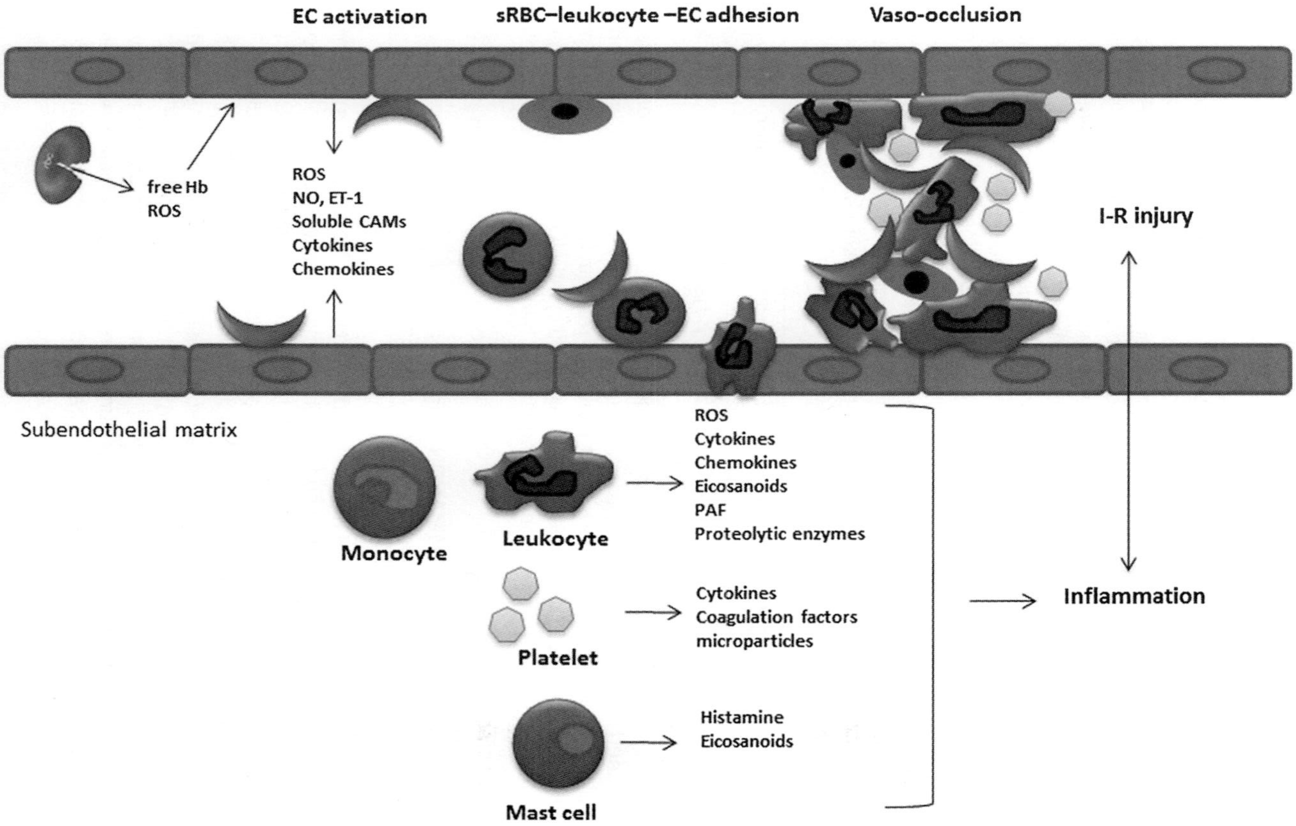

Fig. 1. Role of inflammation in sickle cell vasoocclusion. CAM, cellular adhesion molecules; Hb, hemoglobin; I-R, ischemia-reperfusion; sRBC, sickled RBC.

elevation in ET-1 precedes the development of clinical symptoms, blockade of this endogenous vasoconstrictor may ameliorate the disease process. Treatment with HU has also been shown to down-regulate ET-1 gene expression in vitro and is independently associated with a decrease in circulating ET-1 levels in children with SCD.[58,59]

Adenosine

Adenosine is an endogenous nucleoside that acts to reduce adherence and emigration of leukocytes in inflamed postcapillary venules.[60] The antiinflammatory effects of adenosine have been attributed to the stimulation of the adenosine 2A receptor (A2AR) subtype, expressed on neutrophils, macrophages, platelets, and ECs.[61] Adenosine 2A receptor agonists inhibit oxidative activity and degranulation in neutrophils as well as TNF-α release by monocytes. In preclinical models of SCD, activation of the A2AR in natural killer T cells (NKTs) was shown to reduce NKT-related inflammatory lung injury.[62] In contrast, activation of the adenosine 2B receptor (A2BR) increases RBC 2,3-diphosphoglycerate levels, leading to increased sickling in vitro and to hemolysis, vasoocclusion, and organ failure in sickle mice.[63] Inhibition of the A2BR with an experimental A2BR antagonist, PAB1115, or pegylated adenosine deaminase decreased hypoxia-induced sickling in vitro. These agents produced similar results, with inhibition of sickling, vasoocclusion, and organ damage in sickle mice.[63]

Heme oxygenase-1

Free heme and iron released by hemolyzed RBCs promote inflammatory injury via activation of innate immune responses in macrophages and monocytes. Heme oxygenase and biliverdin reductase signaling detoxify heme and iron and provide catalytic antioxidant, antiproliferative, and antiinflammatory protective signaling.[64] Expression of HO-1 is increased in sickle mice and in SCD patients, in response to heme-induced oxidative stress. By increasing ET-1 expression or administering biliverdin, vasoocclusion and subsequent ischemia-reperfusion injury could be prevented in sickle mice.[65] SCD patients have insufficient HO-1 activity, however, required to handle the excessive heme produced by hemolysis and prevent oxidative stress.

SOLUBLE MEDIATORS OF INFLAMMATION
Histamine, Leukotrienes, and Secretory Phospholipase A2

Histamine
Histamine, a potent inflammatory agent stored in mast cells and basophils, is rapidly released via degranulation in response to proinflammatory stimuli. Under physiologic flow conditions in vitro, histamine can induce the adhesion of sickle RBC to vascular endothelium via H_2 and H_4 receptor–mediated expression of P-selectin.[66] The elevated histamine levels observed in SCD patients at baseline and during morphine administration suggest that the activating effect of histamine on the endothelium may have a significant influence on initiating and propagating pain episodes in SCD.[66–68] In addition, selective blockade of H_2 and/or H_4 receptors has been shown to prevent sickle RBC adhesion, suggesting that concurrent treatment with histamine antagonists may minimize the adverse histaminic effects produced by opioid analgesics.

Leukotrienes
LTs are inflammatory chemokines released by membrane phospholipids via the 5-lipoxygenase (5-LPO) pathway (**Fig. 2**). Dihydroxy LT (LTB4) and the cysteinyl LTs (CysLTs)—LTC4, LTD4, and LTE4—induce proinflammatory signaling through activation of specific LT receptors on inflammatory cells and the vessel wall. LTB4 induces

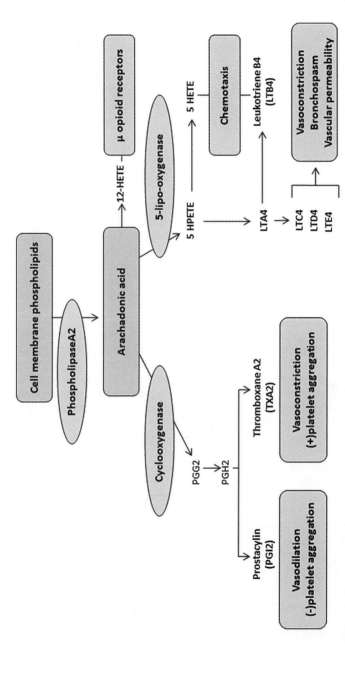

Fig. 2. Lipid metabolites and inflammation. 5-HPETE, 5-hydroperoxyeicosatetraenoic acid; PG, prostaglandin.

adhesion of sickle RBCs and recruitment of neutrophils to the endothelium in sickle mice.[38] Plasma LTB4 levels are markedly elevated in SCA patients at baseline and increase further during vasoocclusive pain episodes and ACS.[69] These neutrophil-derived LTB4 effects on RBC-endothelial adhesion are also supported by prior studies documenting an LTB4-associated increase in the ratio of plasma levels of thromboxane A_2 to prostacyclin and the platelet metabolite, 12-hydroxyeicosatetraenoic acid, as well as up-regulation of endothelial vitronectin receptor expression.[70,71]

LTB4 is also produced by monocytes to stimulate neutrophil chemotaxis and endothelial adhesion. Monocytes from SCD patients have greater expression of the key catalytic molecules in the LT pathway, 5-LPO and its activating protein (FLAP), than monocytes from healthy controls.[72] This increase in monocyte LT production is mediated by placenta growth factor, indicating another mechanism for the chronic inflammation and increased airway hyperreactivity associated with SCD.[73,74]

The CysLTs are known for their bronchoconstrictive effects but also potentiate edema, inflammation, and mucus secretion. In children with SCD, urinary LTE4 levels were found elevated and associated with an increased rate of hospitalizations for vasoocclusive pain.[75] A subsequent study confirmed the observed elevation in baseline LTE4 levels and documented further increases in LTE4 levels during acute pain events, suggesting that the proinflammatory and vasoconstrictive effects of LTE4 may be plausibly related to vasoocclusion.[76] Recent studies also suggest that LT and prostaglandins mediate neuropathic pain in SCD.[77] Stimulated and released during vasoocclusive episodes, LTs facilitate the activation of primary afferent nociceptors, resulting in exaggerated pain sensitization.

sPLA2

sPLA2 represents a class of enzymes that hydrolyze phospholipids from cellular membranes and lipoproteins and is implicated in the pathology of a variety of inflammatory conditions, including arthritis, sepsis, and multiorgan failure.[78,79]

sPLA2 is induced by TNF-α and IL-1 to generate arachidonic acid, lysophophatidic acid, and platelet activating factor (PAF). As such, sPLA2 mediates both proximal and distal effectors of inflammation by catalyzing the production of these compounds and independently inducing ECs and monocytes to release proinflammatory cytokines. In neonates with acute respiratory distress syndrome, sPLA2 levels correlate with alveolar-arterial oxygen gradient, severity of lung injury, and mortality.[80–82] Styles and colleagues[83] found that baseline levels of sPLA2 are increased in SCD and are further elevated at the onset of ACS, indicating that sPLA2 may play a key role in vascular endothelial damage. Because sPLA2 levels rise 24 to 48 hours before ACS is diagnosed clinically, sequential measurements of sPLA2 can be used to predict the development of ACS in patients hospitalized for vasoocclusive crisis.[84] In addition, C-reactive protein (CRP) values correlate closely with changes in sPLA2 levels in SCD patients and have been used as a surrogate biomarker for sPLA2.[85]

Coagulation Mediators of Inflammation

Early-response cytokines, in particular IL-1β, TNF-α, and IL-6, induce TF expression on ECs and monocytes and simultaneously down-regulate thrombomodulin, endothelial protein C receptors, and fibrinolysis, thus establishing a procoagulant shift in the hemostatic balance.[23,86] TF expression is increased in pulmonary ECs and circulating monocytes of sickle mice and can be further induced by hypoxia-reoxygenation.[87,88] Knockout of the *TF* gene from ECs in sickle mice led to decreased expression of IL-6 but did not have an impact on coagulation, suggesting that endothelial TF is primarily involved in signaling rather than coagulation.[89] A direct mechanism by which coagulation factors promote inflammation is through binding to protease-activated receptors (PARs) on monocytes and ECs, thereby up-regulating proinflammatory cytokines, such as monocyte chemoattractant protein-1, IL-6, and IL-8.[90,91] Several studies have demonstrated that TF/factor VIIa–dependent activation of PAR-2 promotes inflammation.[92]

Platelet-associated CD40 Ligand

Platelet-associated CD40 ligand (CD40LG), a ligand for the CD40 TNF receptor superfamily protein, has a significant inflammatory and activating effect on ECs.[93] The soluble form of CD40LG has been found elevated and biologically active in individuals with SCA, suggesting a role for platelet-derived mediators in the chronic inflammatory and hypercoagulable state associated with SCD.[94] Elevated CD40LG has been associated with an increased frequency of pain episodes and correlated with leukocyte and platelet counts in patients with SCA.[95]

Platelet-associated TNFSF14

Platelet-associated TNF ligand superfamily 14 (TNFSF14) levels are known to be elevated in SCA patients and induce up-regulation of ICAM-1, VCAM-1, IL-8, and CCL2.[96] Plasma TNFSF14 levels are elevated in SCA patients and correlate with platelet-associated inflammatory markers, CD40LG, IL-8, and ICAM-1.[97] Platelet expression of TNFSF14 is also increased and correlates with platelet activation as measured by P-selectin, suggesting a mechanism by which platelets localize to the vessel wall and release inflammatory mediators. Plasma TNFSF14 has also been associated with elevated tricuspid regurgitant velocity ($\geq$2.5 m/s) in SCA patients and may contribute to the endothelial activation and inflammation associated with pulmonary hypertension in SCA. SCA patients treated with HU had higher levels of plasma TNF receptor superfamily 6B, a soluble receptor that attenuates the effects of TNFSF14, compared with untreated patients, suggesting another beneficial effect conferred by HU.

Cytokines and Chemokines

The interaction of monocytes with the endothelium plays a pivotal role in initiating the inflammatory response by inducing endothelial E-selectin, ICAM, and VCAM and by secreting cytokines, TNF-α and IL-1.[98] These cytokines, together with ROS produced by sickle cell–endothelial interactions, signal the endothelial transcription factor, NF-κB, to produce additional cytokines and chemokines, including IL-8, PAF, and IL-6, all of which contribute to pancellular activation and a second surge of proinflammatory and procoagulant molecules.[98,99] As discussed previously, many of these inflammatory mediators are chronically elevated in SCD patients, becoming further elevated during acute vasoocclusive pain events and ACS.[3,100–103]

A major stimulant of the acute-phase response, IL-6 has been identified as an independent predictor of peripheral vascular disease progression in patients with atherosclerosis.[104,105] In SCD, IL-6 is liberated at sites of vasoocclusion and stimulates hepatic production of acute-phase reactants, such as CRP, fibrinogen, and haptoglobin. The rise in acute-phase proteins is thought to mitigate tissue damage caused by microvascular ischemia.[106]

Neutrophil activation

In a sickle cell mouse model of vasoocclusion triggered by hemolytic transfusion reaction, Jang and colleagues[107] found that acute vasoocclusive episodes were associated with a striking elevation in neutrophil chemokine CXC motif ligand 1 (CXCL1). Injection of recombinant CXCL1 also induced acute vasoocclusion in sickle mice, as demonstrated by a reduction in microvascular blood flow and leukocyte adhesion to RBC and endothelium. Blockade of CXCL1 receptor, CXCR2, prevented acute occlusion and prolonged survival in these mice. These data suggest that targeted inhibiton of CXCL1 and/or CXCR2 may be a potential therapeutic strategy to prevent acute VOC in SCD patients.

Neutrophil adhesion is enhanced by IL-8 through an increase in cyclic adenosine monophosphate–protein kinase A signaling.[108] Neutrophils isolated from sickle cell patients exhibit increased expression of adhesion molecules compared with neutrophils from healthy control subjects, making them more vulnerable to inflammatory stimuli.[109–112] Adhesion assays using immobilized fibronectin and TNF-α–stimulated ECs confirm the heightened adhesive properties of neutrophils observed in sickle cell patients.[113]

In addition to stimulating adhesion, IL-8 promotes neutrophil degranulation, oxidative burst, and lipid mediator synthesis.[30,114,115] Activated neutrophils thus contribute to oxidative stress by releasing proteolytic enzymes and forming ROS,[116] including superoxide and hydrogen peroxide. Myeloperoxidase (MPO) is also released, binds to ECs, and generates oxidants that scavenge NO and impair endothelial function. Elevated plasma MPO levels have been demonstrated in sickle mice and humans with SCD.[117,118] In sickle mice, treatment with a novel MPO inhibitor decreased ROS production and lipid peroxidation, with restoration of endothelial- and eNOS-dependent vascular function.[119] Release of cathepsin G and elastase by neutrophils activates both coagulation and platelets. Increased levels of these neutrophil-derived mediators have been associated with acute pain episodes in SCA patients.[110] Platelet-neutrophil aggregates (PNAs) formed in response to inflammatory stimuli are present in patients with septic shock[120,121] and are elevated in SCD.[122] In sickle mice, PNAs showed greater oxidative activity than activated neutrophils alone. Hypoxia-reoxygenation induced a further increase in PNAs and additional activation of both platelets and neutrophils. Pretreatment with antiplatelet agents, such as clopidogrel or P-selectin antibody, resulted in decreased formation of PNAs, a reduction in neutrophil activation and decreased lung vascular permeability in these mice.

Neutrophil extracellular traps

Activated neutrophils have also been shown to form neutrophil extracellular traps (NETs), a meshwork of nuclear DNA and histones containing granular proteins, such as elastase, cathepsin G, and MPO.[123] NETs formation is mediated by ROS production involving NADPH oxidase and MPO[124] and has been documented in sepsis, malaria, systemic lupus erythematosus, and cystic fibrosis.[125–128] Aberrant NET formation contributes to tissue damage and predicts multiorgan failure and sepsis.[129] In trauma patients, excessive release of extracellular histones and nucleic acids has been associated with impaired thrombin generation, hyperfibrinolysis, and platelet activation.[130] Using plasma levels of circulating nucleosomes and neutrophil elastase–$α_1$-antitrypsin complexes as markers of neutrophil activation and NET formation, Schimmel and colleagues[131] found greater NETs in SCD patients with vasoocclusive pain compared with patients at steady state. The highest nucleosome levels were observed in patients with ACS, paralleling those found in patients with severe sepsis.

Mast cells in inflammation

Mast cells also release inflammatory mediators and proteases, including TNF-α, that contribute to the heightened inflammation observed in SCA.[132] Mast cell activation was associated with increased expression of Fcγ receptor 1 and Toll-like receptor 4 as well as an increase in circulating acute-phase proteins in sickle mice. Mast cell activation also occurs in response to ischemia-reperfusion injury, influencing leuko-cyte adhesion and transmigration. In sickle mice, pharmacologic inhibition of mast cells with cromolyn or imatinib has been shown to reduce hypoxia-induced systemic and neurogenic inflammation.[133]

In a recent exploratory study using carbon-fiber microelectrode amperometry to monitor the impact of sickle cell–induced inflammation on mast cell function, Mann-ing and colleagues[134] found significantly lower serotonin release in sickle mice compared with control mice. The effect of morphine exposure on mast cell opioid re-ceptors was also demonstrated by an increased release of serotonin in normal mice, indicating the potential ability to compensate for sickle cell–induced changes in mast cell function.

Therapeutic implications

Accumulating data from genomic and preclinical studies in SCD have provided new opportunities to develop therapeutic strategies targeting key genetic and cellular mechanisms in the pathogenesis of SCD. Because antisickling agents only partially ameliorate the vasculopathy of SCD, therapeutic agents targeted at pathways involved in inflammation are attractive candidates for further exploration. Pharmaco-therapies currently under investigation include agents that inhibit cellular adhesion and target mediators of inflammation.

Inhibitors of Cellular Adhesion

Intravenous gammaglobulin

Intravenous gammaglobulin is currently under clinical evaluation after 2 studies demonstrated a dose-dependent reduction in RBC leukocyte adhesion, improvement in microcirculatory blood flow, and prevention of vasoocclusion in sickle mice.[135,136] Although intravenous gammaglobulin showed some beneficial effect in reducing dura-tion of pain in a few patients, its safety profile in SCD still needs to be evaluated. A phase 1/2 study is currently evaluating the effect of a single infusion of intravenous gammaglobulin on the duration of sickle cell pain events (http://clinicaltrials.gov/ct2/show/NCT01757418).

Pan-selectin inhibitor (GMI-1070)

GMI-1070 is pan-selectin inhibitor that prevents adhesion between RBCs and circu-lating monocytes and neutrophils. Initial studies of this investigational agent in a sickle cell mouse model of vasoocclusion analyzed by intravital microscopy demonstrated that through inhibition of primarily E-selectin and P-selectin and, to a lesser extent, L-selectin, the drug decreased adhesion of sickle RBCs to both neutrophils and ECs and decreased adhesion of neutrophils to endothelium.[137] These effects were associated with improved microcirculatory blood flow and improved survival in these mice. A phase 2 trial of this drug was recently completed, demonstrating a reduction in the duration of pain events, length of hospitalization, and parenteral opioid require-ment.[138] With these positive results, a phase 3 trial is planned.

Anti–P-selectin monoclonal antibody (SelG1)

P-selectin blockade by the monoclonal antibody, SelG1, inhibited endothelial adhe-sion molecule (VCAM-1 and ICAM-1) expression and abrogated hypoxia-induced vas-oocclusion in sickle mice.[139] A phase 2, multicenter, randomized controlled study assessing the safety and efficacy of this agent in reducing the frequency of vasooclu-sive pain events has recently been initiated (http://clinicaltrials.gov/ct2/show/NCT01895361).

Anti–P-selectin aptamer

Treatment with an anti–P-selectin aptamer almost completely inhibited the adhesion of sickle RBCs and leukocytes in sickle cell mice exposed to hypoxia.[140] Increased microvascular flow velocities and reduced leukocyte rolling flux were also observed in these mice. Anti–P-selectin aptamer may thus be useful as a novel therapeutic agent for SCD and warrants further clinical evaluation.

Platelet ADP receptor antagonist (prasugrel)

Therapies targeting platelet activation and interaction with inflammatory cells may represent another therapeutic avenue to prevent inflammation in SCD. The potential of antiplatelet agents to lessen the incidence and severity of pain in SCD has recently been studied in a randomized phase 2 study of the platelet P2Y12 ADP receptor antagonist, prasugrel, in adult SCD patients.[141,142] Cellular and soluble markers of platelet activation were decreased and in vivo platelet activation was attenuated in the treated group of patients without serious bleeding complications. In addition to confirming safety, the data suggest the efficacy of prasugrel in reducing the rate of pain in SCD. The safety and efficacy of prasugrel for the reduction of vasoocclusive pain events is now being evaluated in children with SCD in a phase 3 trial (http://clinicaltrials.gov/ct2/show/NCT01794000).

Leukotriene Blockade

Targeting inflammatory mediators involved in arachadonic acid metabolism may be a promising approach for the development of novel therapies for the treatment of SCD. Steroids inhibit production of arachidonic acid, thereby blocking synthesis of LTs and prostaglandins. Ketoprophen is believed to block production of 5-LPO and cyclooxygenase. Aspirin and nonsteroidal antiinflammatory drugs block conversion of cyclooxygenase to prostaglandins and thromboxane A_2. Additionally, aspirin has been shown to induce biosynthesis of a group of bioactive eicosanoids known as the 15-epi-lipoxins or aspirin-triggered lipoxins. Lipoxins are potent inhibitors of leukocyte chemotaxis, adhesion, and transmigration induced by LTs and other inflammatory mediators, which suggests that they are part of innate protective pathways dampening the host inflammatory response. A safety trial investigating the effect of aspirin prophylaxis on decreasing the incidence of ischemic cerebrovascular disease in children with SCD was terminated early due to poor enrollment.

5-Lipoxygenase inhibitor (zileuton)

Placenta growth factor, an angiogenic cytokine produced by hyperplastic erythroid marrow cells and found elevated in SCD, contributes to activation of monocytes and ECs by inducing a key LT synthetic enzyme, 5-LPO.[73,143,144] Zileuton is a specific inhibitor of 5-LPO that decreases LT production, and is Food and Drug Administration–approved for treatment of asthma. Administration of zileuton reduced adhesion of neutrophils and sickle RBCs to rat pulmonary vasculature.[145] Zileuton was also found to increase fetal hemoglobin production in erythroid cells in vitro and may have additive/synergistic effects with HU.[146] A phase I study of zileuton in SCD is now being carried out to establish safety and biologic endpoints (http://clinicaltrials.gov/ct2/show/NCT01136941).

NF-κB Inhibition

Many commonly prescribed antiinflammatory drugs, such as aspirin and glucocorticoids, attenuate activation of transcription factors regulating leukocyte adhesion and or cytokine expression. Nonsteroidal antiinflammatory drugs and glucocorticoids exert therapeutic efficacy by preventing the adhesion and influx of leukocytes.

High-dose methylprednisolone decreased the duration of severe pain in children and adolescents with sickle disease, but treatment was associated with rebound pain after discontinuation.[147]

Sickle cell mice treated with the polynitroxyl albumin, an antioxidant that inhibits NF-κB activity, also decreased hepatic and pulmonary endothelial VCAM-1 and ICAM-1 expression, inhibited microvascular leukocyte rolling, and reduced stasis after hypoxia reperfusion. Inhibition of NF-κB activation correlated with reduction in CAM expression.[99]

Additional antiinflammatory drugs that inhibit NF-κB and the up-regulation of adhesion molecules have shown promise in preliminary studies. Transgenic sickle cell mice treated with sulfasalazine showed a reduction in activated circulating ECs, accompanied by a marked decrease in leukocyte adhesion and improved microvascular blood flow disease.[148] In a pilot study, the administration of sulfasalazine to sickle cell patients abrogated the abnormal expression of these adhesion molecules in circulating ECs.[149]

Statins
The 3-hydroxy-3-methylglutaryl coenzyme A reductase inhibitors (statins) have been shown to improve vascular function, independent of their lipid-lowering properties, by restoring NO bioavailability and suppressing the inflammatory response to endothelial injury.[150] Lovastatin inhibited endothelial TF expression in sickle mice after hypoxia-reoxygenation.[88] Treatment with simvastatin prolonged survival in sickle mice after pneumococcal challenge.[151] In vitro studies of simvastatin in SCD indicate that simvastatin reduces endothelial activation and leukocyte adhesion under basal and stimulated inflammatory conditions.[152,153] Specifically, simvastatin decreased VCAM-1 and ICAM-1 mRNA levels, inhibited TNF-α–induced activation of NF-κB, and enhanced expression of peroxisome proliferator-activated receptor alpha in cultured ECs.

In a pilot study of 25 adult SCD patients with underlying vascular dysfunction, atorvastatin had no effect on endothelial-independent vasodilation but led to an increase in NOS-dependent blood flow, suggesting improvement in endothelial NOS function.[154] Another pilot study of 28 SCD patients treated with short-term simvastatin documented an increase in plasma NO products and a reduction in plasma levels of IL-6, high-sensitivity CRP, and the soluble adhesion molecules, VCAM-1, ICAM-1, and E-selectin.[155] Collectively, these studies have provided the basis for an extended phase 1/2 study investigating the potential clinical efficacy of simvastatin in decreasing the frequency of vasoocclusive pain events (http://clinicaltrials.gov/ct2/show/NCT01702246).

Adenosine 2A receptor agonist (regadenosan)
Invariant NKTs (iNKTs), a subset of lymphocytes that act to propagate the inflammation associated with ischemia-reperfusion injury, are both increased in number and activated in sickle cell anemia.[156] These cells express high amounts of A2ARs that, when activated, reduced inflammation and lung injury in sickle mice. In a phase I trial of regadenoson, a selective A2AR agonist, expression of NF-κB and iNKT activation associated with vasoocclusive pain events was reduced in patients with SCD.[157] A phase 2 study was recently initiated to assess the efficacy of regadenoson in treating vasoocclusive pain events and ACS in SCD (http://clinicaltrials.gov/ct2/show/NCT01788631).

Although it remains to be seen whether these potential antiinflammatory agents prove useful in clinical management of SCD, the experimental and preliminary clinical findings from investigations provide valuable insights into relevant endothelial signaling events and inflammatory responses that lead to vascular injury in SCD. Agents with multiple mechanisms of action or a combination of agents that target various aspects of the pathophysiology of SCD, such as NO regulation, oxidative injury, inflammation, and cell adhesion, may ultimately prove the most effective therapeutic approach.

REFERENCES

1. West MS, Wethers D, Smith J, et al. Laboratory profile of sickle cell disease: a cross-sectional analysis. The cooperative study of sickle cell disease. J Clin Epidemiol 1992;45(8):893–909.
2. Vichinsky E. Understanding the morbidity of sickle cell disease. Br J Haematol 1997;99:974–82.
3. Qari MH, Dier U, Mousa SA. Biomarkers of inflammation, growth factor, and coagulation activation in patients with sickle cell disease. Clin Appl Thromb Hemost 2012;18(2):195–200.
4. Miller ST, Sleeper LA, Pegelow CH, et al. Prediction of adverse outcomes in children with sickle cell disease. N Engl J Med 2000;342(2):83–9.
5. Platt OS, Brambilla DJ, Rosse WF, et al. Mortality in sickle cell disease; life expectancy and risk factors for early death. N Engl J Med 1994;330:1639.
6. Tassel C, Arnaud C, Kulpa M, et al. Leukocytosis is a risk factor for lung function deterioration in children with sickle cell disease. Respir Med 2011;105(5):788–95.
7. Castro O, Brambilla DJ, Thorington B, et al. The acute chest syndrome in sickle cell disease: incidence and risk factors. The cooperative study of sickle cell disease. Blood 1994;84(2):643–9.
8. Ohene-Frempong K, Weiner SJ, Sleeper LA, et al. Cerebrovascular accidents in sickle cell disease: rates and risk factors. Blood 1998;91(1):288–94.
9. Charache S, Terrin ML, Moore RD, et al. Effect of hydroxyurea on the frequency of painful crises in sickle cell anemia. N Engl J Med 1995;332(20):1317–22.
10. Ashley-Koch AE, Elliott L, Kail ME, et al. Identification of genetic polymorphisms associated with risk for pulmonary hypertension in sickle cell disease. Blood 2008;111(12):5721–6.
11. Nolan VG, Ma Q, Cohen HT, et al. Estimated glomerular filtration rate in sickle cell anemia is associated with polymorphisms of bone morphogenetic protein receptor 1B. Am J Hematol 2007;82(3):179–84.
12. Sebastiani P, Nolan VG, Baldwin CT, et al. A network model to predict the risk of death in sickle cell disease. Blood 2007;110(7):2727–35.
13. Adewoye AH, Nolan VG, Ma Q, et al. Association of polymorphisms of IGF1R and genes in the transforming growth factor- beta/bone morphogenetic protein pathway with bacteremia in sickle cell anemia. Clin Infect Dis 2006;43(5):593–8.
14. Steinberg MH, Adewoye AH. Modifier genes and sickle cell anemia. Curr Opin Hematol 2006;13(3):131–6.
15. Dworkis DA, Klings ES, Solovieff N, et al. Severe sickle cell anemia is associated with increased plasma levels of TNF-R1 and VCAM-1. Am J Hematol 2011;86(2):220–3.
16. Galarneau G, Coady S, Garrett ME, et al. Gene-centric association study of acute chest syndrome and painful crisis in sickle cell disease patients. Blood 2013;122(3):434–42.
17. Nebor D, Durpes MC, Mougenel D, et al. Association between Duffy antigen receptor for chemokines expression and levels of inflammation markers in sickle cell anemia patients. Clin Immunol 2010;136(1):116–22.

18. Phelan M, Perrine SP, Brauer M, et al. Sickle erythrocytes, after sickling, regulate the expression of the endothelin-1 gene and protein in human endothelial cells in culture. J Clin Invest 1995;96(2):1145–51.

19. Shiu YT, Udden MM, McIntire LV. Perfusion with sickle erythrocytes up-regulates ICAM-1 and VCAM-1 gene expression in cultured human endothelial cells. Blood 2000;95(10):3232–41.

20. Brown MD, Wick TM, Eckman JR. Activation of vascular endothelial cell adhesion molecule expression by sickle blood cells. Pediatr Pathol Mol Med 2001; 20(1):47–72.

21. Jison ML, Munson PJ, Barb JJ, et al. Blood mononuclear cell gene expression profiles characterize the oxidant, hemolytic, and inflammatory stress of sickle cell disease. Blood 2004;104(1):270–80.

22. Solovey A, Lin Y, Browne P, et al. Circulating activated endothelial cells in sickle cell anemia. N Engl J Med 1997;337(22):1584–90.

23. Solovey A, Gui L, Key NS, et al. Tissue factor expression by endothelial cells in sickle cell anemia. J Clin Invest 1998;101(9):1899–904.

24. Nath KA, Grande JP, Haggard JJ, et al. Oxidative stress and induction of heme oxygenase-1 in the kidney in sickle cell disease. Am J Pathol 2001;158(3):893–903.

25. Pober JS, Cotran RS. The role of endothelial cells in inflammation. Transplantation 1990;50(4):537–44.

26. Rodgers GM. Hemostatic properties of normal and perturbed vascular cells. FASEB J 1988;2(2):116–23.

27. Hebbel RP, Vercellotti GM. The endothelial biology of sickle cell disease. J Lab Clin Med 1997;129(3):288–93.

28. Dias-Da-Motta P, Arruda VR, Muscara MN, et al. The release of nitric oxide and superoxide anion by neutrophils and mononuclear cells from patients with sickle cell anaemia. Br J Haematol 1996;93(2):333–40.

29. Hofstra TC, Kalra VK, Meiselman HJ, et al. Sickle erythrocytes adhere to polymorphonuclear neutrophils and activate the neutrophil respiratory burst. Blood 1996;87(10):4440–7.

30. Reiter CD, Wang X, Tanus-Santos JE, et al. Cell-free hemoglobin limits nitric oxide bioavailability in sickle-cell disease. Nat Med 2002;8(12):1383–9.

31. Aslan M, Freeman BA. Oxidases and oxygenases in regulation of vascular nitric oxide signaling and inflammatory responses. Immunol Res 2002;26(1–3): 107–18.

32. Morris CR, Poljakovic M, Lavrisha L, et al. Decreased arginine bioavailability and increased serum arginase activity in asthma. Am J Respir Crit Care Med 2004; 170(2):148–53.

33. Gladwin MT, Crawford JH, Patel RP. The biochemistry of nitric oxide, nitrite, and hemoglobin: role in blood flow regulation. Free Radic Biol Med 2004;36(6): 707–17.

34. Osarogiagbon UR, Choong S, Belcher JD, et al. Reperfusion injury pathophysiology in sickle transgenic mice. Blood 2000;96(1):314–20.

35. Klings ES, Farber HW. Role of free radicals in the pathogenesis of acute chest syndrome in sickle cell disease. Respir Res 2001;2(5):280–5.

36. Hebbel RP. Special issue of microcirculation: examination of the vascular pathobiology of sickle cell anemia. Microcirculation 2004;11(2):99–100.

37. Amer J, Ghoti H, Rachmilewitz E, et al. Red blood cells, platelets and polymorphonuclear neutrophils of patients with sickle cell disease exhibit oxidative stress that can be ameliorated by antioxidants. Br J Haematol 2006;132(1): 108–13.

38. Kaul DK, Hebbel RP. Hypoxia/reoxygenation causes inflammatory response in transgenic sickle mice but not in normal mice. J Clin Invest 2000;106(3):411–20.
39. Hebbel RP, Eaton JW, Steinberg MH, et al. Erythrocyte/endothelial interactions and the vasocclusive severity of sickle cell disease. Prog Clin Biol Res 1981; 55:145–62.
40. Jain SK, Shohet SB. A novel phospholipid in irreversibly sickled cells: evidence for in vivo peroxidative membrane damage in sickle cell disease. Blood 1984; 63(2):362–7.
41. Rank BH, Hebbel RP, Carlsson J. Oxidation of membrane thiols in sickle erythrocytes. Prog Clin Biol Res 1984;165:473–7.
42. Wood KC, Granger DN. Sickle cell disease: role of reactive oxygen and nitrogen metabolites. Clin Exp Pharmacol Physiol 2007;34(9):926–32.
43. Klings ES, Christman BW, McClung J, et al. Increased F2 isoprostanes in the acute chest syndrome of sickle cell disease as a marker of oxidative stress. Am J Respir Crit Care Med 2001;164(7):1248–52.
44. Manfredini V, Lazzaretti LL, Griebeler IH, et al. Blood antioxidant parameters in sickle cell anemia patients in steady state. J Natl Med Assoc 2008;100(8): 897–902.
45. Gizi A, Papassotiriou I, Apostolakou F, et al. Assessment of oxidative stress in patients with sickle cell disease: the glutathione system and the oxidant-antioxidant status. Blood Cells Mol Dis 2011;46(3):220–5.
46. George A, Pushkaran S, Konstantinidis DG, et al. Erythrocyte NADPH oxidase activity modulated by Rac GTPases, PKC, and plasma cytokines contributes to oxidative stress in sickle cell disease. Blood 2013;121(11):2099–107.
47. Kato GJ, Hebbel RP, Steinberg MH, et al. Vasculopathy in sickle cell disease: biology, pathophysiology, genetics, translational medicine, and new research directions. Am J Hematol 2009;84(9):618–25.
48. Chiu D, Lubin B, Roelofsen B, et al. Sickled erythrocytes accelerate clotting in vitro: an effect of abnormal membrane lipid asymmetry. Blood 1981;58(2): 398–401.
49. Manodori AB, Barabino GA, Lubin BH, et al. Adherence of phosphatidylserine-exposing erythrocytes to endothelial matrix thrombospondin. Blood 2000;95(4): 1293–300.
50. Brittain JE, Mlinar KJ, Anderson CS, et al. Activation of sickle red blood cell adhesion via integrin-associated protein/CD47-induced signal transduction. J Clin Invest 2001;107(12):1555–62.
51. Turhan A, Weiss LA, Mohandas N, et al. Primary role for adherent leukocytes in sickle cell vascular occlusion: a new paradigm. Proc Natl Acad Sci U S A 2002; 99(5):3047–51.
52. Frenette PS. Sickle cell vaso-occlusion: multistep and multicellular paradigm. Curr Opin Hematol 2002;9(2):101–6.
53. Wood KC, Hsu LL, Gladwin MT. Sickle cell disease vasculopathy: a state of nitric oxide resistance. Free Radic Biol Med 2008;44(8):1506–28.
54. Prado GN, Romero JR, Rivera A. Endothelin-1 receptor antagonists regulate cell surface-associated protein disulfide isomerase in sickle cell disease. FASEB J 2013;27(11):4619–29.
55. Graido-Gonzalez E, Doherty JC, Bergreen EW, et al. Plasma endothelin-1, cytokine, and prostaglandin E2 levels in sickle cell disease and acute vaso-occlusive sickle crisis. Blood 1998;92(7):2551–5.
56. Rybicki AC, Benjamin LJ. Increased levels of endothelin-1 in plasma of sickle cell anemia patients. Blood 1998;92(7):2594–6.

57. Ergul S, Brunson CY, Hutchinson J, et al. Vasoactive factors in sickle cell disease: in vitro evidence for endothelin-1-mediated vasoconstriction. Am J Hematol 2004;76(3):245–51.
58. Brun M, Bourdoulous S, Couraud PO, et al. Hydroxyurea downregulates endothelin-1 gene expression and upregulates ICAM-1 gene expression in cultured human endothelial cells. Pharmacogenomics J 2003;3(4):215–26.
59. Lapoumeroulie C, Benkerrou M, Odievre MH, et al. Decreased plasma endothelin-1 levels in children with sickle cell disease treated with hydroxyurea. Haematologica 2005;90(3):401–3.
60. Cronstein BN, Levin RI, Belanoff J, et al. Adenosine: an endogenous inhibitor of neutrophil-mediated injury to endothelial cells. J Clin Invest 1986;78(3):760–70.
61. Cronstein BN, Levin RI, Philips M, et al. Neutrophil adherence to endothelium is enhanced via adenosine A1 receptors and inhibited via adenosine A2 receptors. J Immunol 1992;148(7):2201–6.
62. Wallace KL, Linden J. Adenosine A2A receptors induced on iNKT and NK cells reduce pulmonary inflammation and injury in mice with sickle cell disease. Blood 2010;116(23):5010–20.
63. Zhang Y, Dai Y, Wen J, et al. Detrimental effects of adenosine signaling in sickle cell disease. Nat Med 2011;17(1):79–86.
64. Wagener FA, Volk HD, Willis D, et al. Different faces of the heme-heme oxygenase system in inflammation. Pharmacol Rev 2003;55(3):551–71.
65. Belcher JD, Beckman JD, Balla G, et al. Heme degradation and vascular injury. Antioxid Redox Signal 2010;12(2):233–48.
66. Wagner MC, Eckman JR, Wick TM. Histamine increases sickle erythrocyte adherence to endothelium. Br J Haematol 2006;132(4):512–22.
67. Enwonwu CO, Lu M. Elevated plasma histamine in sickle cell anaemia. Clin Chim Acta 1991;203(2–3):363–8.
68. Withington DE, Patrick JA, Reynolds F. Histamine release by morphine and diamorphine in man. Anaesthesia 1993;48(1):26–9.
69. Setty BN, Stuart MJ, Dampier C, et al. Hypoxaemia in sickle cell disease: biomarker modulation and relevance to pathophysiology. Lancet 2003;362(9394):1450–5.
70. Setty BN, Stuart MJ. Eicosanoids in sickle cell disease: potential relevance of neutrophil leukotriene B4 to disease pathophysiology. J Lab Clin Med 2002; 139(2):80–9.
71. Ibe BO, Kurantsin-Mills J, Raj JU, et al. Plasma and urinary leukotrienes in sickle cell disease: possible role in the inflammatory process. Eur J Clin Invest 1994; 24(1):57–64.
72. Knight-Perry J, DeBaun MR, Strunk RC, et al. Leukotriene pathway in sickle cell disease: a potential target for directed therapy. Expert Rev Hematol 2009;2(1): 57–68.
73. Patel N, Gonsalves CS, Yang M, et al. Placenta growth factor induces 5-lipoxygenase-activating protein to increase leukotriene formation in sickle cell disease. Blood 2009;113(5):1129–38.
74. Perelman N, Selvaraj SK, Batra S, et al. Placenta growth factor activates monocytes and correlates with sickle cell disease severity. Blood 2003;102(4):1506–14.
75. Jennings JE, Ramkumar T, Mao J, et al. Elevated urinary leukotriene E4 levels are associated with hospitalization for pain in children with sickle cell disease. Am J Hematol 2008;83(8):640–3.
76. Field JJ, Strunk RC, Knight-Perry JE, et al. Urinary cysteinyl leukotriene E4 significantly increases during pain in children and adults with sickle cell disease. Am J Hematol 2009;84(4):231–3.

77. Wang ZJ, Wilkie DJ, Molokie R. Neurobiological mechanisms of pain in sickle cell disease. Hematology Am Soc Hematol Educ Program 2010;2010:403–8.

78. Boilard E, Lai Y, Larabee K, et al. A novel anti-inflammatory role for secretory phospholipase A2 in immune complex-mediated arthritis. EMBO Mol Med 2010;2(5):172–87.

79. Corke C, Glenister K, Watson T. Circulating secretory phospholipase A2 in critical illness–the importance of the intestine. Crit Care Resusc 2001;3(4):244–9.

80. Chen HL, Hai CX, Liang X, et al. Correlation between sPLA2-IIA and phosgene-induced rat acute lung injury. Inhal Toxicol 2009;21(4):374–80.

81. De Luca D, Minucci A, Piastra M, et al. Ex vivo effect of varespladib on secretory phospholipase A2 alveolar activity in infants with ARDS. PloS One 2012;7(10): e47066.

82. De Luca D, Lopez-Rodriguez E, Minucci A, et al. Clinical and biological role of secretory phospholipase A2 in acute respiratory distress syndrome infants. Crit Care 2013;17(4):R163.

83. Styles LA, Schalkwijk CG, Aarsman AJ, et al. Phospholipase A2 levels in acute chest syndrome of sickle cell disease. Blood 1996;87:2573–8.

84. Styles L, Wager CG, Labotka RJ, et al. Refining the value of secretory phospholipase A2 as a predictor of acute chest syndrome in sickle cell disease: results of a feasibility study (PROACTIVE). Br J Haematol 2012;157(5):627–36.

85. Bargoma EM, Mitsuyoshi JK, Larkin SK, et al. Serum C-reactive protein parallels secretory phospholipase A2 in sickle cell disease patients with vasoocclusive crisis or acute chest syndrome. Blood 2005;105(8):3384–5.

86. Key NS, Slungaard A, Dandelet L, et al. Whole blood tissue factor procoagulant activity is elevated in patients with sickle cell disease. Blood 1998;91:4216–23.

87. Solovey A, Kollander R, Milbauer LC, et al. Endothelial nitric oxide synthase and nitric oxide regulate endothelial tissue factor expression in vivo in the sickle transgenic mouse. Am J Hematol 2010;85(1):41–5.

88. Solovey A, Kollander R, Shet A, et al. Endothelial cell expression of tissue factor in sickle mice is augmented by hypoxia/reoxygenation and inhibited by lovastatin. Blood 2004;104(3):840–6.

89. Chantrathammachart P, Mackman N, Sparkenbaugh E, et al. Tissue factor promotes activation of coagulation and inflammation in a mouse model of sickle cell disease. Blood 2012;120(3):636–46.

90. Camerer E, Huang W, Coughlin SR. Tissue factor- and factor X-dependent activation of protease-activated receptor 2 by factor VIIa. Proc Natl Acad Sci U S A 2000;97(10):5255–60.

91. Rao LV, Pendurthi UR. Tissue factor-factor VIIa signaling. Arterioscler Thromb Vasc Biol 2005;25(1):47–56.

92. Rothmeier AS, Ruf W. Protease-activated receptor 2 signaling in inflammation. Semin Immunopathol 2012;34(1):133–49.

93. Henn V, Slupsky JR, Grafe M, et al. CD40 ligand on activated platelets triggers an inflammatory reaction of endothelial cells. Nature 1998;391(6667):591–4.

94. Lee SP, Ataga KI, Orringer EP, et al. Biologically active CD40 ligand is elevated in sickle cell anemia: potential role for platelet-mediated inflammation. Arterioscler Thromb Vasc Biol 2006;26(7):1626–31.

95. Ataga KI, Brittain JE, Desai P, et al. Association of coagulation activation with clinical complications in sickle cell disease. PloS One 2012;7(1):e29786.

96. Otterdal K, Smith C, Oie E, et al. Platelet-derived LIGHT induces inflammatory responses in endothelial cells and monocytes. Blood 2006;108(3): 928–35.

97. Garrido VT, Proenca-Ferreira R, Dominical VM, et al. Elevated plasma levels and platelet-associated expression of the pro-thrombotic and pro-inflammatory protein, TNFSF14 (LIGHT), in sickle cell disease. Br J Haematol 2012;158(6): 788–97.

98. Belcher JD, Marker PH, Weber JP, et al. Activated monocytes in sickle cell disease: potential role in the activation of vascular endothelium and vaso-occlusion. Blood 2000;96(7):2451–9.

99. Sultana C, Shen Y, Rattan V, et al. Interaction of sickle erythrocytes with endothelial cells in the presence of endothelial cell conditioned medium induces oxidant stress leading to transendothelial migration of monocytes. Blood 1998;92(10): 3924–35.

100. Pathare A, Al Kindi S, Alnaqdy AA, et al. Cytokine profile of sickle cell disease in Oman. Am J Hematol 2004;77(4):323–8.

101. Duits AJ, Schnog JB, Lard LR, et al. Elevated IL-8 levels during sickle cell crisis. Eur J Haematol 1998;61(5):302–5.

102. Conran N, Oresco-Santos C, Acosta HC, et al. Increased soluble guanylate cyclase activity in the red blood cells of sickle cell patients. Br J Haematol 2004;124(4):547–54.

103. Lanaro C, Franco-Penteado CF, Albuqueque DM, et al. Altered levels of cytokines and inflammatory mediators in plasma and leukocytes of sickle cell anemia patients and effects of hydroxyurea therapy. J Leukoc Biol 2009;85(2): 235–42.

104. Tzoulaki I, Murray GD, Lee AJ, et al. C-reactive protein, interleukin-6, and soluble adhesion molecules as predictors of progressive peripheral atherosclerosis in the general population: Edinburgh artery study. Circulation 2005;112(7): 976–83.

105. Castell JV, Gomez-Lechon MJ, David M, et al. Recombinant human interleukin-6 (IL-6/BSF-2/HSF) regulates the synthesis of acute phase proteins in human hepatocytes. FEBS Lett 1988;232(2):347–50.

106. Baumann H, Gauldie J. The acute phase response. Immunol Today 1994;15(2): 74–80.

107. Jang JE, Hod EA, Spitalnik SL, et al. CXCL1 and its receptor, CXCR2, mediate murine sickle cell vaso-occlusion during hemolytic transfusion reactions. J Clin Invest 2011;121(4):1397–401.

108. Canalli AA, Franco-Penteado CF, Traina F, et al. Role for cAMP-protein kinase A signalling in augmented neutrophil adhesion and chemotaxis in sickle cell disease. Eur J Haematol 2007;79(4):330–7.

109. Okpala I, Daniel Y, Haynes R, et al. Relationship between the clinical manifestations of sickle cell disease and the expression of adhesion molecules on white blood cells. Eur J Haematol 2002;69(3):135–44.

110. Lard LR, Mul FP, de Haas M, et al. Neutrophil activation in sickle cell disease. J Leukoc Biol 1999;66(3):411–5.

111. Fadlon E, Vordermeier S, Pearson TC, et al. Blood polymorphonuclear leukocytes from the majority of sickle cell patients in the crisis phase of the disease show enhanced adhesion to vascular endothelium and increased expression of CD64. Blood 1998;91(1):266–74.

112. Lum AF, Wun T, Staunton D, et al. Inflammatory potential of neutrophils detected in sickle cell disease. Am J Hematol 2004;76(2):126–33.

113. Finnegan EM, Turhan A, Golan DE, et al. Adherent leukocytes capture sickle erythrocytes in an in vitro flow model of vaso-occlusion. Am J Hematol 2007; 82(4):266–75.

114. Baggiolini M, Dewald B, Moser B. Interleukin-8 and related chemotactic cytokines–CXC and CC chemokines. Adv Immunol 1994;55:97–179.

115. Aslan M, Canatan D. Modulation of redox pathways in neutrophils from sickle cell disease patients. Exp Hematol 2008;36(11):1535–44.

116. Nur E, Biemond BJ, Otten HM, et al. Oxidative stress in sickle cell disease; pathophysiology and potential implications for disease management. Am J Hematol 2011;86(6):484–9.

117. Mohamed AO, Hashim MS, Nilsson UR, et al. Increased in vivo activation of neutrophils and complement in sickle cell disease. Am J Trop Med Hyg 1993;49(6): 799–803.

118. Bergeron MF, Cannon JG, Hall EL, et al. Erythrocyte sickling during exercise and thermal stress. Clin J Sport Med 2004;14(6):354–6.

119. Zhang H, Xu H, Weihrauch D, et al. Inhibition of myeloperoxidase decreases vascular oxidative stress and increases vasodilatation in sickle cell disease mice. J Lipid Res 2013;54(11):3009–15.

120. Gawaz M, Fateh-Moghadam S, Pilz G, et al. Platelet activation and interaction with leucocytes in patients with sepsis or multiple organ failure. Eur J Clin Invest 1995;25(11):843–51.

121. Kirschenbaum LA, Adler D, Astiz ME, et al. Mechanisms of platelet-neutrophil interactions and effects on cell filtration in septic shock. Shock 2002;17(6): 508–12.

122. Polanowska-Grabowska R, Wallace K, Field JJ, et al. P-selectin-mediated platelet-neutrophil aggregate formation activates neutrophils in mouse and human sickle cell disease. Arterioscler Thromb Vasc Biol 2010;30(12):2392–9.

123. Brinkmann V, Reichard U, Goosmann C, et al. Neutrophil extracellular traps kill bacteria. Science 2004;303(5663):1532–5.

124. Fuchs TA, Abed U, Goosmann C, et al. Novel cell death program leads to neutrophil extracellular traps. J Cell Biol 2007;176(2):231–41.

125. Clark SR, Ma AC, Tavener SA, et al. Platelet TLR4 activates neutrophil extracellular traps to ensnare bacteria in septic blood. Nat Med 2007;13(4):463–9.

126. Baker VS, Imade GE, Molta NB, et al. Cytokine-associated neutrophil extracellular traps and antinuclear antibodies in Plasmodium falciparum infected children under six years of age. Malar J 2008;7:41.

127. Hakkim A, Furnrohr BG, Amann K, et al. Impairment of neutrophil extracellular trap degradation is associated with lupus nephritis. Proc Natl Acad Sci U S A 2010;107(21):9813–8.

128. Marcos V, Zhou Z, Yildirim AO, et al. CXCR2 mediates NADPH oxidase-independent neutrophil extracellular trap formation in cystic fibrosis airway inflammation. Nat Med 2010;16(9):1018–23.

129. Margraf S, Logters T, Reipen J, et al. Neutrophil-derived circulating free DNA (cf-DNA/NETs): a potential prognostic marker for posttraumatic development of inflammatory second hit and sepsis. Shock 2008;30(4):352–8.

130. Johansson PI, Windelov NA, Rasmussen LS, et al. Blood levels of histone-complexed DNA fragments are associated with coagulopathy, inflammation and endothelial damage early after trauma. J Emerg Trauma Shock 2013;6(3): 171–5.

131. Schimmel M, Nur E, Biemond BJ, et al. Nucleosomes and neutrophil activation in sickle cell disease painful crisis. Haematologica 2013;98(11):1797–803.

132. Ansel JC, Brown JR, Payan DG, et al. Substance P selectively activates TNF-alpha gene expression in murine mast cells. J Immunol 1993;150(10): 4478–85.

133. Vincent L, Vang D, Nguyen J, et al. Mast cell activation contributes to sickle cell pathobiology and pain in mice. Blood 2013;122(11):1853–62.
134. Manning BM, Hebbel RP, Gupta K, et al. Carbon-fiber microelectrode amperometry reveals sickle-cell-induced inflammation and chronic morphine effects on single mast cells. ACS Chem Biol 2012;7(3):543–51.
135. Turhan A, Jenab P, Bruhns P, et al. Intravenous immune globulin prevents venular vaso-occlusion in sickle cell mice by inhibiting leukocyte adhesion and the interactions between sickle erythrocytes and adherent leukocytes. Blood 2004; 103(6):2397–400.
136. Chang J, Shi PA, Chiang EY, et al. Intravenous immunoglobulins reverse acute vaso-occlusive crises in sickle cell mice through rapid inhibition of neutrophil adhesion. Blood 2008;111(2):915–23.
137. Chang J, Patton JT, Sarkar A, et al. GMI-1070, a novel pan-selectin antagonist, reverses acute vascular occlusions in sickle cell mice. Blood 2010;116(10):1779–86.
138. Wun T, De Castro L, Styles L, et al. Effects of GMI-1070, a pan-selectin inhibitor, on leukocyte adhesion in sickle cell disease: results from a phase 1/2 study. Blood 2010;116(21):262a.
139. Kutlar A, Ataga KI, McMahon L, et al. A potent oral P-selectin blocking agent improves microcirculatory blood flow and a marker of endothelial cell injury in patients with sickle cell disease. Am J Hematol 2012;87(5):536–9.
140. Gutsaeva DR, Parkerson JB, Yerigenahally SD, et al. Inhibition of cell adhesion by anti-P-selectin aptamer: a new potential therapeutic agent for sickle cell disease. Blood 2011;117(2):727–35.
141. Frelinger AL 3rd, Jakubowski JA, Brooks JK, et al. Platelet Activation and Inhibition iN Sickle cell disease (PAINS) study. Platelets 2013;24(8):1–9.
142. Wun T, Soulieres D, Frelinger AL, et al. A double-blind, randomized, multicenter phase 2 study of prasugrel versus placebo in adult patients with sickle cell disease. J Hematol Oncol 2013;6:17.
143. Selvaraj SK, Giri RK, Perelman N, et al. Mechanism of monocyte activation and expression of proinflammatory cytochemokines by placenta growth factor. Blood 2003;102(4):1515–24.
144. Brittain JE, Hulkower B, Jones SK, et al. Placenta growth factor in sickle cell disease: association with hemolysis and inflammation. Blood 2010;115(10):2014–20.
145. Kuvibidila S, Baliga BS, Gardner R, et al. Differential effects of hydroxyurea and zileuton on interleukin-13 secretion by activated murine spleen cells: implication on the expression of vascular cell adhesion molecule-1 and vasoocclusion in sickle cell anemia. Cytokine 2005;30(5):213–8.
146. Haynes J Jr, Baliga BS, Obiako B, et al. Zileuton induces hemoglobin F synthesis in erythroid progenitors: role of the L-arginine-nitric oxide signaling pathway. Blood 2004;103(10):3945–50.
147. Griffin TC, McIntire D, Buchanan GR. High-dose intravenous methylprednisolone therapy for pain in children and adolescents with sickle cell disease. N Engl J Med 1994;330(11):733–7.
148. Kaul DK, Liu XD, Choong S, et al. Anti-inflammatory therapy ameliorates leukocyte adhesion and microvascular flow abnormalities in transgenic sickle mice. Am J Physiol Heart Circ Physiol 2004;287(1):H293–301.
149. Solovey AA, Solovey AN, Harkness J, et al. Modulation of endothelial cell activation in sickle cell disease: a pilot study. Blood 2001;97(7):1937–41.
150. Jasinska M, Owczarek J, Orszulak-Michalak D. Statins: a new insight into their mechanisms of action and consequent pleiotropic effects. Pharmacol Rep 2007;59(5):483–99.

151. Rosch JW, Boyd AR, Hinojosa E, et al. Statins protect against fulminant pneumococcal infection and cytolysin toxicity in a mouse model of sickle cell disease. J Clin Invest 2010;120(2):627–35.

152. Canalli AA, Franco-Penteado CF, Saad ST, et al. Increased adhesive properties of neutrophils in sickle cell disease may be reversed by pharmacological nitric oxide donation. Haematologica 2008;93(4):605–9.

153. Canalli AA, Proenca RF, Franco-Penteado CF, et al. Participation of Mac-1, LFA-1 and VLA-4 integrins in the in vitro adhesion of sickle cell disease neutrophils to endothelial layers, and reversal of adhesion by simvastatin. Haematologica 2011;96(4):526–33.

154. Bereal-Williams C, Machado RF, McGowan V 2nd, et al. Atorvastatin reduces serum cholesterol and triglycerides with limited improvement in vascular function in adults with sickle cell anemia. Haematologica 2012;97(11):1768–70.

155. Hoppe C, Kuypers F, Larkin S, et al. A pilot study of the short-term use of simvastatin in sickle cell disease: effects on markers of vascular dysfunction. Br J Haematol 2011;153(5):655–63.

156. Field JJ, Nathan DG, Linden J. Targeting iNKT cells for the treatment of sickle cell disease. Clin Immunol 2011;140(2):177–83.

157. Field JJ, Lin G, Okam MM, et al. Sickle cell vaso-occlusion causes activation of iNKT cells that is decreased by the adenosine A2A receptor agonist regadenoson. Blood 2013;121(17):3329–34.

The Role of Adenosine Signaling in Sickle Cell Therapeutics

Joshua J. Field, MD, MS[a,b,*], David G. Nathan, MD[c,d,e],
Joel Linden, PhD[f]

KEYWORDS

- Sickle cell disease • Adenosine • Adenosine A_{2A} receptor • Adenosine A_{2B} receptor
- NKT cells

KEY POINTS

- Activation of adenosine A_{2A} receptor ($A_{2A}R$) on invariant natural killer T (iNKT) cells decreases inflammation in a transgenic mouse model of sickle cell disease (SCD). The effects of regadenoson, an $A_{2A}R$ agonist, are currently being examined in patients with SCD.
- The adenosine A_{2B} receptor ($A_{2B}R$) on red blood cells and corpus cavernosal cells of the penis has been implicated in the formation of sickle erythrocytes and priapism, respectively.
- These 2 independent lines of research examining the roles of $A_{2A}R$ and $A_{2B}R$ signaling in SCD may provide opportunities for new therapies.

INTRODUCTION

SCD is characterized by rigid, sickle-shaped erythrocytes, microvascular occlusion, and tissue ischemia.[1] Sickle erythrocytes initiate the development of vasoocclusion that ultimately leads to tissue ischemia in a complex multicellular process. Tissue ischemia promotes an inflammatory response that is further amplified by ischemia reperfusion injury.[2] Thereafter, a vicious cycle of vasoocclusion, tissue injury, and inflammation is set into motion, promoting further erythrocyte sickling.[1,2] The consequences of vasoocclusion are pain, end-organ damage, and often premature death.[3,4]

Disclosure: J.J. Field and D.G. Nathan were consultants for NKT Therapeutics.
[a] Blood Research Institute, BloodCenter of Wisconsin, 8733 Watertown Plank Road, Milwaukee, WI 53226, USA; [b] Department of Medicine, Medical College of Wisconsin, 9200 West Wisconsin Avenue, Milwaukee, WI 53226, USA; [c] Department of Pediatric Oncology, Dana-Farber Cancer Institute, 450 Brookline Avenue, Boston, MA 02215, USA; [d] Division of Pediatric Hematology and Oncology, Boston Children's Hospital, 300 Longwood Avenue, Boston, MA 02115, USA; [e] Department of Pediatrics, Harvard Medical School, 25 Shattuck Street, Boston, MA 02115, USA; [f] Inflammation Biology, La Jolla Institute for Allergy and Immunology, 9420 Athena Circle, San Diego, CA 92037, USA
* Corresponding author. BloodCenter of Wisconsin, 8733 Watertown Plank Road, Milwaukee, WI 53226.
E-mail address: joshua.field@bcw.edu

Hematol Oncol Clin N Am 28 (2014) 287–299
http://dx.doi.org/10.1016/j.hoc.2013.11.003
0889-8588/14/$ – see front matter © 2014 Elsevier Inc. All rights reserved.
hemonc.theclinics.com

Therapies for preventing or treating sickle cell vasoocclusion are limited. Broadly, treatments either prevent the formation of sickle erythrocytes (eg, hydroxyurea) or interrupt the cellular interactions that follow red cell sickling and lead to vasoocclusion.[5] Hydroxyurea stimulates fetal hemoglobin synthesis in a variable fraction of erythroblasts and thereby inhibits polymerization of sickle hemoglobin and, to date, is the only Food and Drug Administration (FDA)-approved therapy for the prevention of painful vasoocclusive crises (pVOCs).[6] Patient and provider barriers have limited the widespread use of hydroxyurea in patients with SCD, affecting the impact of the drug.[7] Hematopoietic stem cell transplantation is a potential cure; however, it is an option for only a few patients with SCD.[8]

This review examines the role of adenosine signaling in SCD pathogenesis. There are opportunities to modulate adenosine pathways using therapies to prevent or treat SCD complications. As evidence has emerged about the importance of adenosine in SCD, separate lines of investigation have demonstrated protective and detrimental effects of adenosine in regard to disease severity. Recent data suggest that actions of adenosine mediated through the $A_{2A}R$ decrease inflammation, largely by selectively inhibiting the activation of a subset of lymphocytes, called iNKT cells.[9–11] In contrast, other studies have shown that adenosine signaling through the $A_{2B}R$ may contribute to the adverse processes of erythrocyte sickling[12] and priapism.[13–15] Although much additional work is needed to fully elucidate the roles of adenosine signaling in SCD, targeting these pathways may produce novel therapeutic approaches.

ADENOSINE SIGNALING PATHWAY
Adenosine Physiology

Adenosine signaling protects tissues by promoting vasodilation as well as by decreasing heart rate and inflammation.[16] During periods of cellular hypoxia or stress, adenosine is released from cells along with the adenine nucleotides, ATP, ADP, and AMP, which are converted to adenosine by ectonucleotidases. Binding of adenosine to 4 receptor subtypes, A_1, A_{2A}, A_{2B}, and A_3, elicits responses that are dependent on the receptor subtypes found in various tissues (**Table 1**). Adenosine receptors are 7-transmembrane, G-coupled receptors that signal through adenylyl cyclase, affecting the production of cyclic AMP (cAMP) and calcium or the conductance of ion channels. A_1 and A_3 receptors couple to inhibitory G receptors (Gi) and decrease adenylyl cyclase activity, whereas A_{2A} and A_{2B} increase adenylyl cyclase activity by coupling to stimulatory G receptors (Gs or Go).[16] The affinity for adenosine also differs among the receptor subtypes, affecting the concentration of adenosine necessary for activation. A_1 and A_{2A} are high-affinity receptors, activating at lower concentrations of adenosine (approximately 0.01 μM–1 μM). A_{2B} is a low-affinity receptor requiring 10- to 1000-fold higher levels of adenosine (approximately 10 μM) for activation.[17] Downstream from adenylyl cyclase and cAMP, adenosine signaling modifies the activity of nuclear factor κB (NF-κB), JAK-STAT, and ERK pathways, regulating transcription and ultimately cellular functions.[18] Adenosine that accumulates during cellular stress is removed by uptake into cells and converted to AMP or inosine by adenosine kinase and adenosine deaminase (ADA), respectively. In patients with SCD, tissue injury may increase levels of plasma adenosine, suggesting that adenosine pathways may influence SCD pathogenesis.[12]

Current Therapeutic Uses of Adenosine and Adenosine Derivatives

Drugs that target adenosine receptors are part of current standard practice. Adenosine, dipyridamole, and adenosine $A_{2A}R$ agonists (eg, regadenoson) are used clinically

Table 1
Adenosine receptor subtypes

	Adenosine Receptor Subtypes			
Characteristics	**A_1**	**A_{2A}**	**A_{2B}**	**A_3**
Predominant tissue/cell expression	• Lung • Heart • Brain • Leukocytes	• Lung • Brain • Vasculature • Leukocytes	• Lung • Colon • Vasculature • Leukocytes • Erythrocytes • Penis	• Lung • Liver • Heart • Brain • Leukocytes
Actions	• Negative chronotropic • ↑Inflammation	• Vasodilation • ↓Inflammation	• ↑Inflammation in lung and colon	• ↓Inflammation
Affinity for adenosine	High	High	Low	High
Major disease associations	• Sepsis	• SCD • Ischemia • Arthritis • Wound healing	• SCD • Asthma • COPD • IBD	• Asthma • Arthritis

Data from Hasko G, Linden J, Cronstein B, et al. Adenosine receptors: therapeutic aspects for inflammatory and immune diseases. Nat Rev Drug Discov 2008;7:759–70; and Haskó G, Csóka B, Németh ZH, et al. A_{2B} adenosine receptors in immunity and inflammation. Trends Immunol 2009;30:263–70.

to induce cardiac hyperemia during myocardial stress testing via activation of coronary artery A_{2A}Rs. Adenosine-mediated activation of A_1 receptors in the heart is a treatment of tachyarrhythmias. Theophylline, either alone or in complex with ethylenediame (aminophylline), nonselectively blocks A_1, A_{2A}, and A_{2B} receptors and is used as a therapy for asthma.[16] A limitation of these therapies is lack of selectivity for the adenosine receptor subtypes, sometimes resulting in unwanted and potentially dangerous side effects. These include hypotension and tachycardia from A_{2A}R activation, bradycardia or heart block from A_1 activation and bronchospasm from A_{2B}R activation in patients with asthma. Newer-generation adenosine agonists and antagonists have greater receptor subtype selectivity, thereby minimizing toxicities.[16] There are emerging cellular, animal, and human data suggesting a role for the A_{2A} and A_{2B} receptors in the pathogenesis of SCD (**Table 2**). Adenosine-based therapies are currently being examined in patients with SCD (Clinicaltrials.gov #01788631).

ROLE OF A_{2A}R IN SICKLE CELL DISEASE
A_{2A}R

A_{2A}R activation is well known for producing vasodilation due to effects on vascular smooth muscle and some endothelial cells. In addition, A_{2A}R has a central role in the regulation of inflammation and immunity.[17] Ubiquitously expressed on neutrophils, monocytes, macrophages, T cells, natural killer cells, and iNKT cells, adenosine signaling through the A_{2A}R has been shown to suppress key inflammatory and immune responses, including leukocyte activation, recruitment, and cytokine production.[18] These immune suppressive effects of A_{2A}R activation are mediated by cAMP and protein kinase A.[18] Protein kinase A signaling can inhibit other signaling pathways that activate inflammation mediated by NF-κB or the JAK-STAT pathway and serves to decrease transcription of key inflammatory genes.[19] The NF-κB pathway deserves

Table 2
Comparison of $A_{2A}R$ and $A_{2B}R$ data in sickle cell disease

Reference	Type of Study	Transgenic SCD Model	No. SCD Patients	Agents Evaluated	Key Findings
$A_{2A}R$					
VOC					
Wallace & Linden,[10] 2010	Investigation of transgenic SCD mice	NY1DD	—	$A_{2A}R$ agonist ATL146e	• SCD causes induction of $A_{2A}R$ on iNKT cells • $A_{2A}R$ agonist ATL146e reverses pulmonary dysfunction in SCD mice
Field et al,[11] 2013	Phase 1 clinical study	—	27	$A_{2A}R$ agonist regadenoson	• $A_{2A}R$ agonist regadenoson decreases activation of iNKT cells in patients with SCD during VOC • $A_{2A}R$ agonist regadenoson is safe in patients with SCD
Lin et al,[19] 2013	Investigation of transgenic SCD mice	NY1DD	8	—	• VOC causes further induction of $A_{2A}R$ on iNKT cells • $A_{2A}R$ expression on iNKT cells is mediated through NF-κB
$A_{2B}R$					
Red blood cell sickling					
Zhang et al,[12] 2011	Investigation of transgenic SCD mice, cultured human red blood cells and SCD patient blood samples	Berkley	12	PEG-ADA, theophylline, $A_{2B}R$ antagonist MRS1754	• Adenosine is elevated in the plasma of mice and patients with SCD • $A_{2B}R$ on erythrocytes mediates sickling via decreasing hemoglobin oxygen-binding affinity
Priapism					
Mi et al,[15] 2008	Investigation of ADA-deficient and transgenic SCD mice	Berkley	—	PEG-ADA, theophylline, $A_{2B}R$ antagonist MRS1706	• Priapism is present in $ADA^{-/-}$ mice and corrected by PEG-ADA • Interruption of $A_{2B}R$ activity on corpus cavernosal cells decreases priapism
Wen et al,[14] 2010	Investigation of ADA-deficient and transgenic SCD mice	Berkley	—	PEG-ADA	• PEG-ADA therapy prevented episodes of priapism in SCD mice
Wen et al,[13] 2010	Investigation of ADA-deficient and transgenic SCD mice	Berkley	—	PEG-ADA, $A_{2B}R$ antagonist MRS1706	• PEG-ADA therapy prevented penile fibrosis in SCD mice • Interruption of $A_{2B}R$ in corpus cavernosal fibroblast cells prevents penile fibrosis

Abbreviation: VOC, vasooclusion.

special attention because it has been used as a marker of iNKT cell activity in clinical trials of the $A_{2A}R$ agonist, regadenoson, in patients with SCD.[11]

NF-κB is a critically important transcription factor that generally enhances inflammation.[20] Comprised of a dimer of transcription factors from the RelA family of proteins (p50 or p52 and p65), NF-κB resides in the cytoplasm of cells bound to the inhibitory protein, IκB. On activation of the NF-κB by numerous inflammatory mediators, including tumor necrosis factor α or interleukin (IL)-1, IκB is phosphorylated by IκB kinase, ubiquinated, and degraded, thus liberating NF-κB to translocate into the nucleus and promote the transcription of proinflammatory genes. When NF-κB is released from IκB, the 65-kDa subunit (p65) can be phosphorylated on several sites, including Ser536. The phosphorylation of p65 (phospho-p65) serves as a marker of NF-κB activity used in flow cytometry assays.[11] In cased of $A_{2A}R$ activation, in vitro data suggest that agonists of the $A_{2A}R$ reduce IκB degradation, decreasing the ability of NF-κB to promote a proinflammatory cellular response.[21] NF-κB has also been shown to mediate the up-regulation of $A_{2A}R$ in iNKT cells after activation.[19]

$A_{2A}R$ Agonist Decreases Inflammation After Ischemia-Reperfusion Injury by Interfering with iNKT-Cell Activation

Murine models of liver and kidney transplant demonstrated that activation of $A_{2A}Rs$ by adenosine analogs administered during or after ischemia reperfusion injury markedly inhibit inflammation and secondary injury.[22] An investigation of the cell type primarily responsible for the protective effect of $A_{2A}R$ activation implicated the iNKT cell as the primary target.[22] Although iNKT cells normally constitute less than 1% of the lymphocyte population, iNKT cells can rapidly release large amounts of proinflammatory cytokines, giving them a critical role in inflammation, despite representing only a small proportion of lymphocytes.[23] Similar to B cells and T cells that produce adaptive immune responses, iNKT-cell activation requires the engagement of an antigen presented on an antigen-presenting cell.[24] Unlike B cell and T cell populations, which express diverse receptors that recognize various peptides, iNKT cells express a semi-invariant T-cell receptor that nonspecifically binds to lipid antigens presented on CD1d, an major histocompatibility complex class I–like molecule. Different lipids (glycolipids and phospholipids) have been shown to activate iNKT cells.[24,25] The activation of iNKT cells is enhanced by cytokines produced by antigen-presenting cells in response to Toll-like receptor activation.[26] Thus, the activation of iNKT cells is facilitated by innate immune responses stimulated by pathogen-associated molecular patterns or danger-associated molecular patterns. On CD1d-restricted activation, iNKT cells rapidly make mRNAs and release large quantities of interferon-γ (IFN-γ), tumor necrosis factor α, IL-2, and IL-4.[27] IFN-γ stimulates the production in many cells of interferon-inducible CXCR3 chemokines, CXCL9, CXCL10, and CXCL11.[28] IL-2 is known to induce CXCR3 receptors on lymphocytes.[28] Thus, through rapid activation and generation of copious amounts of cytokines and chemokines, iNKT cells stimulate a proinflammatory cascade that may promote and sustain vasoocclusion.[9,10] Activation of $A_{2A}Rs$, abundantly expressed on activated iNKT cells, reduces this inflammatory response and is critical to modulating the immune functions of iNKT cells.[10,11]

$A_{2A}R$ Agonists Decrease iNKT-Cell Activation and Reduce Inflammation in SCD Mice

In a series of experiments in an NY1DD mouse model of SCD, Wallace and colleagues[9,10] generated several lines of evidence implicating iNKT cells as critical to the process of sickle cell vasoocclusion. Lung inflammation and injury were reduced (1) when iNKT cells were antibody depleted or genetically knocked out, (2) when activation or chemotaxis was inhibited, and (3) on administration of $A_{2A}R$ agonists.[9]

NY1DD mice treated with a continuous subcutaneous infusion of the $A_{2A}R$ agonist ATL146e demonstrated a maximal improvement in lung function, histology, and inflammatory cell infiltrate in 3 days at an infusion rate of 10 ng/kg/min. The improvement was sustained up to the end of infusion at 7 days.[10] The infused dose of ATL146e only achieved plasma concentrations of approximately 1 nM, and the mice did not demonstrate cardiovascular toxicities.[10] The absence of toxicity is in accord with prior studies demonstrating that the antiinflammatory effects of $A_{2A}R$ agonists occur at 10- to 100-fold lower concentrations compared with the cardiovascular effects.[22] Blockade or depletion of iNKT cells mitigated the beneficial effects of the $A_{2A}R$ agonist, providing evidence that the antiinflammatory actions of $A_{2A}R$ activation are mediated largely through iNKT cells.[9,10]

In the plasma of adult patients with SCD, circulating iNKT cells were also more likely to be activated and expanded compared with healthy controls.[9] There is selective expansion of iNKT cells among lymphocytes, from less than 1% in control blood to an average of approximately 5% in the blood of SCD patients, whose iNKT cells were also more likely to express the activation markers, CD69, intracellular IFN-γ, and CXCR3.[9]

Phase 1 Study of the $A_{2A}R$ Agonist Regadenoson in Patients with SCD: Study Design and Rationale

Based on the promising data from mice and patients with SCD suggesting that $A_{2A}R$ agonists may interrupt activation of iNKT cells and potentially decrease sickle cell complications, a phase 1 trial was conducted of the $A_{2A}R$ agonist, regadenoson.[29] FDA approved for inducing cardiac hyperemia during myocardial imaging, regadenoson is a selective $A_{2A}R$ agonist with 10-fold greater affinity for A_{2A} versus A_1 and few, if any, effects on A_{2B} or A_3.[30,31] When used for myocardial imaging, regadenoson is administered as a 400-μg bolus over 10 seconds.[30] Bolus injection induces vasodilation and hyperemia in a time frame appropriate for capturing images before blood flow reverts to normal.[31] If the goal of administering regadenoson is to dampen the severity of a pVOC over several days, a continuous infusion is necessary, given its terminal half-life of 2 hours. When designing the study, 3 relatively low doses of regadenoson were selected based on data extrapolated from animal models.[29] All of these doses produced the desired antiinflammatory effects while avoiding cardiovascular toxicities.[29] Using a traditional 3 + 3 study design, the dose levels were examined during a 12-hour infusion of regadenoson while patients with SCD were at steady state.[29] Once the highest dose of infusional regadenoson (1.44 μg/kg/h) was found safe, SCD subjects were examined during a 24- or 48-hour infusion at steady state and then during a pVOC.[29]

To evaluate the effects of regadenoson on iNKT-cell activation, various activation markers were examined. Phospho-p65 NF-κB was identified as the most promising marker of iNKT-cell activation because, as opposed to cell surface markers or cytokines, changes in phosphorylation are pretranscriptional and thus occur quickly.

Phase 1 Study of the $A_{2A}R$ Agonist Regadenoson in Patients with SCD: Study Results

Twenty-seven adult patients with SCD were administered regadenoson, 21 at steady state and 6 during pVOCs.[11] Circulating iNKT cells from adults with SCD during pVOC showed increased phospho-p65 NF-κB activation compared with steady state or healthy controls. When adults with SCD were administered a 24-hour infusion of the $A_{2A}R$ agonist regadenoson during pVOC, the percentage of iNKT cells expressing increased phospho-p65 NF-κB decreased to levels similar to steady state patients and healthy controls. The effects of regadenoson were achieved at plasma concentrations that peaked at 2 ng/mL and were devoid of effects on heart rate or blood pressure. Three children with SCD above the age of assent were also administered regadenoson without toxicity (unpublished data). A large, randomized, controlled, phase 2 trial is in progress to evaluate the clinical efficacy of regadenoson during pVOC (Clinicaltrials.gov #01788631).

ROLE OF $A_{2B}R$ IN SICKLE CELL DISEASE
$A_{2B}R$

The $A_{2B}R$ is a lower-affinity receptor that has well-described proinflammatory roles in the pathogenesis of asthma, chronic obstructive pulmonary disease, and inflammatory bowel disease.[32] Higher levels of adenosine are necessary to activate the $A_{2B}R$ (10–100 fold > $A_{2A}R$) and, therefore, signaling through $A_{2B}R$ occurs selectively in stressed cells when adenosine is generated by ischemia, injury, or inflammation.[17] Although the distribution of the $A_{2B}R$ is widespread on cells and tissues, including smooth muscle cells, endothelial cells, and macrophages, pathogenic inflammation is most notably promoted by the actions of the $A_{2B}R$ on mast cells and intestinal epithelial cells.[32] Recent data suggest that activation of $A_{2B}R$ on mast cells results in the production of cytokines with important roles in asthma pathogenesis, such as IL-4 and IL-13, and stimulates B cells to produce IgE.[33] The role of $A_{2B}R$ in asthma is also supported by data demonstrating increased inflammation in asthma patients after inhalation of adenosine.[34,35] The nonselective adenosine receptor antagonist, theophylline, has a long-standing role in the management of asthma in part working through blockade of the $A_{2B}R$,[36] although its lack of selectivity is associated with side effects. $A_{2B}R$ expression on intestinal epithelial cells is also important in disease pathogenesis, promoting IL-6 production and resulting in intestinal inflammation, potentially contributing to the process of inflammatory bowel disease.[37] More recently, $A_{2B}R$ activation in the corpus cavernosum of the penis and erythrocytes has been shown to promote priapism[13–15] and red cell sickling,[12] respectively, in a murine model of SCD.

Adenosine Signaling Through $A_{2B}R$ is Implicated in Priapism and Penile Fibrosis

Studies in non-SCD mouse models demonstrating that intracavernosal injections of adenosine provoked priapism provided preliminary evidence for a role for adenosine signaling in the pathogenesis of priapism.[38,39] More recent work has found that the actions of adenosine are mediated through $A_{2B}R$ signaling on corpus cavernosum smooth muscle cells within the penis.[40] In a series of experiments, investigators determined that ADA-deficient mice had higher intrapenile adenosine levels, leading to cavernosal smooth muscle relaxation and priapism.[15] Administration of ADA or the $A_{2B}R$ antagonists, theophylline or MRS1706, antagonized the effects of excess adenosine and reversed priapism.[14,15] $ADA^{-/-}/A_{2B}R^{-/-}$ mice were also protected from priapic episodes.[15] Many of the same findings were recapitulated in a transgenic SCD mouse model. SCD mice had higher plasma levels of adenosine than controls and similarly their episodes of priapism were counteracted by decreasing adenosine levels with ADA or administration of an $A_{2B}R$ antagonist.[15] In SCD mice, there is also evidence that adenosine signaling through the $A_{2B}R$ contributes to penile fibrosis, a consequence of priapism episodes that contributes to erectile dysfunction.[13] Taken together, these data suggest that interruption of adenosine signaling through $A_{2B}R$ may have a role in the treatment of priapism and prevention of penile fibrosis in SCD.

Sickle Erythrocyte Formation Promoted Through $A_{2B}R$

Recently, another detrimental effect of $A_{2B}R$ activation was described when Zhang and colleagues[12] reported a novel mechanism of erythrocyte sickling in transgenic SCD mice caused by high plasma adenosine and activation of $A_{2B}Rs$ expressed on red cells. These investigators first discovered that, in transgenic SCD mice, a reduction in circulating adenosine levels after pegylated (PEG)-ADA administration was associated with a decreased number of sickle erythrocytes. To identify the adenosine receptor subtype responsible for promoting sickle cell formation, red cells from mice genetically deficient in 1 of the 4 receptor subtypes were activated with an adenosine analog. The deleterious effects of adenosine were found to be mediated through the $A_{2B}R$ due to an increase in intraerythrocyte 2,3-diphospho-glycerate (DPG) levels and a decreased hemoglobin-oxygen affinity. The resulting increased formation of deoxyhemoglobin provides an explanation for the increased erythrocyte sickling. Translating these findings to humans, levels of plasma adenosine were found higher in patients with SCD versus healthy controls as were intra-erythrocyte 2,3-DPG levels (the latter more likely due to the effects of anemia). In vitro treatment of erythrocytes from patients with SCD with PEG-ADA or $A_{2B}R$ antagonists reduced red cell sickling, consistent with the findings from the murine model.

CAN ADENOSINE HAVE BOTH PROTECTIVE AND DELETERIOUS ROLES IN SCD?

Recent data describing the role of adenosine signaling in SCD suggest discrepant effects on morbidity when the actions of adenosine are medicated through the $A_{2A}R$ versus $A_{2B}R$.[41] On one hand, data show that activation of $A_{2A}R$ decreases inflammation, largely through the inhibition of iNKT-cell activation, potentially dampening the severity of pVOCs.[10,11] On the other hand, a separate line of research suggests that adenosine signaling through $A_{2B}R$ promotes priapism[13–15] and erythrocyte sickling.[12] Although further studies are needed to fully understand the seemingly conflicting roles of adenosine signaling in SCD, differences in adenosine receptor expression and affinity along with a better understanding of in vivo levels of adenosine in patients with SCD may help to reconcile the confusion.

Effects of Adenosine Levels and Receptor Density on $A_{2A}R$ Versus $A_{2B}R$ Signaling in SCD

Under steady state conditions and potentially during pVOCs, levels of adenosine may be sufficient to signal through the $A_{2A}R$ yet not high enough to trigger $A_{2B}R$ signaling. In comparison with $A_{2B}R$, affinity of adenosine for $A_{2A}R$ is 10 to 1000 times greater than $A_{2B}R$.[17] Moreover, the effects of adenosine are further potentiated in cells or tissue densely expressing adenosine receptors, as is the case for $A_{2A}R$ expression on activated iNKT cells. Compared with CD4+ T cells, iNKT cells express 10 times more $A_{2A}R$ and receptor expression increases further (100-fold) during pVOCs.[10,19] Thus, iNKT cells are exquisitely sensitive to inhibition through adenosine signaling due to dense expression of the high-affinity receptor, $A_{2A}R$. Based on receptor affinity and density, a model for adenosine signaling emerges whereby differing levels of adenosine in a localized area may produce actions through $A_{2A}R$ and/or $A_{2B}R$. Potentially, under conditions where levels of adenosine in SCD are not extremely high, the effects of adenosine are mediated through the $A_{2A}R$ and only during the more extreme conditions of pVOC would the deleterious effects of the $A_{2B}R$ activation be observed (**Fig. 1**).

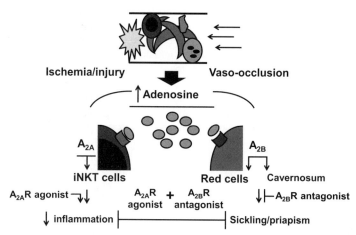

Fig. 1. The proposed roles of the $A_{2A}R$ and the $A_{2B}R$ in the pathogenesis of SCD. Sickle cell vasoocclusion leads to tissue injury and liberation of adenosine. (*Left side of schema*) Expression of $A_{2A}R$ is increased on iNKT cells and activation of $A_{2A}R$ on iNKT cells leads to a reduction in proinflammatory mediators (IFN-γ and IL-4) and dampening in the severity of vasoocclusion. $A_{2A}R$ agonists (eg, regadenoson) may promote the antiinflammatory effects of the $A_{2A}R$. (*Right side of schema*) Activation of $A_{2B}R$ on erythrocytes results in increased levels of 2,3 DPG decreasing hemoglobin affinity for oxygen and contributing to red cell sickling. On corpus cavernosal cells of the penis, activation of $A_{2B}R$ promotes priapism. Antagonists to $A_{2B}R$ may decrease the formation of sickle erythrocytes and prevent priapic episodes. Potentially, dual therapy with an $A_{2A}R$ agonist/$A_{2B}R$ antagonist would have beneficial effects on inflammation, sickling and priapism in patients with SCD.

Adenosine Measurements Have Limitations

Levels of adenosine in patients with SCD have been shown higher than in healthy controls and, likely, levels rise further during pVOCs.[12] Adenosine measurements in the extracellular space reflect the sum of adenosine's formation, transport, and degradation.[42] During periods of microvascular occlusion and tissue ischemia, extracellular concentrations of adenosine may increase and activate adenosine signaling pathways to counteract further tissue damage by increasing blood flow and reducing heart rate and inflammation. Unfortunately, rapid cellular uptake and degradation cause adenosine to have a half-life of approximately 5 seconds, creating challenges to obtaining accurate measurements.[42] Further compounding errors in measurement is the compartmentalization of adenosine between the intravascular and interstitial spaces and the restricted tissue-specific rise that may occur in adenosine levels after ischemia and injury.[42] Thus, measurement of adenosine levels in blood from the right arm may not accurately reflect the physiologic effects of adenosine in a patient who is experiencing ongoing vasoocclusion in the vasculature of the left leg. A final consideration in the interpretation of adenosine levels in the preceding studies is the differences in adenosine biology between people and mice. Adenosine's half-life is longer in mice than in people, and, therefore, blood levels are also higher in mice.[41] Under these conditions, adenosine signaling through $A_{2B}R$ may be more pronounced in mouse models than in patients. A better understanding of adenosine levels in patients with SCD may clarify the role of $A_{2A}R$ and $A_{2B}R$ signaling under varied conditions and the contribution of this signaling to SCD morbidities.

LIMITATIONS OF ADENOSINE THERAPEUTICS IN SCD

The main challenges for using adenosine analogs to treat and prevent vasoocclusion are the need for a continuous intravenous infusion and unwanted side effects. The short half-life of regadenoson necessitates a continuous infusion, which requires stable intravenous access and limits the role of regadenoson to the treatment of acute crises. Regadenoson has multiphasic pharmacokinetics, but the terminal half-life is still only 2 hours.[30] Current conceptual models of SCD describe ongoing vasoocclusion with inflammation and end-organ damage that is punctuated by severe pVOCs that result in a hospitalization. Treatments aimed to shorten the duration of hospitalizations, such as regadenoson, have value because there is a higher risk of death during these acute events[4]; however, they do not affect the continuing daily damage that culminates in organ dysfunction. Preventing a major crisis is a better strategy to decease morbidity and mortality than treating one. To this end, a humanized monoclonal antibody that targets iNKT cells independently of the adenosine signaling pathways is currently under investigation in a phase 1 study (Clinicaltrials.gov #01783691). This investigational agent could potentially deplete iNKT cells on a longer-term basis than the effects of regadenoson and prevent crises. Another challenge to the use of adenosine signaling in the treatment of SCD is unwanted side effects due to a lack of adenosine receptor selectivity. Adenosine and dipyridamole cause activation of all adenosine receptor subtypes and are associated with severe side effects, such as heart block and hypotension. The $A_{2A}R$ agonist regadenoson has been administered to patients with SCD without toxicity due to a high degree of selectivity for the $A_{2A}R$, along with the fact that lower concentrations of the drug are still able to achieve antiinflammatory effects.[11]

FUTURE DIRECTIONS: COMBINED $A_{2A}R$ AND $A_{2B}R$ THERAPIES FOR SCD?

Modulating the adenosine signaling pathway holds promise as a treatment of patients with SCD. Independent lines of investigation have provided evidence that the $A_{2A}R$ and $A_{2B}R$ are, respectively, protective and deleterious in the pathogenesis of vasoocclusion. The combination of an $A_{2A}R$ agonist with an $A_{2B}R$ antagonist may be an ideal treatment in SCD. Thus far, the $A_{2A}R$ agonist regadenoson is the only adenosine-based therapeutic that has been studied in patients with SCD.[11] Another approach that has been suggested is PEG-ADA infusions to lower circulating adenosine levels and minimize signaling through the $A_{2B}R$. ADA is an FDA-approved therapy for patients with ADA deficiency.[43] The possible shortcoming of this approach is that positive effects from adenosine signaling through the $A_{2A}R$ might be negated with ADA therapy. A more novel and potentially effective approach to prevent and treat vasoocclusion is dual therapy with $A_{2B}R$ antagonists to prevent erythrocyte sickling and $A_{2A}R$ agonists to decrease inflammation and dampen the severity of pVOCs (see **Fig. 1**).[44] Highly selective $A_{2B}R$ antagonists are currently in development for maintenance treatment of asthma.[16,44] Rigorously designed clinical trials demonstrating the clinical efficacy of $A_{2A}R$ agonists and/or $A_{2B}R$ antagonists need to be conducted prior to considering combination therapy; however, innovative approaches are needed in the treatment of SCD and multimodal therapies may be necessary to demonstrate clinical benefit.

REFERENCES

1. Hebbel RP, Osarogiagbon R, Kaul D. The endothelial biology of sickle cell disease: inflammation and a chronic vasculopathy. Microcirculation 2004;11: 129–51.

2. Kaul DK, Hebbel RP. Hypoxia/reoxygenation causes inflammatory response in transgenic sickle mice but not in normal mice. J Clin Invest 2000;106:411–20.
3. Platt OS, Thorington BD, Brambilla DJ, et al. Pain in sickle cell disease. rates and risk factors. N Engl J Med 1991;325:11–6.
4. Platt OS, Brambilla DJ, Rosse WF, et al. Mortality in sickle cell disease. Life expectancy and risk factors for early death. N Engl J Med 1994;330:1639–44.
5. Vichinsky E. Emerging 'A' therapies in hemoglobinopathies: agonists, antagonists, antioxidants, and arginine. Hematology Am Soc Hematol Educ Program 2012;2012:271–5.
6. Ware RE, Aygun B. Advances in the use of hydroxyurea. Hematology Am Soc Hematol Educ Program 2009;62–9.
7. Lanzkron S, Haywood C Jr, Hassell KL, et al. Provider barriers to hydroxyurea use in adults with sickle cell disease: a survey of the Sickle Cell Disease Adult Provider Network. J Natl Med Assoc 2008;100:968–73.
8. Dew A, Collins D, Artz A, et al. Paucity of HLA-identical unrelated donors for African-Americans with hematologic malignancies: the need for new donor options. Biol Blood Marrow Transplant 2008;14:938–41.
9. Wallace KL, Marshall MA, Ramos SI, et al. NKT cells mediate pulmonary inflammation and dysfunction in murine sickle cell disease through production of IFN-gamma and CXCR3 chemokines. Blood 2009;114:667–76.
10. Wallace KL, Linden J. Adenosine A_{2A} receptors induced on iNKT and NK cells reduce pulmonary inflammation and injury in mice with sickle cell disease. Blood 2010;116:5010–20.
11. Field JJ, Lin G, Okam MM, et al. Sickle cell vaso-occlusion causes activation of iNKT cells that is decreased by the adenosine A_{2A} receptor agonist regadenoson. Blood 2013;121:3329–34.
12. Zhang Y, Dai Y, Wen J, et al. Detrimental effects of adenosine signaling in sickle cell disease. Nat Med 2011;17:79–86.
13. Wen J, Jiang X, Dai Y, et al. Increased adenosine contributes to penile fibrosis, a dangerous feature of priapism, via A_{2B} adenosine receptor signaling. FASEB J 2010;24:740–9.
14. Wen J, Jiang X, Dai Y, et al. Adenosine deaminase enzyme therapy prevents and reverses the heightened cavernosal relaxation in priapism. J Sex Med 2010;7: 3011–22.
15. Mi T, Abbasi S, Zhang H, et al. Excess adenosine in murine penile erectile tissues contributes to priapism via A_{2B} adenosine receptor signaling. J Clin Invest 2008; 118:1491–501.
16. Jacobson KA, Gao ZG. Adenosine receptors as therapeutic targets. Nat Rev Drug Discov 2006;5:247–64.
17. Hasko G, Linden J, Cronstein B, et al. Adenosine receptors: therapeutic aspects for inflammatory and immune diseases. Nat Rev Drug Discov 2008;7:759–70.
18. Milne GR, Palmer TM. Anti-inflammatory and immunosuppressive effects of the A_{2A} adenosine receptor. ScientificWorldJournal 2011;11:320–39.
19. Lin G, Field JJ, Yu JC, et al. NF-kB is activated in CD4+ iNKT cells by sickle cell disease and mediates rapid induction of adenosine A_{2A} receptors. PLoS One 2013;8(10):e74664.
20. Karin M, Ben-Neriah Y. Phosphorylation meets ubiquitination: the control of NF-[kappa]B activity. Annu Rev Immunol 2000;18:621–63.
21. Lukashev D, Ohta A, Apasov S, et al. Cutting edge: physiologic attenuation of proinflammatory transcription by the Gs protein-coupled A_{2A} adenosine receptor in vivo. J Immunol 2004;173:21–4.

22. Lappas CM, Day YJ, Marshall MA, et al. Adenosine A$_{2A}$ receptor activation reduces hepatic ischemia reperfusion injury by inhibiting CD1d-dependent NKT cell activation. J Exp Med 2006;203:2639–48.

23. Matsuda JL, Mallevaey T, Scott-Browne J, et al. CD1d-restricted iNKT cells, the 'Swiss-Army knife' of the immune system. Curr Opin Immunol 2008;20: 358–68.

24. Van Kaer L, Parekh VV, Wu L. Invariant natural killer T cells: bridging innate and adaptive immunity. Cell Tissue Res 2011;343:43–55.

25. Gumperz JE, Roy C, Makowska A, et al. Murine CD1d-restricted T cell recognition of cellular lipids. Immunity 2000;12:211–21.

26. Salio M, Speak AO, Shepherd D, et al. Modulation of human natural killer T cell ligands on TLR-mediated antigen-presenting cell activation. Proc Natl Acad Sci U S A 2007;104:20490–5.

27. Kronenberg M, Gapin L. The unconventional lifestyle of NKT cells. Nat Rev Immunol 2002;2:557–68.

28. Singh UP, Venkataraman C, Singh R, et al. CXCR3 axis: role in inflammatory bowel disease and its therapeutic implication. Endocr Metab Immune Disord Drug Targets 2007;7:111–23.

29. Field JJ, Nathan DG, Linden J. Targeting iNKT cells for the treatment of sickle cell disease. Clin Immunol 2011;140:177–83.

30. Astellas Pharma. Lexiscan [package insert]. Northbrook (IL): Astellas Pharma; 2009.

31. Buhr C, Gossl M, Erbel R, et al. Regadenoson in the detection of coronary artery disease. Vasc Health Risk Manag 2008;4:337–40.

32. Haskó G, Csóka B, Németh ZH, et al. A$_{2B}$ adenosine receptors in immunity and inflammation. Trends Immunol 2009;30:263–70.

33. Ryzhov S, Goldstein AE, Matafonov A, et al. Adenosine-activated mast cells induce IgE synthesis by B lymphocytes: an A$_{2B}$-mediated process involving Th2 cytokines IL-4 and IL-13 with implications for asthma. J Immunol 2004;172: 7726–33.

34. Cushley MJ, Tattersfield AE, Holgate ST. Inhaled adenosine and guanosine on airway resistance in normal and asthmatic subjects. Br J Clin Pharmacol 1983; 15:161–5.

35. Holgate ST. The Quintiles Prize Lecture 2004. The identification of the adenosine A$_{2B}$ receptor as a novel therapeutic target in asthma. Br J Pharmacol 2005;145: 1009–15.

36. Wilson CN. Adenosine receptors and asthma in humans. Br J Pharmacol 2008; 155:475–86.

37. Kolachala VL, Bajaj R, Chalasani M, et al. Purinergic receptors in gastrointestinal inflammation. Am J Physiol Gastrointest Liver Physiol 2008;294:G401–10.

38. Lin CS, Lin G, Lue TF. Cyclic nucleotide signaling in cavernous smooth muscle. J Sex Med 2005;2:478–91.

39. Noto T, Inoue H, Mochida H, et al. Role of adenosine and P2 receptors in the penile tumescence in anesthetized dogs. Eur J Pharmacol 2001;425: 51–5.

40. Faria M, Magalhaes-Cardoso T, Lafuente-de-Carvalho JM, et al. Corpus cavernosum from men with vasculogenic impotence is partially resistant to adenosine relaxation due to endothelial A$_{2B}$ receptor dysfunction. J Pharmacol Exp Ther 2006;319:405–13.

41. Gladwin MT. Adenosine receptor crossroads in sickle cell disease. Nat Med 2011;17:38–40.

42. Ramakers BP, Pickkers P, Deussen A, et al. Measurement of the endogenous adenosine concentration in humans in vivo: methodological considerations. Curr Drug Metab 2008;9:679–85.

43. Gaspar HB, Aiuti A, Porta F, et al. How I treat ADA deficiency. Blood 2009;114: 3524–32.

44. Haas MJ. Two edges of sickle cell disease. Science-Business eXchange 2011; 4(3).

Alterations of the Arginine Metabolome in Sickle Cell Disease

A Growing Rationale for Arginine Therapy

Claudia R. Morris, MD

KEYWORDS

- Arginine • Arginase • Hemolysis • Nitric oxide • Sickle cell disease
- Vasoocclusive pain episodes

KEY POINTS

- Low global arginine bioavailability is associated with severe pain, pulmonary hypertension risk, and early mortality in sickle cell disease (SCD).
- Mechanisms of arginine dysregulation in SCD involve a complex paradigm of excess arginase activity, elevated levels of asymmetric dimethylarginine (an arginine analogue and nitric oxide synthase inhibitor), altered intracellular arginine transport, renal dysfunction (which disrupts normal de novo arginine synthesis in the kidneys), and nitric oxide synthase dysfunction.
- Arginine therapy shows promise for the treatment of leg ulcers, pulmonary hypertension, and vasoocclusive pain episodes in patients with SCD in preliminary studies.
- Parenteral arginine (100 mg/kg per dose 3 times a day) decreased total opioid use by more than 50% and was associated with lower pain scores at discharge in children with SCD hospitalized for pain compared with placebo in a recently published randomized placebo-controlled trial of arginine therapy.

AN ALTERED ARGININE METABOLOME IN SICKLE CELL DISEASE

Normal arginine metabolism is impaired in sickle cell disease (SCD)[1] for a variety of reasons discussed in this review that contribute to endothelial dysfunction, vasoocclusion, pulmonary complications, and early mortality (**Fig. 1**). The altered arginine metabolome

Disclosure Statement: There are no conflicts of interest relevant to this review article. Claudia R. Morris, MD is the inventor or co-inventor of several Children's Hospital & Research Center Oakland (CHRCO) patents/pending patent applications that include biomarkers and treatments of cardiovascular disease and low arginine bioavailability. She has also received royalties from a patent-pending omega-3/antioxidant nutritional supplement licensed by CHRCO to Nourish Life.

Division of Emergency Medicine, Department of Pediatrics, Emory-Children's Center for Cystic Fibrosis and Airways Disease Research, Emory University School of Medicine, 1645 Tullie Circle Northeast, Atlanta, GA 30329, USA

E-mail address: claudia.r.morris@emory.edu

differs in children compared with adult patients.[2] Adults with SCD are arginine deficient at steady state,[1-3] whereas children tend to have plasma levels that are similar to normal controls. An arginine deficiency develops over time and is influenced by acute events and chronic end-organ damage. Plasma arginine concentration decreases significantly, however, in both adults and children during vasoocclusive pain episodes (VOE) and acute chest syndrome (ACS)[2,4] and is associated with low plasma nitric oxide (NO) metabolite (NO$_x$) levels.[2,4-6] Low plasma arginine levels predicted the need for hospitalization in children evaluated in an emergency department for pain[2] and normalized with clinical recovery.[2] Although mechanisms of arginine dysregulation are complex and multifactorial,[7,8] they can be overcome through arginine supplementation, a phenomenon known as the "arginine paradox."[9] Short-term oral arginine therapy significantly improved estimated pulmonary artery systolic pressures in patients with SCD at risk for pulmonary hypertension in a small pilot study,[10] whereas parenteral arginine significantly decreased total opioid use and improved pain scores in children with SCD hospitalized for VOE compared with placebo in a recently published

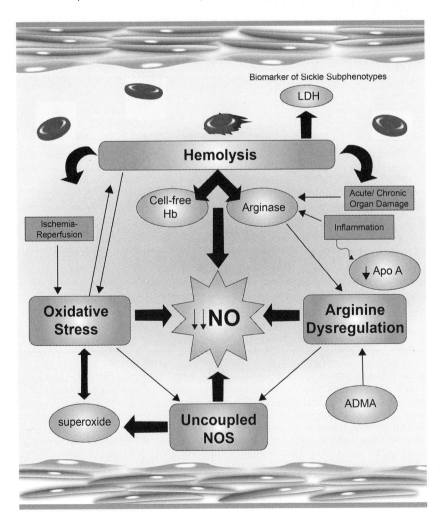

randomized controlled trial.[11] Case reports also suggest a potential role of arginine for the treatment of leg ulcers.[10,12–15] Addressing the alterations in arginine metabolism may result in new strategies for the treatment of SCD.

ALTERED NO HOMEOSTASIS

NO has been well described in the literature as an important signaling molecule involved in the regulation of many mammalian physiologic and pathophysiologic processes. As one of the most potent vasodilators known,[16] NO is essential to vascular homeostasis. It plays a critical role in the maintenance of vasomotor tone, limits platelet aggregation[16–18] and ischemia-reperfusion injury,[19] modulates endothelial proliferation,[20] and has antiinflammatory properties.[21]

NO is produced by a family of NO synthase (NOS) enzymes that metabolize L-arginine through the intermediate N-hydroxy-L-arginine (NOHA) to form NO and L-citrulline using oxygen and nicotinamide adenine dinucleotide phosphate as cosubstrates. NO causes vasodilation through the activation of soluble guanylate cyclase to produce the intracellular messenger cyclic guanylate monophosphate.[16–18] Increased consumption and decreased production of both NO and arginine contribute to complications associated with SCD.[2,7,22,23]

Hemolysis will significantly compromise NO bioavailability in SCD with the release of cell-free hemoglobin (Hb) that rapidly scavenges NO.[24–27] Under normal conditions, Hb is safely packaged within the erythrocyte plasma membrane; however, during hemolysis it is decompartmentalized and released into plasma where it rapidly reacts with and destroys NO.[24] This process results in abnormally high NO consumption and the formation of reactive oxygen species, ultimately inhibiting vasodilation. This phenomenon has also been implicated as a mechanism of NO depletion in the red

Fig. 1. Mechanisms of arginine dysregulation in SCD. Hemolysis, arginine dysregulation, oxidative stress, and uncoupled nitric oxide synthase (NOS) are key mechanisms that contribute to the complex vascular pathophysiology of SCD. These events limits nitric oxide (NO) bioavailability through several paths that ultimately provoke increased consumption and decreased production of the potent vasodilator, NO. Although often discussed independently, there is significant overlap closely linking these pathways of endothelial dysfunction that prohibit determining cause and effect. Inflammation coupled with antioxidant depletion, ischemia-reperfusion injury, and acute as well as chronic end-organ damage obscure mechanistic boundaries further. Endogenous synthesis of arginine from citrulline may be compromised by renal dysfunction, commonly associated with SCD. The bioavailability of arginine is further decreased by elevated ornithine levels because ornithine and arginine compete for the same transporter system for cellular uptake. Asymmetric dimethyl arginine (ADMA) is an arginine analogue and NOS inhibitor that is elevated in SCD that will further diminish global arginine bioavailability. Despite an increase in NOS in SCD, NO bioavailability is paradoxically low because of the low substrate availability; NO scavenging by cell-free hemoglobin (Hb) released during hemolysis; and through reactions with free radicals, such as superoxide. Superoxide is elevated in SCD because of the low superoxide dismutase activity, high xanthine oxidase activity, and potentially as a result of uncoupled NOS in an environment of low arginine and/or tetrahydrobiopterin concentration. Apolipoprotein A1 (Apo-A) is an antiathertogenic lipoprotein that is decreased through inflammation. During hemolysis, cell-free Hb and arginase are simultaneously released from the erythrocyte and profoundly contribute to low NO bioavailability. Lactate dehydrogenase (LDH) is also released from the erythrocyte and represents a convenient biomarker of hemolysis that delineates the subphenotypes of SCD. This new disease paradigm is now recognized as an important mechanism in the pathophysiology of SCD. (*From* Morris CR. Mechanisms of vasculopathy in sickle cell disease and thalassemia. Hematology Am Soc Hematol Educ Program 2008;2008:177–85; with permission.)

cell storage lesion[28,29] and other hemolytic conditions, such as paroxysmal nocturnal hemoglobinuria[30] and malaria.[31] The simultaneous release of the arginine-consuming enzyme arginase also found within human erythrocytes will further compromise the obligate substrate for NO production during hemolysis, as arginase is released into circulation in active form, shifting metabolism of L-arginine to L-ornithine and urea.[1]

ALTERED ARGININE HOMEOSTASIS

As the obligate substrate for NOS, L-arginine bioavailability plays a key role in determining NO production and depends on pathways of biosynthesis, cellular uptake, and catabolism by several distinct enzymes (**Fig. 2**), including those from the NOS and arginase enzyme families. Little is known about arginine metabolism to creatine and agmatine in SCD.

Biosynthesis of the semiessential amino acid occurs in a stepwise fashion though what is called the *intestinal-renal axis*. L-glutamine is absorbed from the small intestine and converted to L-citrulline by the enterocytes. L-citrulline is also synthesized from L-ornithine by ornithine carbamoyl transferase and carbamoyl phosphate synthetase 1 in hepatocytes as part of the urea cycle, as well as in the intestine. L-arginine is produced from L-citrulline by cytosolic enzymes argininosuccinate synthetase 1 and argininosuccinate lyase in kidneys. When L-arginine is subsequently metabolized to NO via NOS, L-citrulline is again produced and can be used for recycling back to L-arginine, which may be an important source of L-arginine during prolonged NO synthesis by inducible nitric oxide synthase.[32]

Arginine becomes an essential amino acid under conditions involving an increased catabolic state, such as sepsis, burn injury, and trauma, when the capacity of endogenous arginine synthesis is surpassed.[33] It is likely that SCD represents another catabolic state whereby the body's ability to maintain an arginine balance is disrupted, with several mechanisms involved summarized in **Box 1**. In addition to acute pain events, low global arginine bioavailability is also found in adults at steady state with a hemolytic subphenotype that includes risk for leg ulcers, pulmonary hypertension risk, and

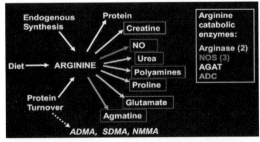

Fig. 2. Sources and metabolic fates of L-arginine. Arginine is produced through de novo synthesis from citrulline primarily in the proximal tubules of the kidney, through protein turnover, or via uptake from the diet. Four enzymes use arginine as their substrate: the NOS, arginases, arginine decarboxylase (ADC), and arginine/glycine amidinotransferase (AGAT). The action of these 4 sets of enzymes ultimately results in production of the 7 products depicted in the figure. Putrescine, spermine, and spermidine are the polyamines produced as downstream byproducts of arginase activity. Turnover of proteins containing methylated arginine residues release asymmetric dimethyl arginine (ADMA), symmetric dimethylarginine (SMMA), and N-methylarginine (NMMA), which are potent inhibitors of NOS. (*Adapted from* Morris SM Jr. Arginine: beyond protein. Am J Clin Nutr 2006; 83(2):508S–12S; with permission.)

> **Box 1**
> **Mechanisms of arginine dysregulation**
>
> - Excess arginase concentration and activity
> - Intracellular arginine transport dysfunction
> - Renal dysfunction
> - Exogenous NOS inhibitors (arginine analogues)

priapism[1,34] and is associated with high plasma lactate dehydrogenase levels.[1,35] Of concern, low arginine bioavailability is associated with early mortality in both adults[1] and children with SCD.[36] Accumulating data also support its role as a biomarker of vasculopathy that goes beyond SCD, associated with malaria-related mortality[27]; diabetes control[37]; severe asthma[38,39]; pulmonary hypertension risk[8,40,41]; coronary artery disease; and major adverse cardiovascular events, including stroke and mortality in patients screened for cardiovascular disease.[42–45] Coined the *global arginine bioavailability ratio*,[1,42–44] this biomarker, defined as the ratio of arginine/(ornithine + citrulline), has emerged as a more robust predictor of cardiovascular disease than cholesterol. These findings suggest that adequate arginine bioavailability is critical for survival and provide clinicians with an objective index of disease severity.[1,36]

Increased Arginase Activity and Concentration

Arginase is an essential enzyme in the urea cycle, responsible for the conversion of arginine to ornithine and urea. The NOS and arginase enzymes can be expressed simultaneously under a wide variety of inflammatory conditions, resulting in competition for their common substrate.[46] Although the affinity (the Michaelis constant K_m) of L-arginine for arginase is in the low micromolar range compared with the low millimolar range for NOS, substrate competition does occur between arginase and NOS because the maximum rate achieved (Vmax) of arginase is 1000-fold higher.[47] Two forms of arginase have been identified: type 1, a cytosolic enzyme highly expressed in the liver, and type 2, a mitochondrial enzyme found predominantly in the kidney, prostate, testis, and small intestine.[46] Arginase-1 is also present in human red blood cells. Plasma arginase activity is elevated in SCD as a consequence of inflammation; liver dysfunction; and, most significantly, by the release of erythrocyte arginase during intravascular hemolysis, which has been demonstrated by the strong correlation between plasma arginase levels and cell-free Hb levels and other markers of increased hemolytic rate.[1] In addition, arginase activity is higher in the erythrocytes of patients with SCD compared with normal controls and strongly correlates to plasma arginase activity.[1] Upregulated expression of arginase-1 also results in increased proliferation rates of vascular smooth muscle and endothelial cells[46] and, in this capacity, may further contribute to vasculopathy in addition to its unique role during hemolysis. When arginine is catalyzed to NO, NOS produces the intermediate product NOHA.[48] NOHA is a potent arginase inhibitor, reflecting complicated feedback mechanisms in place to maintain homeostasis, with both NOS and arginase playing a regulatory role in NO production.[46] Because there is only limited arginase-1 found in the murine erythrocyte compared with human red blood cells, the major sources of increased arginase activity in the sickle cell mouse[49] originate from cells other than the erythrocyte. It is unfortunately not feasible to extrapolate the contribution of erythrocyte arginase release to complications of hemolysis in human SCD from the sickle cell mouse model.

Whether inflammatory or hemolytic in origin, arginase will redirect the metabolism of arginine to ornithine and the formation of polyamines and proline,[50] which are essential for smooth muscle cell growth and collagen synthesis.[51] By creating a shift toward ornithine metabolism, arginase can trigger a process that contributes to the vascular smooth muscle proliferation and airway remodeling that occur in pulmonary hypertension and asthma,[1,52–55] common comorbidities in SCD.

Intracellular Arginine Transport

The primary source of L-arginine for most cells is cellular uptake via the Na-independent cationic amino acid transporter (CAT) proteins of the y^+-system. L-arginine uptake via the y^+-system can be inhibited by other amino acids, such as L-ornithine and L-lysine.[56–58] Therefore, an arginase-triggered increase in ornithine will further impact arginine transport and bioavailability. Plasma arginine concentration in adults with SCD is approximately 40 to 50 µM at baseline,[1,2] well less than the K_m for CAT (100–150 µM). Even modest fluctuations in extracellular arginine concentration, may significantly impact cellular arginine uptake and bioavailability. Alterations in arginine transport have been demonstrated in several disease states, including septic shock, hypertension, diabetes mellitus,[59] and asthma,[60,61] although little is known about CAT and arginine transport in SCD.

Renal Dysfunction

Renal dysfunction is common in SCD[62,63] and will further diminish global arginine bioavailability through the loss of de novo arginine synthesis from citrulline, which occurs primarily in the kidney.[32] Renal dysfunction impairs the major route for endogenous arginine biosynthesis, thereby contributing to a global reduction in arginine bioavailability.

Endogenous NOS Inhibitors

Low arginine bioavailability may be exacerbated further by the presence of elevated asymmetric dimethylarginine (ADMA), an endogenous NOS inhibitor that competes with L-arginine for binding to NOS.[64] Well established as a biomarker of cardiovascular disease and endothelial dysfunction,[7] it may also contribute to inflammation, collagen deposition, and nitrosative stress in SCD. Circulating ADMA levels are elevated in SCD[65–67] and have been implicated in the pathophysiology of asthma,[68,69] systemic and pulmonary hypertension,[70–74] and risk of early mortality.[42,45,75] The most elevated ADMA level occurred in patients with SCD with the highest hemolytic rate and was associated with pulmonary hypertension risk reflected by a high tricuspid regurgitant jet velocity (TRV) and mortality.[65,76] High levels of ADMA can also contribute to NOS uncoupling.[77] Landburg and colleagues[67] recently demonstrated that elevated ADMA levels in patients with SCD did not increase over baseline during VOE. Although they conclude that there is no primary role for ADMA during acute pain,[67] given that arginine bioavailability decreases significantly during VOE and ACS,[2] an increase in the ratio of ADMA to arginine may have some impact on global arginine bioavailability and endothelial dysfunction that should be explored further.

IMPACT OF ARGININE THERAPY ON NO PRODUCTION: A POTENTIAL EXPLANATION FOR A VARIED RESPONSE TO THERAPY

Mechanistically, oral arginine (100 mg/kg per dose) acutely increases both plasma and exhaled NO when administered to African American healthy control subjects within 2 hours.[78–80] When arginine is given to patients with SCD at steady state, however, a paradoxic decrease in plasma NO_x occurs that is not overcome by higher doses,[78] clearly indicating that arginine is metabolized differently in SCD compared with control subjects. However, when arginine is given during VOE, a condition associated with an acute arginine deficiency,[2,4] a robust dose-dependent increase in NO_x occurs.[78]

These early observations may account for the negative outcome of the Comprehensive Sickle Cell Centers' (CSCC) arginine trial that targeted patients with SCD at steady state, particularly because the primary outcome measure of that study was an increase in plasma NO_x,[81] despite preliminary data showing a paradoxic decrease in NO_x when oral arginine is given to patients with SCD at steady state. Also, low-dose arginine therapy is likely to be subtherapeutic in SCD and may represent an additional flaw in the CSCC prophylactic arginine trial design[81] because doses used were close to placebo based on the cardiovascular literature.[82,83] Previous studies have shown that low-dose arginine is unlikely to impact NO synthesis,[83] an observation confirmed in the CSCC study.[81]

Based on preliminary pharmacokinetic studies,[78,79] peak plasma arginine concentration after oral arginine (100 mg/kg) is significantly higher during SCD steady state compared with VOE, although levels are similar by 4 hours. Healthy controls reach a peak arginine level between 1 to 2 hours that is maintained at 4 hours and does not trend down as in SCD.[78] Accelerated arginine metabolism or consumption occurs during VOE compared with steady state despite the same oral arginine dose given. The author also found that the capacity of arginine to increase NO_x production in patients with SCD with pain is dose dependent.[78] Higher concentrations of plasma arginine are likely needed to overcome multifactorial effects, including the impact of arginase and ADMA on global arginine bioavailability. Therefore, low doses are unlikely to achieve a maximal benefit. However, the long-term safety of doses greater than 100 mg/kg per dose 3 times per day is unknown in SCD, even though a 1-time dose of 30 g is commonly used for growth hormone stimulation testing with an excellent safety profile.[84,85] Because the arginine formula generally available is L-arginine hydrochloride, the wisdom of higher doses is questionable given the potential to induce acidosis with repeated dosing over time and must be taken into consideration. However, a single loading dose of 200 to 300 mg/kg may provide an additional benefit during VOE given the pharmacokinetics data showing increased arginine consumption in patients with pain compared with steady state and warrants further study. However, to date, the safety of 100 mg/kg per dose 3 times a day (300 mg/kg/d total) has been well established in the literature and has been found efficacious in the author's experiences with SCD.[10,11]

These data highlight the importance of careful identification of ideal outcome measures, optimal study drug dosing, and enrollment of targeted clinical phenotypes to insure comparison of apples to apples in light of growing evidence of metabolic variations among patients with SCD that may manifest with a specific clinical profile.

In transgenic mouse models of SCD, L-arginine supplementation inhibits the red cell Gardos channels[86]; reduces red cell density[86]; improves perfusion; and reduces lung injury, microvascular vasoocclusion, and mortality.[49,87–89] Arginine also increases erythrocyte glutathione levels in both mouse[88] and human trials[90] and may downregulate inflammatory pathways.[91] In addition, arginine is a key substrate in creatine synthesis, an important metabolic pathway not yet sufficiently studied in SCD that may be impacted by an arginine-deficient state. Although the role of NO in SCD has become controversial,[92,93] these studies demonstrate that the mechanistic impact of arginine goes beyond NO.

ARGININE COADMINISTRATION WITH HYDROXYUREA

Coadministration of oral arginine with hydroxyurea (HU) ameliorated the paradoxic decrease in plasma NO_x observed in patients with SCD at steady state compared with arginine monotherapy.[79] A recently published study performed in Brazil adds to the growing body of literature in support of arginine coadministration with HU. Twenty-one adult patients with SCD were randomized to receive HU alone (500–1500 mg/d; n = 9) or HU + arginine (250 mg/d; n = 12) for 12 weeks. An increase in levels of nitrite and fetal Hb was observed in the arginine/HU arm compared with patients receiving HU alone,[94] despite the low dose of arginine used. Arginine therapy together with HU may be superior to either single intervention.

ARGININE THERAPY FOR CLINICAL COMPLICATIONS OF SCD
Leg Ulcers

Chronic refractory leg ulcers are a debilitating and painful complication of SCD. To date, there is no specific Food and Drug Administration (FDA)–approved therapy for leg ulcers, and most patients undergo multiple treatments of surgical debridement and grafting and courses of topical and systemic treatments with only anecdotal evidence of improvement. Rapid healing of leg ulcers was initially reported with parenteral *arginine* butyrate in both SCD and thalassemia.[12,13,95,96] Although improvement of leg ulcers occurred in patients despite little change in fetal hemoglobin,[12] considered to be butyrate's mechanism of action,[97,98] it is not possible to determine from these observations whether the benefits were in fact from the butyrate or arginine component of treatment. Rapid healing of chronic recalcitrant leg ulcers was also observed after 5 days of oral L-arginine-hydrochloride (100 mg/kg 3 times a day) in a pilot study treating patients with SCD with pulmonary hypertension risk,[10] suggesting a therapeutic potential for the arginine component. A randomized-controlled phase II trial of parenteral arginine butyrate confirmed the initial anecdotal observations.[14] Eligible patients included adults with SCD suffering from extremity ulcers refractory to standard care for at least 6 months. Many of the enrolled patients had suffered from refractory ulcers for many years and had tried multiple therapies. Twenty-three patients with 25 refractory leg ulcers present were randomized to receive standard local care alone (the control arm, n = 12) or standard care together with parenteral arginine butyrate administered 5 days per week for 12 weeks (n = 11, patients with 37 leg ulcers). A higher percentage of ulcer proportions healed after 3 months in the treatment arm compared with the control arm (78% vs 24%, P<.001). Additional case reports of oral arginine therapy anecdotally improving recalcitrant leg ulcers in SCD support the need for further study.[15]

Pulmonary Hypertension Risk

The cause of pulmonary hypertension is multifactorial; however, there is growing evidence that the disease process, in part, involves altered arginine metabolism or decreased bioavailability. Several human studies have demonstrated therapeutic benefits of arginine therapy for both idiopathic and secondary pulmonary hypertension,[99,100] although other studies have demonstrated little effect. A single arginine infusion (500 mg/kg over 30 minutes) decreased pulmonary vascular resistance and improved blood oxygenation in infants with persistent pulmonary hypertension of the newborn.[101] Mehta and colleagues[100] found that an infusion of arginine (500 mg/kg over 30 minutes) reduced mean pulmonary artery pressures by nearly 16% and pulmonary vascular resistance by 27.6% in 10 patients with pulmonary hypertension of various origins. Nagaya and colleagues[99] demonstrated that oral arginine (50 mg/kg) produced a 9% decrease in mean pulmonary artery pressure and a 16% decrease in pulmonary vascular resistance 60 minutes after supplementation in 10 patients with pulmonary hypertension of mixed cause compared with 9 patients receiving placebo. One-week continued supplementation of arginine (150 mg/kg 3 times a day) resulted in a significant improvement in cardiopulmonary exercise testing; however, the impact on hemodynamics was not reassessed. In contrast, an acute arginine infusion (12.6 g over 90 minutes) in 4 patients with idiopathic pulmonary artery hypertension demonstrated little impact on pulmonary hemodynamics and a significant decrease in systemic resistance in 2 of the patients,[102] whereas an arginine infusion (500 mg/kg over 30 minutes) given to 5 controls and 5 patients with systemic sclerosis and pulmonary artery hypertension demonstrated no significant effect on systemic or pulmonary hemodynamics in either group.[103]

Pulmonary hypertension is a common complication in hemoglobinopathies.[104] A similar pattern of altered arginine metabolism is seen in both SCD[1] and thalassemia.[52,53,105] The prevalence of pulmonary hypertension in SCD has generated a great deal of controversy[92,93]; however, recent screening studies in SCD that include right heart catheterization (RHC) for patients at an increased risk of pulmonary hypertension based on an elevated TRV on Doppler echocardiography demonstrate that 6% to 11% of adults with SCD have pulmonary hypertension defined by a mean pulmonary artery pressure greater than or equal to 25 mm Hg.[106–110] This prevalence of 6% to 11% pulmonary hypertension in SCD is much higher than the prevalence of 0.0015% in the general population, 0.5% in patients with human immunodeficiency virus, and 7.8% in patients with scleroderma.[108] Given the global burden of SCD affecting millions of patients, SCD is one of the most common causes of pulmonary hypertension worldwide. In light of the high mortality risk associated with pulmonary hypertension in SCD,[62,106,108,109,111] novel therapies are needed, although studies to date with traditional FDA-approved pulmonary artery hypertension medications, including bosentan and sildenafil, have been disappointing.[112–114] In order to provide some recommendations for clinicians, consensus-based guidelines for the diagnosis and treatment of pulmonary hypertension of SCD have recently been created.[115]

Similar to the original observations with respect to leg ulcers, anecdotal improvement in estimated pulmonary artery pressure was observed after treatment with *arginine* butyrate in patients with SCD and pulmonary hypertension risk who were on HU therapy.[116] In a later study of 10 patients with SCD and high risk for pulmonary hypertension determined by an elevated TRV, oral L-arginine hydrochloride supplementation (100 mg/kg 3 times a day) produced a 15.2% mean reduction in pulmonary artery pressures estimated by Doppler echocardiography and improved venous oxygen saturation measured by co-oximetry after 5 days of treatment (**Fig. 3**).[10] Plasma arginine concentration more than doubled in all compliant patients. Only one patient did not demonstrate a change in pulmonary artery systolic pressure after supplemental arginine; however, noncompliance was indicated by a low plasma arginine concentration at the end of the study in addition to the patient's admission to not taking the study drug. Arginase activity was also found to be high in this cohort of patients,[10] a phenomenon observed in pulmonary hypertension of various causes.[1,117,118]

In contrast, a lack of therapeutic effect on estimated pulmonary artery pressures was found in a study that combined arginine therapy (100–200 mg/kg divided 3 times a day) with HU in 6 adults with SCD and an elevated TRV. Twelve weeks of oral arginine did increase plasma glutathione levels in these patients, suggesting that arginine increases antioxidants, a finding anticipated in studies of murine models of SCD.[88] One significant difference between these 2 arginine studies that could help explain the discrepant findings is the level of risk of pulmonary hypertension based on the TRV measurement of the patients enrolled. In the study by Little and colleagues,[90] the mean TRV for patients receiving arginine was 2.57 ± 0.32 m/s compared with 3.47 ± 0.5 m/s in the earlier study. An elevated TRV 2.5 m/s or more is one of the

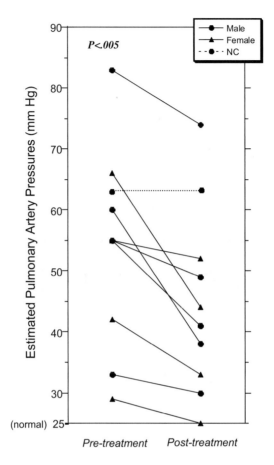

Arginine Therapy

Fig. 3. Changes in estimated mean pulmonary artery systolic pressures (millimeters of mercury) measured by Doppler echocardiography in patients with SCD and pulmonary hypertension risk. Measurements are taken before arginine therapy is started (*pretreatment*) and after completion of 15 doses of arginine (*posttreatment*). Male patients are represented by circles, and female patients are represented by triangles. The dotted line represents the only patient found to be noncompliant based on posttreatment plasma arginine levels. Arginine supplementation significantly decreases estimated pulmonary artery systolic pressures (n = 10; P<.005). NC, non compliant. (Reprinted with permission of the American Thoracic Society. Copyright © 2014 American Thoracic Society. *From* Morris CR, Morris SM Jr, Hagar W, et al. Arginine therapy: a new treatment for pulmonary hypertension in sickle cell disease? Am J Respir Crit Care Med 2003;168:63–9. Official Journal of the American Thoracic Society.)

most robust biomarkers of early mortality in SCD described to date,[62] yet whether this is a reflection of systemic vasculopathy and disease severity versus true pulmonary hypertension defined by RHC fuels the controversy that has recently surrounded this topic.[92,93,108,119,120] Not all patients with an elevated TRV have RHC-defined pulmonary hypertension. Parent and colleagues[109] demonstrate RHC-defined pulmonary hypertension in 25% and 64% of patients with SCD and a TRV of 2.5 m/s or more and a TRV of 2.9 m/s or more, respectively. Similar results were found in the National

Institutes of Health cohort,[111] with 65.5% of patients with a TRV of 2.8 m/s or more diagnosed with pulmonary hypertension by RHC. It is likely that most patients in the arginine study with a mean TRV of 3.5 m/s had pulmonary hypertension,[10] compared with a low risk of pulmonary hypertension in the alternate study.[90] Because global arginine bioavailability decreases significantly in patients with a TRV of 3.0 m/s or more compared with those with a TRV less than 3.0 m/s,[1] it is intuitive that patients with marked TRV elevation are more likely to demonstrate a clinical response to arginine therapy than those who are less arginine deficient. In addition, the arginine dosage used in the study by Little and colleagues[90] (100–200 mg/kg/d) was less than the dosage used by Morris and colleagues[10] (300 mg/kg/d) and may have been subtherapeutic.

Priapism

Priapism is a serious complication associated with SCD resulting from either increased arterial inflow (high flow) or, more commonly, the failure of venous outflow (low flow), resulting in blood trapping within the erectile bodies of the penis. Approximately 30% of males with SCD under the age of 20 years report at least one episode of priapism, with frequencies of 30% to 45% estimated for adult men.[121] An association of priapism with increased hemolysis has been reported[122]; together with leg ulcers and pulmonary hypertension, this complication is included in the hemolytic subphenotype of SCD.[34] Case reports describe a therapeutic benefit of sildenafil in humans,[123] whereas a recent study demonstrates that sildenafil citrate prevents priapism by restoring normal endothelial nitric oxide synthase (eNOS) function through reversed uncoupling in a sickle cell mouse model.[124] Although studies of arginine use for priapism have not yet been performed, this author anecdotally used parenteral arginine-hydrochloride (100 mg/kg per dose intravenously [IV]) in an adolescent with Hb-SS and recurrent priapism during his third visit to the emergency department in 4 days. As his priapism crisis was approaching 4 hours without signs of improvement, and access to a urologist was limited, a decision with the hematology team was made to use arginine therapy in the emergency department. Successful resolution of priapism occurred within 20 minutes of infusion, and the patient was discharged shortly thereafter. Although anecdotal, arginine is a safe option during a time when a treating emergency department physician may have few alternatives.

VOE: Results of a Randomize Double-Blinded Placebo-Controlled Trial

Pain is the leading cause of hospitalizations and emergency department visits in SCD and is associated with increased mortality.[125,126] Low NO bioavailability contributes to vasculopathy in SCD. Because arginine is the obligate substrate for NO production, and an acute deficiency is associated with VOE,[2,4] arginine represents a promising treatment of SCD-associated pain. Thirty-eight children with SCD hospitalized for 56 episodes of VOE were randomized into this single-center, double-blinded placebo-controlled trial. Patients received L-arginine (100 mg/kg 3 times per day) or placebo for 5 days or until discharge. A significant reduction in total parenteral opioid use by 54% (1.9 ± 2.0 mg/kg vs 4.1 ± 4.1 mg/kg, $P = .02$) and lower pain scores at discharge (1.9 ± 2.4 vs 3.9 ± 2.9, $P = .01$) were observed in the treatment arm receiving arginine compared with placebo (**Fig. 4**). There was no significant difference in hospital length of stay (4.1 ± 01.8 vs 4.8 ± 2.5 days, $P = .34$), although a trend favored the arginine arm, and total opioid use correlated strongly to length of admission ($r = 0.86$, $P<.0001$; **Fig. 5**). In future studies, delivering arginine therapy as early as possible in the emergency department or clinic may have a greater impact on length of stay (**Fig. 6**) because many patients received their first dose of study medication more than 24 hours after presenting the emergency department in pain.

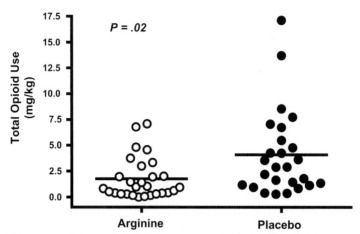

Fig. 4. Impact of arginine therapy on total opioid use (milligrams per kilograms) during hospital stay. Arginine supplementation (*unfilled circles*) led to a significant and clinically relevant reduction in total opioid use by 54% over the course of the hospital stay compared with total opioid use in the placebo group (*filled circles*). The difference remains significant even when the 2 outliers with the largest total opioid use in the placebo arm are excluded from the analysis (P = .04). (*From* Morris CR, Kuypers FA, Lavrisha L, et al. A randomized, placebo-control trial of arginine therapy for the treatment of children with sickle cell disease hospitalized with vaso-occlusive pain episodes. Haematologica 2013;98:1375–82; with permission.)

No drug-related adverse events were observed. One patient experienced clinical deterioration associated with ACS requiring emergent transfusion and a transfer to the pediatric intensive care unit (PICU) in the placebo arm. No clinical deterioration or PICU transfers occurred in the arginine arm.[11] Although a large-scale multicenter trial is needed to confirm these observations, arginine may be a beneficial adjunct

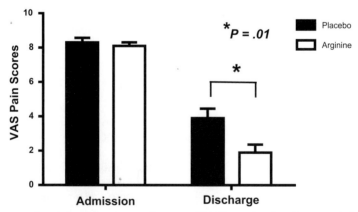

Fig. 5. Impact of arginine therapy on pain scores. The 10-cm visual analogue scale (VAS) pain scores were similar at the time of admission in both groups but were significantly lower at discharge in the arginine group compared with placebo by 2 cm (P = .01). (*From* Morris CR, Kuypers FA, Lavrisha L, et al. A randomized, placebo-control trial of arginine therapy for the treatment of children with sickle cell disease hospitalized with vaso-occlusive pain episodes. Haematologica 2013;98:1375–82; with permission.)

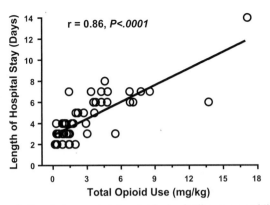

Fig. 6. Pearson correlation between total opioid use (milligram per kilogram) and total length of hospital stay (days). Total opioid use (milligram per kilogram) is directly correlated to length of hospital stay ($r = 0.86$, $P<.0001$). Total opioid use may be a surrogate for length of hospital stay as an outcome measure for patients with SCD and pain. (*From* Morris CR, Kuypers FA, Lavrisha L, et al. A randomized, placebo-control trial of arginine therapy for the treatment of children with sickle cell disease hospitalized with vaso-occlusive pain episodes. Haematologica 2013;98:1375–82; with permission.)

to standard pain therapy for VOE that could reduce suffering and improve emergency care. Plans for such a trial by this author are underway.

SAFETY DATA FOR ARGININE SUPPLEMENTATION

Typical daily human arginine consumption is from 2 to 7 g. L-arginine is one of the least toxic of all amino acids, with its efficacy tested in hundreds of human and animal trials. It has been shown that high dosages of supplemental arginine (30–60 g/d) are well tolerated in humans.[127,128] Previous studies have shown that low dosages of oral arginine are essentially ineffective in providing clinical benefits.[83] The lowest effective dosage for L-arginine for an endothelial dysfunction-related condition is 6 to 8 g/d for adults, but a daily dose of 18 to 20 g is likely to provide a maximal benefit without significant side effects.[83] Compliance with these higher oral doses over extended periods of time is poor because of the large number of capsules necessary. This factor was a hurdle also in the recent arginine trial for treatment of SCD-related pain; IV administration was preferred by patients and improved feasibility of the study drug delivery compared with oral administration in the acute setting.[11] Arginine can be given both orally and via IV. Side effects attributable to arginine have largely been seen in patients who were given rapid IV infusions of large doses of arginine (30 g). Nausea, vomiting, flushing, and headache have occurred with rapid IV infusion.[129] In patients with advanced renal or hepatic insufficiency, hyperkalemia may develop with arginine administration.[128–130] A fatal medication error was reported in a 3-year-old child receiving a 10-fold overdose of a 10% arginine hydrochloride injection during outpatient growth hormone stimulation testing.[131] Caution around parenteral dosage calculations are essential especially when treating children. Allergic reactions to arginine are very rare[129] but have been reported. After oral administration, only gastrointestinal upset and headaches have been reported with long-term use. Notably, the potential mild hypotensive effect of high-dose IV arginine has not been observed in human studies using oral L-arginine, although a normalization of blood pressure in hypertensive patients has been reported. Experience with arginine therapy in SCD has grown over the last decade[10,11,41,78,79,88,132,133]; to date, no serious adverse events have been reported.

WHY ARGININE THERAPY WHEN OTHER NO-BASED THERAPIES HAVE FAILED IN SCD?

Hemolysis and inflammation will drive arginine consumption, which will ultimately exacerbate NO sequestration and decreased NO synthesis.[7] Under conditions of hypoxia, high ADMA, low arginine, or low essential NOS cofactors,[134] NOS will uncouple, producing reactive oxygen species in lieu of NO, further reducing NO bioavailability and adding the milieu of oxidative stress (see **Fig. 1**). An imbalance between eNO synthase-derived NO and superoxide generation exists in SCD.[135] Upregulation of NOS would, therefore, enhance oxidative stress when the local milieu favors NOS uncoupling. Indeed, studies in transgenic sickle cell mice demonstrate that NOS activity is paradoxically increased and uncoupled while NO bioavailability is low.[49] With NOS uncoupling, inhaled NO gas will be rapidly sequestered by superoxide, forming peroxynitrite known to cause lung damage and cell death. It is plausible that the provision of NO excess in SCD may lack a therapeutic benefit in the absence of sufficient L-arginine bioavailability. This lack of benefit is a potential pitfall of sildenafil therapy[112] as well as inhaled NO gas,[136] both with disappointing results in randomized clinical trials targeting SCD.

THE ARGININE METABOLOME: A NOVEL THERAPEUTIC TARGET FOR SCD

Global disruption of the arginine-NO pathway occurs in SCD through multiple mechanisms discussed in detail throughout this review. Therefore, restoration of arginine bioavailability to NOS through exogenous supplementation of L-arginine is an intriguing potential therapeutic target.[137] The exact mechanism of action for arginine in SCD remains unknown but is likely multifactorial. As early as the 1970s, it was suggested that arginine has a stabilizing effect on sickle-hemoglobin.[138] Since then, accumulating clinical and biologic data support further consideration of arginine therapy in SCD.

REFERENCES

1. Morris CR, Kato GJ, Poljakovic M, et al. Dysregulated arginine metabolism, hemolysis-associated pulmonary hypertension and mortality in sickle cell disease. JAMA 2005;294:81–90.
2. Morris CR, Kuypers FA, Larkin S, et al. Patterns of arginine and nitric oxide in sickle cell disease patients with vaso-occlusive crisis and acute chest syndrome. J Pediatr Hematol Oncol 2000;22:515–20.
3. Enwonwu CO, Xu X, Turner E. Nitrogen metabolism in sickle cell anemia: Free amino acids in plasma and urine. Am J Med Sci 1990;300:366–71.
4. Lopez B, Kreshak A, Morris CR, et al. L-arginine levels are diminished in adult acute vaso-occlusive sickle cell crisis in the emergency department. Br J Haematol 2003;120:532–4.
5. Lopez B, Davis-Moon L, Ballas S. Sequential nitric oxide measurements during the emergency department treatment of acute vasoocclusive sickle cell crisis. Am J Hematol 2000;64:15–9.
6. Lopez BL, Barnett J, Ballas SK, et al. Nitric oxide metabolite levels in acute vaso-occlusive sickle-cell crisis. Acad Emerg Med 1996;3:1098–103.
7. Morris CR. Mechanisms of vasculopathy in sickle cell disease and thalassemia. Hematology Am Soc Hematol Educ Program 2008;2008:177–85.

8. Morris CR, Gladwin MT, Kato G. Nitric oxide and arginine dysregulation: a novel pathway to pulmonary hypertension in hemolytic disorders. Curr Mol Med 2008; 8:81–90.
9. Gornik HL, Creager MA. Arginine and endothelial and vascular health. J Nutr 2004;134(Suppl 10):2880S–7S [discussion: 95S].
10. Morris CR, Morris SM Jr, Hagar W, et al. Arginine therapy: a new treatment for pulmonary hypertension in sickle cell disease? Am J Respir Crit Care Med 2003;168:63–9.
11. Morris CR, Kuypers FA, Lavrisha L, et al. A randomized, placebo-control trial of arginine therapy for the treatment of children with sickle cell disease hospitalized with vaso-occlusive pain episodes. Haematologica 2013;98:1375–82.
12. Sher GD, Olivieri NG. Rapid healing of leg ulcers during arginine butyrate therapy in patients with sickle cell disease and thalassemia. Blood 1994;84:2378–80.
13. Koshy M, Askin M, McMahon L, et al, editors. Arginine butyrate in sickle cell leg ulcers: interim findings of a phase II trial. 24th Annual Meeting of the National Sickle Cell Disease Program. Philadelphia, PA, April 9–12, 2000.
14. McMahon L, Tamary H, Askin M, et al. A randomized phase II trial of arginine butyrate with standard local therapy in refractory sickle cell leg ulcers. Br J Haematol 2010;151(5):516–24.
15. Novelli E, Delaney K, Axelrod K, et al, editors. Arginine therapy in a patient with Hb-SS disease and refractory leg ulcers. Sickle Cell Disease Association of America Annual Convention. Baltimore, MD, September 25–29, 2012.
16. Moncada S, Higgs A. The L-arginine-nitric oxide pathway. N Engl J Med 1993; 329:2002–12.
17. Palmer RM, Ferrige AG, Moncada S. Nitric oxide release accounts for the biological activity of endothelium-derived relaxing factor. Nat Med 1987;327: 524–6.
18. Ignarro LJ. Heme-dependent activation of soluble guanylate cyclase by nitric oxide: regulation of enzyme activity by porphyrins and metalloporphyrins. Semin Hematol 1989;26:63–76.
19. Kaul DK, Hebbel RP. Hypoxia/reoxygenation causes inflammatory response in transgenic sickle mice but not in normal mice. J Clin Invest 2000;106:411–20.
20. Hebbel RP, Osarogiagbon KD. The endothelial biology of sickle cell disease: inflammation and a chronic vasculopathy. Microcirculation 2004;11:129–51.
21. Peng HB, Spiecker M, Liao J. Inducible nitric oxide: an autoregulatory feedback inhibitor of vascular inflammation. J Immunol 1998;161:1970–6.
22. Reiter CD, Gladwin MT. An emerging role for nitric oxide in sickle cell disease vascular homeostasis and therapy. Curr Opin Hematol 2003;10:99–107.
23. Gladwin M, Schechter A, Ognibene F, et al. Divergent nitric oxide bioavailability in men and women with sickle cell disease. Circulation 2003;107:271–8.
24. Reiter C, Wang X, Tanus-Santos J, et al. Cell-free hemoglobin limits nitric oxide bioavailability in sickle cell disease. Nat Med 2002;8:1383–9.
25. Minneci PC, Deans KJ, Zhi H, et al. Hemolysis-associated endothelial dysfunction mediated by accelerated NO inactivation by decompartmentalized oxyhemoglobin. J Clin Invest 2005;115(12):3409–17.
26. Deonikar P, Kavdia M. Low micromolar intravascular cell-free hemoglobin concentration affects vascular NO bioavailability in sickle cell disease: a computational analysis. J Appl Physiol 2012;112(8):1383–92.
27. Omodeo-Sale F, Cortelezzi L, Vommaro Z, et al. Dysregulation of L-arginine metabolism and bioavailability associated to free plasma heme. Am J Physiol Cell Physiol 2010;299(1):C148–54.

28. Donadee C, Raat NJ, Kanias T, et al. Nitric oxide scavenging by red blood cell microparticles and cell-free hemoglobin as a mechanism for the red cell storage lesion. Circulation 2011;124(4):465–76.

29. Baron DM, Beloiartsev A, Nakagawa A, et al. Adverse effects of hemorrhagic shock resuscitation with stored blood are ameliorated by inhaled nitric oxide in lambs. Crit Care Med 2013;41(11):2492–501.

30. Hill A, Rother RP, Wang X, et al. Effect of eculizumab on haemolysis-associated nitric oxide depletion, dyspnoea, and measures of pulmonary hypertension in patients with paroxysmal nocturnal haemoglobinuria. Br J Haematol 2010; 149(3):414–25.

31. Yeo TW, Lampah DA, Gitawati R, et al. Impaired nitric oxide bioavailability and L-arginine reversible endothelial dysfunction in adults with falciparum malaria. J Exp Med 2007;204(11):2693–704.

32. Morris SM Jr. Arginine: beyond protein. Am J Clin Nutr 2006;83(2):508S–12S.

33. Hallemeesch MM, Lamers WH, Deutz NE. Reduced arginine availability and nitric oxide production. Clin Nutr 2002;21(4):273–9.

34. Kato GJ, Gladwin MT, Steinberg MH. Deconstructing sickle cell disease: reappraisal of the role of hemolysis in the development of clinical subphenotypes. Blood Rev 2007;21(1):37–47.

35. Kato GJ, McGowan V, Machado RF, et al. Lactate dehydrogenase as a biomarker of hemolysis-associated nitric oxide resistance, priapism, leg ulceration, pulmonary hypertension, and death in patients with sickle cell disease. Blood 2006;107(6):2279–85.

36. Cox SE, Makani J, Komba AN, et al. Global arginine bioavailability in Tanzanian sickle cell anaemia patients at steady-state: a nested case control study of deaths versus survivors. Br J Haematol 2011;155(4):522–4.

37. Tripolt NJ, Meinitzer A, Eder M, et al. Multifactorial risk factor intervention in patients with type 2 diabetes improves arginine bioavailability ratios. Diabet Med 2012;29(10):e365–8.

38. Lara A, Khatri SB, Wang Z, et al. Alterations of the arginine metabolome in asthma. Am J Respir Crit Care Med 2008;178(7):673–81.

39. Morris CR, Poljakovic M, Lavisha L, et al. Decreased arginine bioavailability and increased arginase activity in asthma. Am J Respir Crit Care Med 2004;170:148–53.

40. Morris CR, Teehankee C, Kato G, et al, editors. Decreased arginine bioavailability contributes to the pathogenesis of pulmonary artery hypertension. American College of Cardiology Annual Meeting. Orlando (FL), March 6–9, 2005.

41. Morris CR. New strategies for the treatment of pulmonary hypertension in sickle cell disease: the rationale for arginine therapy. Treat Respir Med 2006;5(1): 31–45.

42. Tang WH, Wang Z, Cho L, et al. Diminished global arginine bioavailability and increased arginine catabolism as metabolic profile of increased cardiovascular risk. J Am Coll Cardiol 2009;53(22):2061–7.

43. Tang WH, Shrestha K, Wang Z, et al. Diminished global arginine bioavailability as a metabolic defect in chronic systolic heart failure. J Card Fail 2013;19(2):87–93.

44. Sourij H, Meinitzer A, Pilz S, et al. Arginine bioavailability ratios are associated with cardiovascular mortality in patients referred to coronary angiography. Atherosclerosis 2011;218(1):220–5.

45. Wang Z, Tang WH, Cho L, et al. Targeted metabolomic evaluation of arginine methylation and cardiovascular risks: potential mechanisms beyond nitric oxide synthase inhibition. Arterioscler Thromb Vasc Biol 2009;29(9):1383–91.

46. Morris SM Jr. Enzymes of arginine metabolism. J Nutr 2004;134:2743S–7S.

47. Wu G, Morris SM. Arginine metabolism: nitric oxide and beyond. Biochem J 1998;336:1–17.
48. Stuehr DJ, Kwon N, Nathan CF, et al. N-Hydroxyl-L-arginine is an intermediate in the biosynthesis of nitric oxide for L-arginine. J Biol Chem 1991;266:6259–63.
49. Hsu LL, Champion HC, Campbell-Lee SA, et al. Hemolysis in sickle cell mice causes pulmonary hypertension due to global impairment in nitric oxide bioavailability. Blood 2007;109:3088–98.
50. Li H, Meininger CJ, Hawker JR, et al. Regulatory role of arginase I and II in nitric oxide, polyamine, and proline syntheses in endothelial cells. Am J Physiol 2002; 282:R64–9.
51. Durante W, Johnson FK, Johnson RA. Arginase: a critical regulator of nitric oxide synthesis and vascular function. Clin Exp Pharmacol Physiol 2007;34(9):906–11.
52. Morris CR, Kuypers FA, Kato GJ, et al. Hemolysis-associated pulmonary hypertension in thalassemia. Ann N Y Acad Sci 2005;1054:481–5.
53. Morris CR, Vichinsky E, Singer ST. Pulmonary hypertension in thalassemia: association with hemolysis, arginine metabolism dysregulation and a hypercoagulable state. Advances Pulmonary Hypertension 2007;6:31–8.
54. Morris CR. Asthma management: reinventing the wheel in sickle cell disease. Am J Hematol 2009;84(4):234–41.
55. Morris CR. Role of arginase in sickle cell lung disease and hemolytic anemias. Open Nitric Oxide J 2010;2:41–54.
56. Messeri-Dreissig MD, Hammermann R, Mossner J, et al. In rat alveolar macrophages lipopolysaccharides exert divergent effects on the transport of the cationic amino acids L-arginine and L-ornithine. Naunyn Schmiedbergs Arch Pharmacol 2000;361:621–8.
57. Bogle RG, Baydoun AR, Pearson JD, et al. L-arginine transport is increased in macrophages generating nitric oxide. Biochem J 1992;284:15–8.
58. Hammermann R, Hirschmann J, Hey C, et al. Cationic proteins inhibit L-arginine uptake in rat alveolar macrophages and tracheal epithelial cells. Implications for nitric oxide synthesis. Am J Respir Cell Mol Biol 1999;21:155–62.
59. Mendes Ribeiro AC, Brunini TM. L-arginine transport in disease. Curr Med Chem Cardiovasc Hematol Agents 2004;2:123–31.
60. Meurs H, Schuurman FE, Duyvendak M, et al. Deficiency of nitric oxide in polycation-induced airway hyperreactivity. Br J Pharmacol 1999;126:559–62.
61. Yahata T, Nishimura Y, Maeda H, et al. Modulation of airway responsiveness by anionic and cationic polyelectrolyte substances. Eur J Pharmacol 2002;434:71–9.
62. Gladwin M, Sachdev V, Jison M, et al. Pulmonary hypertension as a risk factor for death in patients with sickle cell disease. N Engl J Med 2004;350:22–31.
63. De Castro LM, Jonassaint JC, Graham FL, et al. Pulmonary hypertension associated with sickle cell disease: clinical and laboratory endpoints and disease outcomes. Am J Hematol 2008;83(1):19–25.
64. Vallance P. The asymmetrical dimethylarginine/dimethylarginine dimethylaminohydrolase pathway in the regulation of nitric oxide generation. Clin Sci 2001;100: 159–60.
65. Kato GJ, Wang Z, Machado RF, et al. Endogenous nitric oxide synthase inhibitors in sickle cell disease: abnormal levels and correlations with pulmonary hypertension, desaturation, haemolysis, organ dysfunction and death. Br J Haematol 2009;145(4):506–13.
66. Schnog JB, Teerlink T, van der Dijs FP, et al. Plasma levels of asymmetric dimethylarginine (ADMA), an endogenous nitric oxide synthase inhibitor, are elevated in sickle cell disease. Ann Hematol 2005;84(5):282–6.

67. Landburg PP, Teerlink T, Muskiet FA, et al. Plasma concentrations of asymmetric dimethylarginine, an endogenous nitric oxide synthase inhibitor, are elevated in sickle cell patients but do not increase further during painful crisis. Am J Hematol 2008;83(7):577–9.

68. Scott JA, North ML, Rafii M, et al. Asymmetric dimethylarginine is increased in asthma. Am J Respir Crit Care Med 2011;184(7):779–85.

69. Riccioni G, Bucciarelli V, Verini M, et al. ADMA, SDMA, L-Arginine and nitric oxide in allergic pediatric bronchial asthma. J Biol Regul Homeost Agents 2012; 26(3):561–6.

70. Gorenflo M, Zheng C, Werle E, et al. Plasma levels of asymmetrical dimethyl-L-arginine in patients with congenital heart disease and pulmonary hypertension. J Cardiovasc Pharmacol 2001;37(4):489–92.

71. Kielstein JT, Bode-Boger SM, Hesse G, et al. Asymmetrical dimethylarginine in idiopathic pulmonary arterial hypertension. Arterioscler Thromb Vasc Biol 2005; 25(7):1414–8.

72. Millatt LJ, Whitley GS, Li D, et al. Evidence for dysregulation of dimethylarginine dimethylaminohydrolase I in chronic hypoxia-induced pulmonary hypertension. Circulation 2003;108(12):1493–8.

73. Pullamsetti S, Kiss L, Ghofrani HA, et al. Increased levels and reduced catabolism of asymmetric and symmetric dimethylarginines in pulmonary hypertension. FASEB J 2005;19(9):1175–7.

74. Perticone F, Sciacqua A, Maio R, et al. Asymmetric dimethylarginine, L-arginine, and endothelial dysfunction in essential hypertension. J Am Coll Cardiol 2005; 46(3):518–23.

75. Meinitzer A, Seelhorst U, Wellnitz B, et al. Asymmetrical dimethylarginine independently predicts total and cardiovascular mortality in individuals with angiographic coronary artery disease (the Ludwigshafen risk and cardiovascular health study). Clin Chem 2007;53(2):273–83.

76. El-Shanshory M, Badraia I, Donia A, et al. Asymmetric dimethylarginine levels in children with sickle cell disease and its correlation to tricuspid regurgitant jet velocity. Eur J Haematol 2013;91(1):55–61.

77. Sydow K, Munzel T. ADMA and oxidative stress. Atheroscler Suppl 2003;4(4): 41–51.

78. Morris CR, Kuypers FA, Larkin S, et al. Arginine therapy: a novel strategy to increase nitric oxide production in sickle cell disease. Br J Haematol 2000;111: 498–500.

79. Morris CR, Vichinsky EP, van Warmerdam J, et al. Hydroxyurea and arginine therapy: impact on nitric oxide production in sickle cell disease. J Pediatr Hematol Oncol 2003;25:629–34.

80. Sullivan KJ, Kissoon N, Sandler E, et al. Effect of oral arginine supplementation on exhaled nitric oxide concentration in sickle cell anemia and acute chest syndrome. J Pediatr Hematol Oncol 2010;32(7):e249–58.

81. Styles L, Kuypers F, Kesler K, et al, editors. Arginine therapy does not benefit children with sickle cell anemia: results of the comprehensive sickle cell center multi-center study. 35th Convention of the National Sickle Cell Disease Program and the Sickle Cell Disease Association of America. Washington, DC, September 17–22, 2007.

82. Morris CR. Reduced global arginine bioavailability: a common mechanism of vasculopathy in sickle cell disease and pulmonary hypertension [e-letter]. Blood. Available at: http://bloodjournal.hematologylibrary.org/cgi/eletters/blood-2010-02-268193v1. Accessed April 22, 2010.

83. Maxwell AJ, Cooke JP. Cardiovascular effects of L-arginine. Curr Opin Nephrol Hypertens 1998;7:63–70.
84. Merimee TJ, Rabinowitz D, Riggs L, et al. Plasma growth hormone after arginine infusion. N Engl J Med 1967;276:434–9.
85. Merimee TJ, Rabinowitz D, Fineberg S. Arginine-initiated release of human growth hormone. N Engl J Med 1969;28:1434–8.
86. Romero J, Suzuka S, Nagel R, et al. Arginine supplementation of sickle trans-genic mice reduces red cell density and Gardos channel activity. Blood 2002; 99:1103–8.
87. Sinden RE, Barker GC, Paton MJ, et al. Factors regulating natural transmission of Plasmodium berghei to the mosquito vector, and the cloning of a transmission-blocking immunogen. Parassitologia 1993;35(Suppl):107–12.
88. Dasgupta T, Hebbel RP, Kaul DK. Protective effect of arginine on oxidative stress in transgenic sickle mouse models. Free Radic Biol Med 2006;41(12):1771–80.
89. Kaul DK, Zhang X, Dasgupta T, et al. Arginine therapy of transgenic-knockout sickle mice improves microvascular function by reducing non-nitric oxide vaso-dilators, hemolysis, and oxidative stress. Am J Physiol Heart Circ Physiol 2008; 295(1):H39–47.
90. Little JA, Hauser KP, Martyr SE, et al. Hematologic, biochemical, and cardiopul-monary effects of L-arginine supplementation or phosphodiesterase 5 inhibition in patients with sickle cell disease who are on hydroxyurea therapy. Eur J Hae-matol 2009;82(4):315–21.
91. Archer DR, Stiles JK, Newman GW, et al. C-reactive protein and interleukin-6 are decreased in transgenic sickle cell mice fed a high protein diet. J Nutr 2008; 138(6):1148–52.
92. Gladwin MT, Barst RJ, Castro OL, et al. Pulmonary hypertension and NO in sickle cell. Blood 2010;116(5):852–4.
93. Bunn HF, Nathan DG, Dover GJ, et al. Pulmonary hypertension and nitric oxide depletion in sickle cell disease. Blood 2010;116(5):687–92.
94. Elias DB, Barbosa MC, Rocha LB, et al. L-arginine as an adjuvant drug in the treatment of sickle cell anaemia. Br J Haematol 2013;160(3):410–2.
95. Perrine SP, Ginder GD, Faller DV, et al. A short-term trial of butyrate to stimulate fetal-globin-gene expression in the beta-globin disorders. N Engl J Med 1993; 328(2):81–6.
96. Sutton LL, Castro O, Cross DJ, et al. Pulmonary hypertension in sickle cell dis-ease. Am J Cardiol 1994;74:626–8.
97. Sher GD, Ginder GD, Little J, et al. Extended therapy with intravenous arginine butyrate in patients with b-hemoglobinopathies. N Engl J Med 1995;332: 1606–10.
98. Perrine SP, Olivieri NF, Faller DV, et al. Butyrate derivatives. New agents for stim-ulating fetal globin production in the beta-globin disorders. Am J Pediatr Hem-atol Oncol 1994;16:67–71.
99. Nagaya N, Uematsu M, Oya H, et al. Short-term oral administration of L-arginine improves hemodynamics and exercise capacity in patients with precapillary pulmonary hypertension. Am J Respir Crit Care Med 2001;163:887–91.
100. Mehta S, Stewart D, Langleben D, et al. Short-term pulmonary vasodilation with L-arginine in pulmonary hypertension. Circulation 1995;92:1539–45.
101. McCaffrey M, Bose C, Reiter P, et al. Effect of L-arginine infusion on infants with persistent pulmonary hypertension of the newborn. Biol Neonate 1995;67:240–3.
102. Surdacki A, Zmudka K, Bieron K, et al. Lack of beneficial effects of L-arginine infu-sion in primary pulmonary hypertension. Wien Klin Wochenschr 1994;106:521–6.

103. Baudouin SV, Bath P, Martin JF, et al. L-arginine infusion has no effect on systemic haemodynamics in normal volunteers, or systemic and pulmonary haemodynamics in patients with elevated pulmonary vascular resistance. Br J Clin Pharmacol 1993;36:45–9.

104. Farmakis D, Aessopos A. Pulmonary hypertension associated with hemoglobinopathies: prevalent but overlooked. Circulation 2011;123(11):1227–32.

105. Morris CR, Vichinsky EP. Pulmonary hypertension in thalassemia. Ann N Y Acad Sci 2010;1202:205–13.

106. Gladwin MT, Vichinsky E. Pulmonary complications of sickle cell disease. N Engl J Med 2008;359(21):2254–65.

107. Bachir D, Parent F, Hajji L, et al. Prospective multicentric survey on pulmonary hypertension (PH) in adults with sickle cell disease. Blood 2009;114 [abstract 572].

108. Gladwin MT. Prevalence, risk factors and mortality of pulmonary hypertension defined by right heart catheterization in patients with sickle cell disease. Expert Rev Hematol 2011;4(6):593–6.

109. Parent F, Bachir D, Inamo J, et al. A hemodynamic study of pulmonary hypertension in sickle cell disease. N Engl J Med 2011;365(1):44–53.

110. Fonseca GH, Souza R, Salemi VC, et al. Pulmonary hypertension diagnosed by right heart catheterization in sickle cell disease. Eur Respir J 2012;39(1):112–8.

111. Mehari A, Gladwin MT, Tian X, et al. Mortality in adults with sickle cell disease and pulmonary hypertension. JAMA 2012;307(12):1254–6.

112. Machado RF, Barst RJ, Yovetich NA, et al. Hospitalization for pain in patients with sickle cell disease treated with sildenafil for elevated TRV and low exercise capacity. Blood 2011;118(4):855–64.

113. Morris CR, Gladwin MT. Pulmonary hypertension in sickle cell disease and thalassemia. In: Peacock A, Naeije R, Rubin L, editors. Pulmonary circulation. 3rd edition. London: Hodder Arnold; 2011. p. 271–87.

114. Barst RJ, Mubarak KK, Machado RF, et al. Exercise capacity and haemodynamics in patients with sickle cell disease with pulmonary hypertension treated with bosentan: results of the ASSET studies. Br J Haematol 2010;149(3): 426–35.

115. Klings E, Machado R, Barst R, et al. Consensus-based guidelines for the diagnosis and treatment of pulmonary hypertension of sickle cell disease. Am J Respir Crit Care Med, in press.

116. Sutton M, Weinberg R, Padilla M, et al, editors. Development of pulmonary hypertension in sickle cell disease in spite of a response to hydroxyurea. 24th Annual Meeting of the National Sickle Cell Disease Program. Philadelphia, PA, April 9–12, 2000.

117. Xu W, Kaneko TF, Zheng S, et al. Increased arginase II and decreased NO synthesis in endothelial cells of patients with pulmonary arterial hypertension. FASEB J 2004;18:1746–8.

118. Morris CR, Kim HY, Wood J, et al. Sildenafil therapy in thalassemia patients with Doppler-defined risk of pulmonary hypertension. Haematologica 2013;98(9): 1359–67.

119. Morris CR. Vascular risk assessment in patients with sickle cell disease. Haematologica 2011;96(1):1–5.

120. Hebbel RP. Reconstructing sickle cell disease: a data-based analysis of the "hyperhemolysis paradigm" for pulmonary hypertension from the perspective of evidence-based medicine. Am J Hematol 2011;86(2):123–54.

121. Kato GJ. Priapism in sickle-cell disease: a hematologist's perspective. J Sex Med 2012;9(1):70–8.

122. Nolan VG, Wyszynski DF, Farrer LA, et al. Hemolysis-associated priapism in sickle cell disease. Blood 2005;106(9):3264–7.
123. Bialecki ES, Bridges KR. Sildenafil relieves priapism in patients with sickle cell disease. Am J Med 2002;113(3):252.
124. Bivalacqua TJ, Musicki B, Hsu LL, et al. Sildenafil citrate-restored eNOS and PDE5 regulation in sickle cell mouse penis prevents priapism via control of oxidative/nitrosative stress. PLoS One 2013;8(7):e68028.
125. Bunn HF. Pathogenesis and treatment of sickle cell disease. N Engl J Med 1997; 337(11):762–9.
126. Brousseau DC, Owens PL, Mosso AL, et al. Acute care utilization and rehospitalizations for sickle cell disease. JAMA 2010;303(13):1288–94.
127. Barbul A, Rettura G, Levenson SM, et al. Wound healing and thymotropic effects of arginine: a pituitary mechanism of action. Am J Clin Nutr 1983;37:786–94.
128. Barbul A. Arginine: biochemistry, physiology and therapeutic implications. JPEN J Parenter Enteral Nutr 1986;10:227–38.
129. McEvoy G. American Society of Health-System Pharmacists. 1996.
130. Hertz P, Richardson J. Arginine-induced hyperkalemia in renal failure patients. Arch Intern Med 1972;130:778–80.
131. Medication error causes death of boy, 3. Florida Today. Oct 25, 2007.
132. Morris C, Ansari M, Lavrisha L, et al. Arginine therapy for vaso-occlusive pain episodes in sickle cell disease. Blood 2009;114 [abstract 573].
133. Little JA, McGowan VR, Kato GJ, et al. Combination erythropoietin-hydroxyurea therapy in sickle cell disease: experience from the National Institutes of Health and a literature review. Haematologica 2006;91(8):1076–83.
134. Berka V, Yeh HC, Gao D, et al. Redox function of tetrahydrobiopterin and effect of L-arginine on oxygen binding in endothelial nitric oxide synthase. Biochemistry 2004;43(41):13137–48.
135. Wood KC, Hebbel RP, Lefer DJ, et al. Critical role of endothelial cell-derived nitric oxide synthase in sickle cell disease-induced microvascular dysfunction. Free Radic Biol Med 2006;40(8):1443–53.
136. Gladwin MT, Kato GJ, Weiner D, et al. Nitric oxide for inhalation in the acute treatment of sickle cell pain crisis: a randomized controlled trial. JAMA 2011; 305(9):893–902.
137. Vichinsky E. Emerging 'A' therapies in hemoglobinopathies: agonists, antagonists, antioxidants, and arginine. Hematology Am Soc Hematol Educ Program 2012;2012:271–5.
138. Solomons C, Hathaway W, Cotton E. L-arginine, the sickling phenomenon, and cystic fibrosis. Pediatrics 1972;49:933.

Cellular Adhesion and the Endothelium: P-Selectin

Abdullah Kutlar, MD[a], Stephen H. Embury, MD[b,c],*

KEYWORDS

- Sickle cell disease • Impaired blood flow in sickle cell disease
- Sickle red cell adhesion • P-selectin • Pentosan polysulfate sodium
- Microvascular occlusion

KEY POINTS

- Impaired blood flow is the ultimate morbid effect of the canonical sequence deoxygenation → sickle hemoglobin polymerization → erythrocyte sickling.
- Adhesion of sickle red blood cells to the vascular endothelium has been shown to initiate acute vascular occlusion; numerous polymerization-dependent and polymerization-independent mechanisms contribute to its completion.
- Effective correction of abnormal blood flow acting through any mechanism will provide therapeutic benefit.
- Endothelial P-selectin is initiatory and necessary for adhesion of sickle red blood cells to the endothelium.
- Although several selectin-blocking drugs are in their development phase, an orally active agent is preferable for long-term, prophylactic therapy.

INTRODUCTION

The importance of P-selectin to the pathophysiology of sickle cell disease (SCD) is understood through its effect on blood flow. P-selectin is central to the abnormal blood flow in SCD, and abnormal blood flow is paramount to the morbidity and mortality of the disorder. Although the expression of P-selectin makes important contributions to normal platelet activity, hemostasis, coagulation, and inflammation,[1–4] the focus of

Funding Sources: Dr A. Kutlar: Novartis Pharmaceuticals, Inc, Celgene Corporation, Inc, and GlycoMimetics, Inc; Dr S.H. Embury: Consultant for Global Blood Therapeutics, Inc and JUNCTIONRx.
Conflict of Interest: Dr A. Kutlar: None; Dr S.H. Embury: Executive of Vanguard Therapeutics, Inc.
[a] Sickle Cell Center, Department of Medicine, Georgia Regents University, 1120 15th Street, Augusta, GA 30912, USA; [b] Department of Medicine, University of California San Francisco School of Medicine, 505 Parnassus Avenue, San Francisco, CA 94143, USA; [c] Vanguard Therapeutics, Inc, 108 Eagle Trace Drive, Half Moon Bay, CA 94019-2286, USA
* Corresponding author. Vanguard Therapeutics, Inc, 108 Eagle Trace Drive, Half Moon Bay, CA 94019-2286.
E-mail address: shembury@gmail.com

this review is the detrimental effect of endothelial P-selectin–mediated sickle red cell adhesion on sickle cell blood flow.

ABNORMAL BLOOD FLOW IN SICKLE CELL DISEASE

Abnormal blood flow is responsible for most of the morbidity associated with SCD.[5–9] Stroke,[10,11] acute painful episodes,[12–14] splenic sequestration and infarcts, osteonecrosis, acute chest syndrome, and priapism are among the clinical events caused by or significantly contributed to by impaired blood flow. Stroke is an important cause of disability and death[15,16]; pain crises are major determinants of the quality of life[17] and have been associated with increased mortality.[18] In this regard, deficient blood flow can be regarded as the principal defect of SCD.

Microvascular blood flow has been found to be consistently abnormal in sickle cell patients even when they are not experiencing pain crises, independent of the technique used for measurement (nail-bed microscopy, laser Doppler measurement, or ocular computer-assisted intravital microscopy).[19–22] During acute pain crises, additional flow changes are detected using these same methods.[20–22]

The contribution of numerous polymerization-independent processes to impaired sickle cell blood flow[23–33] provides several therapeutic targets for remedying abnormal sickle cell blood flow as alternatives to unraveling the paradigmatic Gordian knot of deoxygenation → sickle hemoglobin (HbS) polymerization → sickle red blood cell (SRBC) rigidification and sickling.[34] This understanding suggests that genetic diseases do not necessarily require genetic treatments. The primacy of abnormal blood flow to these complex interrelated pathophysiologies is revealed by the dependence of polymerization-independent mechanisms on ischemia/reperfusion.[35,36]

DETERMINANTS OF SICKLE CELL BLOOD FLOW

The flow of sickle cell blood is influenced by classical descriptors of Newtonian fluid flow, as well as by additional determinants that pertain to its non-Newtonian nature, unique properties as sickle cell blood, and exogenous influences to which it is singularly susceptible.[32,37] The relative influences of these myriad factors vary in different parts of the circulation and variable conditions affecting those vessels.[38]

It has been reasoned that blood viscosity is a more important determinant of blood flow in large vessels and that individual SRBC deformability is of greater consequence to microcirculatory flow, and that this accounts for the contrasting clinical effects of RBC transfusion that differ according to the conflicting influences on the two circulations.[39–43] In this analysis the importance of SRBC folding to squeeze through small vessels is paramount in the microcirculation where rigidification of SRBC is highly detrimental.[9,39,44–47] Most critical to the present discussion, the tight squeeze of flowing cells through the smallest vessels exposes the entire circumference of these cells to endothelial cell adhesion molecules, which renders microcirculatory flow more susceptible than large-vessel flow to the detrimental effects of cell adhesion.[30] This concept was illustrated clearly by Hebbel,[30] as shown in **Fig. 1**.

IMPORTANCE OF SRBC ADHESION TO BLOOD FLOW

Awareness of the potential importance of SRBC adhesivity to microcirculatory blood flow began with the initial reports of abnormal SRBC adhesivity to cultured endothelial cells in comparison with normal RBC.[48,49] Evidence for the clinical importance of this

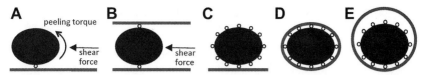

Fig. 1. Conceptual models illustrating the significance of circumferential contact between a red cell and vascular wall. Here, the red cell is conceived as being sufficiently rounded (rendered as a *black oval*) so that adhesion can represent a single point-of-contact phenomenon. Blood flow is from right to left in *A* and *B*, and is perpendicular to the plane of the page in *C* to *E*. In large vessels precluding circumferential contact (*A*), detachment forces countering the adhesive bond are derived from shear flow and a peeling torque. If the vessel is small enough to allow adhesive contacts on opposite sides of the red cell (*B*), the effect of the peeling torque is lost. Also, because twice as many attachments to endothelium exist in *B*, the avidity of each can be lower than in *A* to still allow the red cell to maintain endothelial adhesion. The potential influence of multiple adhesion molecules is not realized as long as the red cell makes contact in a large vessel (*C*), so adhesion there is most likely to develop via high-affinity mechanisms. However, in a microcirculatory vessel that allows complete (*D*) or partial (*E*) circumferential contact, the forces promoting detachment can be countered by development of multiple contacts, even if they individually are of much lower affinity than that required to allow attachment via a single point. In the case of complete circumferential contact (*D*), the effect of peeling torque is lost as well. This highly simplified model can be greatly complicated by inclusion of a wide variety of parameters relevant to real physiology, but this does not materially change the basic conclusions illustrated here. (*From* Hebbel RP. Adhesive interactions of sickle erythrocytes with endothelium. J Clin Invest 1997;99:2563, Fig. 2. © the American Society for Clinical Investigation; with permission.)

adhesion followed promptly, with the determination that the degree of SRBC adhesivity correlates with vaso-occlusive severity of disease.[50] It subsequently was demonstrated that acute vaso-occlusion occurs as a 2-step process initiated by the adhesion of a stickier subset of SRBC and completed by the physical trapping of a more rigid, polymerization-prone subset.[51,52] In these studies, human SRBC were separated according to density and fractions studied in an ex vivo rat mesocecum flow system, in which intravital microscopy was used to assess the adherence of SRBC and the pressure resistance units were measured to detect flow obstruction in the microcirculation. Infusion of low-density SRBC resulted in adherence but not obstruction of flow; infusion of high-density SRBC resulted in neither adherence nor obstruction of flow; and sequential infusion of low-density followed by high-density SRBC resulted in both adherence and obstruction of flow. This discovery suggested that the preceding 79 years of sickle cell research had been focused on the second step of vaso-occlusion and established SRBC adhesion as a valid initial target for sickle cell research and therapy. In this regard, therapies that abrogate SRBC adhesion have a major impact on SRBC flow in vitro, ex vivo, in mouse models of SCD, and in patients with SCD.[32,53–55] The chronic expression of an SRBC-binding adhesion molecule, P-selectin,[56] on the vascular endothelium in sickle cell mouse models[57] and human endothelial cells from sickle cell patients[58] supports the notion that adhesion-mediated chronic drag on SRBC flow might account for the chronically abnormal microcirculatory blood flow in animal models and patients with SCD.[19–22,59]

CELLULAR MECHANISMS OF SRBC ADHESION

Based on results from experiments using bone marrow transplantation of sickle cell mouse bone marrow[60] to C57BL control mice and aggressive methods of endothelial activation with high doses of tumor necrosis factor (TNF)-α in vivo, it was concluded that leukocyte adhesion to the endothelium precedes and mediates SRBC adhesion.[61] Follow-on considerations posited that heterocellular aggregates also contribute to abnormalities of blood flow.[62] The possible relevance of these adhesion mechanisms to blood rheology notwithstanding, direct adhesion of SRBC to the endothelium independent of leukocytes is well established in the vascular perturbation of SCD,[63–67] and argues against the hypothesis that leukocyte adhesion must precede SRBC adhesion.

MOLECULAR MECHANISMS OF CELL ADHESION

The process of leukocyte adhesion to the endothelium during the inflammation is understood in great detail[4] and serves as a model for deciphering SRBC adhesion to endothelial cells. Pioneering studies disclosed that during inflammation leukocyte adhesion uses a cascade of adhesion molecules, triggered by initial contact with selectins and completed by firm adhesion to molecules of other types.[68–70] Among the selectins, P-selectin has been found to be initiatory in the adhesion cascade,[68] predominant over the other selectins,[71] and essential for a complete inflammatory response.[72] Downstream molecules that mediate firm adhesion and transendothelial migration of leukocytes are members of the integrin family and immunoglobulin superfamily.[4,73] Those molecules have considerable overlap in their function, which makes it unlikely that absence or inhibition of any one of these would abrogate their aggregate function. These considerations define P-selectin as the initiatory linchpin molecule for leukocyte adhesion to the vascular endothelium.

The selectin family of cytoadhesion molecules consist of P-selectin, E-selectin, and L-selectin, each of which mediates cytoadhesion through Ca^{2+}-dependent recognition of specific cell surface carbohydrates.[74,75] P-selectin requires fucose and sialic acid in its recognition determinant; its glycan ligand, PSGL-1, has sialyl Lewis X (sLeX) in close proximity to sulfated tyrosine near the amino terminus of the ligand.[74–77] Adhesion by any of the selectins requires hydrodynamic shear stress and is nonexistent in the absence of flow.[78,79] Expression of P-selectin on the surface of platelets and endothelial cells requires their activation.[74,80] The prompt translocation of P-selectin from α storage granules within platelets to the cell surface is induced by the rapid-acting secretagogue thrombin[81]; thrombin, histamine, complement components, oxygen radicals, phorbol esters, calcium ionophores, hypoxia, hypoxia/reoxygenation, and heme induce the rapid translocation of P-selectin from the Weibel-Palade body storage granules in endothelial cells to the surface of those cells.[74,80,82–86] Constitutive transcription of P-selectin within endothelial cells supplies Weibel-Palade bodies with the molecule, and induction of more rapid transcription[74,82] may overload the Weibel-Palade bodies, resulting in chronic surface expression of P-selectin.[87]

Initial reviews of the therapeutic potential of blocking SRBC adhesion did not include a molecular cascade mechanism,[88,89] as selectins had not been tested for SRBC adhesivity. Subsequent studies established that endothelial P-selectin mediates abnormal static adhesion and rolling adhesion of SRBC in vitro, as shown in **Fig. 2**,[56,90] and that this SRBC adhesion to endothelial P-selectin can be prevented in vitro using approved P-selectin–blocking therapeutic agents.[90,91] Induction of endothelial P-selectin expression with an N-terminal peptide of protease-activated receptor-1, which selectively activates mouse endothelial cells but not mouse platelets,[92] triggered prompt SRBC adhesion and acute stoppage of blood flow in the microcirculation of sickle cell chimeric mice.[66] These in vivo adhesion studies were rigorously controlled by use of a combination of leukocyte adhesion–blocking

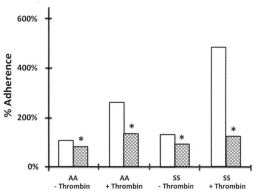

Fig. 2. Effect of P-selectin antibodies on the adherence of nonsickle and sickle erythrocytes to human umbilical vein endothelial cells (HUVEC) treated with or without thrombin. The data shown indicate the static adherence of red blood cells (RBC) to HUVEC that were treated with thrombin or medium alone and then exposed to medium with or without P-selectin–blocking antibody 9E1. The 100% adherence level is the mean number of non-sickle (AA) RBC/field adherent to untreated HUVEC. SS, sickle erythrocytes. The reduction of erythrocyte adherence to untreated or thrombin-treated HUVEC is shown in the presence (*hatched bars*) or absence (*open bars*) of monoclonal antibody (mAb) 9E1. The data are mean percent adherence from 12 replicate experiments. Significant inhibition of adherence (*P*<.05) due to mAb 9E1 is denoted by an asterisk. (*From* Matsui NM, Borsig L, Rosen SD, et al. P-selectin mediates the adhesion of sickle erythrocytes to the endothelium. Blood 2001;98:1957, Fig. 1A. © the American Society of Hematology; with permission.)

antibodies, tagging leukocytes with rhodamine 6G, and careful visual and video monitoring for leukocyte adhesion, which established that leukocyte adhesion was not involved in the SRBC adhesion measured. Preliminary attempts to identify the ligand for P-selectin on SRBC detected no PSGL-1, abnormally increased amounts of sLeX, and an absolute dependence on sLeX for SRBC rolling on immobilized P-selectin, whether the sLeX was on glycolipids or O-linked, N-linked, or PI-linked glycoproteins.[93] Numerous other adhesion molecules also have been described as participants in SRBC adhesion,[27,94,95] which is in accordance with multifactorial completion of SRBC adhesion.[33] The initiatory role of P-selectin in SRBC adhesion to the endothelium suggests a strong therapeutic potential for blocking this molecule.

CHRONIC EXPRESSION OF ENDOTHELIAL P-SELECTIN IN SCD

The rapid transfer of P-selectin to the surface of endothelial cells and initiatory role of P-selectin in SRBC adhesion together suggest a role for endothelial P-selectin in acute vaso-occlusion; the chronic endothelial expression of P-selectin on the endothelium in sickle cell mouse models[57] and circulating endothelial cells in human SCD patients[58] has entirely different rheologic implications. Persistent endothelial presentation of P-selectin likely accounts for the slower microcirculatory flow velocity in sickle cell chimeric mice with sickle cell mouse hosts compared with chimeras with P-selectin knockout mouse hosts, as shown in **Fig. 3**.[66] In addition, intravenous administration of subanticoagulant but P-selectin–blocking doses of heparin[91] to patients with SCD resulted in an immediate and prolonged increase in blood-flow velocity.[55] This evidence from animal SCD models and human SCD patients of endothelial P-selectin causing a chronic drag on microcirculatory flow, a circulation particularly susceptible to the influence of adhesion processes,[30] has been challenged by the notion that

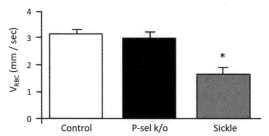

Fig. 3. Baseline red blood cell (RBC) velocity (VRBC) of substituted rhodamine isothiocyanate (XRITC)-labeled sickle RBC injected into mouse recipients expected to have different levels of endothelial P-selectin expression. Computer-assisted intravital microscopy flow data from visualization of 20- to 40-μm diameter mucosal-intestinal venules are represented as the average VRBC of XRITC-labeled RBC. Labeled sickle RBC were injected intravenously into C57BL/6 (Control; n = 24), P-selectin knockout (P-sel k/o; n = 9), and sickle cell mice (Sickle; n = 10). The error bars indicate the standard error of the mean. Asterisk indicates a statistically significant difference (P<.05) from the other groups. (*From* Embury SH, Matsui NM, Ramanujam S, et al. The contribution of endothelial cell P-selectin to the microvascular flow of mouse sickle erythrocytes in vivo. Blood 2004;104:3380, Fig. 1. © the American Society of Hematology; with permission.)

human endothelial cells are incapable of transcriptionally regulated expression of P-selectin.[96] That claim is based on results using tumor necrosis factor α, interleukin-1β, or lipopolysaccharide as human endothelial cell agonists. Because P-selectin transcription in human endothelial cells is driven successfully by interleukin-3, interleukin-4, or oncostatin M,[97,98] a group of cytokine agonists that also are germane to SCD, this challenge does not invalidate the concept that chronic P-selectin expression on human endothelium slows microcirculatory SRBC flow in SCD patients. Moreover, persistent cycling of P-selectin translocation, endocytosis, and reexpression on the cell surface[99] can be driven by rapid-acting P-selectin agonists, such as thrombin and reactive oxygen species (ROS), which are increased in patients with SCD.[8,26,85] Moreover, the adhesion of SRBC to endothelial cells results in increased levels of ROS within the endothelial cells,[100] and increased ROS within endothelial cells upregulates the expression of P-selectin on the cell surface.[85] In this regard, the mere act of SRBC adhesion creates a positive feedback cycle of SRBC-endothelial adhesion. Detectable evidence of this perturbation evolves from the increased transcription of soluble vascular cell adhesion molecule 1 (sVCAM-1) resulting from the increased endothelial ROS,[101] and the predicted increased plasma levels of sVCAM-1.

P-selectin on the microvascular endothelium of patients with SCD presents an opportunity for therapeutic intervention.

THERAPEUTIC AND COMMERCIAL POTENTIAL OF P-SELECTIN BLOCKING

The foregoing discussion presents a coherent background for the application of adhesion-blocking agents for the treatment of SCD. Antiadhesion therapy is also justified by numerous reports and reviews on the subject,[102–104] and by inclusion of this mechanism in discussions of other therapeutic strategies such as overcoming arginase effects,[105] improving redox abnormalities with L-glutamine,[106] and the use of statins[107] or nitric oxide.[108] The commercial potential in the sickle cell space is demonstrated by the recent exclusive licensing agreement between Pfizer and Glycomimetics worth up to $340 million for a selectin-blocking agent, exclusive option for Novartis to acquire Selexys and their P-selectin monoclonal antibody for $665 million, and the $47 million investment by Third Rock Ventures in Global Blood Therapeutics.

CONSIDERATIONS FOR DEVELOPMENT OF ANTIADHESION THERAPIES

Considerations for the development of pharmaceutical agents include the therapeutic target and route of delivery for new agents. A basic decision for developing antiadhesion agents for SCD therapy is whether to treat vaso-occlusive pain crises or prevent them. The multiple mechanisms involved once vaso-occlusion is completed[27,33] argue against the use of a monospecific adhesion-blocking agent for the treatment of established pain crises. Based on this thinking, another cautionary argument can be made against the use of agents that block only the initiatory molecules, the selectins, for the treatment of established pain crises. The dependence of selectin adhesivity on shear stress[78,79] suggests that blocking these molecules for the treatment of an event caused by stoppage of blood flow has questionable potential. Treatment of established pain crises with a nonspecific adhesion blocker would redress more of the adhesive processes that initiate vaso-occlusion, but an effect on the physical trapping of rigid SRBC is unlikely. Testing the efficacy of agents that target the treatment of established SCD pain crises uses measurements of the duration and intensity of pain, duration of hospitalization, and opioid use.

The use of antiadhesion therapy for prophylaxis of pain crisis has much to recommend it, particularly blocking P-selectin, which is chronically expressed and initiates acute vaso-occlusion. A possible exception to targeting only selectins for prophylaxis of vaso-occlusion derives from a study in sickle cell mice in which platelet-activating factor–induced SRBC adhesion and vaso-occlusion was prevented by pretreatment with a monoclonal antibody against $\alpha V\beta 3$ integrin.[53] To the extent that leukocyte-endothelial adhesion and heterocellular aggregates contribute to impaired blood flow, both processes involve P-selectin–mediated adhesion,[36,71,109–113] which suggests that their possible detrimental effects would likely be overcome by P-selectin–blocking drugs.[114]

Regarding routes of administration, parenteral administration is well suited for inpatient treatment of pain crises, but less so for outpatient pain management. Prophylactic therapy is necessarily conducted in an outpatient setting, the success of which is strongly dependent on patient adherence.[115,116] Patients prefer oral administration to injections or infusions for outpatient therapy,[115–118] and programs for enhancing patient adherence to oral outpatient therapy have been developed.[115] Patients adhere more to once-daily oral therapy than to divided oral doses.[116] Testing the efficacy of antiadhesion agents used for the prophylaxis of SCD pain crises uses measurements of the frequency of pain and possibly also of daily pain scores, health care utilization, opioid use, microvascular blood flow, and markers of vascular injury. In the last regard, the plasma level of sVCAM-1 is an especially sensitive and robust marker for antiadhesion agents, as blocking SRBC adhesion to endothelial cells reduces levels of ROS within endothelial cells[100] and consequent P-selectin on endothelial cell surfaces[85] and VCAM-1 synthesis.[101]

ANTIADHESIVE AGENTS UNDER DEVELOPMENT OR CONSIDERATION FOR TREATING SCD

Several antiadhesive agents have been created for use in treating SCD, and other P-selectin blockers have such potential.

GMI-1070 is a small molecule glycomimetic compound that was synthesized using a rational design strategy intended to block selectin-mediated adhesion.[119] This compound, which must be administered by injection, is being applied to the treatment of established acute pain crises in patients with SCD. The drug inhibits adhesion of sLeA or sLeX to E-, P- and L-selectins with IC_{50}s of 4.3, 423, and 337 mM, respectively.[120] Its negligible effect on P-selectin may be a consideration for this drug if leukocyte adhesion is important to vaso-occlusion, because it has been shown in a mouse SCD model that leukocyte-endothelial adhesion is mediated by P-selectin but not E-selectin.[36] GMI-1070 had no detectable effect on blood flow in patients with SCD.[121] A phase 2 clinical trial with end points of reducing the severity and duration of pain crises and duration of hospitalization was encouraging, and the drug will therefore undergo phase 3 study.

SelG1 is a humanized P-selectin monoclonal antibody[122] that has a $t_{1/2}$ in the circulation of 2 weeks. It must be administered intravenously. SelG1 is being applied to the prophylaxis of acute pain crises in patients with SCD. No phase 1 results are available as of the time of this writing. A multicenter phase 2 trial is being planned, in which the drug will be administered as a 100-mL infusion monthly for 1 year, with an end point of reducing the frequency of pain crises.

MST-188 is a nonionic block copolymer surfactant that binds to hydrophobic surfaces of damaged cells to block cell-cell adhesion through a broadly specific mechanism.[123,124] It is administered by 48-hour intravenous infusion and is being applied to the treatment of established acute pain crises in patients with SCD. Results from a phase 3 clinical trial demonstrated improved microvascular blood flow[125] and more rapid resolution of pain crises in comparison with placebo, particularly in children.[126] This drug will undergo a second phase 3 trial in pediatric SCD patients.

Heparin is an injectable anticoagulant that had been in the clinic for decades before it was found to have effective P- and L-selectin–blocking activity.[127] Subsequent studies revealed that unfractionated heparin blocked L-selectin at concentrations one-tenth that of anticoagulant concentrations, and P-selectin at one-tenth yet lower concentrations.[91] Thus there is a large therapeutic window that avoids hemorrhagic risks. These studies also revealed that unfractionated heparin had 100-fold greater P-selectin–blocking activity than 2 commercially available low molecular weight heparins. Intravenous administration of subanticoagulant but P-selectin–blocking doses of unfractionated heparin to patients with SCD resulted in prompt sustained increases in velocity of microvascular blood flow.[55] The low concentrations of heparin needed for P-selectin blocking support its use as prophylactic therapy, but its requirement for injectable administration hinders this application. In this regard, an oral formulation called SNAC heparin showed anticoagulant and antithrombotic activity when administered orally,[128] and could have been a candidate for prophylactic therapy for SCD. However, it did not meet its primary end point in a phase 3 clinical trial for the prevention of postoperative thrombosis,[129] and its development was not continued. Low molecular weight heparins are under consideration for the treatment of SCD[130] (ClinTrials.gov: NCT01419977).

Pentosan polysulfate sodium (PPS) is a semisynthetic hypersulfated polyxylan[131] that has been approved in the United States for use as an oral agent since 1996. It is an effective blocker of cell adhesion to P-selectin[132] and is more effective than heparin as a blocker of molecular P-selectin adhesion.[55] Its safety in humans has been established by 17 years on the market and no requirement for change in its Food and Drug Administration safety information since 2008.[133] Administered as a single oral dose, PPS has normalized microvascular blood flow in patients with SCD for a period of 8 but not 24 hours, a duration of activity commensurate with the reported 2-hour T_{max} of PPS[134]; administered as single daily doses it reduced plasma levels of sVCAM-1, a reliable marker of vascular injury, in SCD patients who took the drug for at least 8 weeks.[55]

PSI-697 is an orally available noncarbohydrate and nonantibody inhibitor of P-selectin that, curiously, has little blocking activity in vitro and greater activity in vivo.[135,136] Its clinical trials as an antithrombotic were not positive, and its clinical development is not active at present. A similar compound, PSI-421, had certain advantages as a P-selectin blocker,[137] but its development also is not active.

ARC-5690, a single-stranded oligonucleotide aptamer that binds P-selectin with high affinity and specificity, inhibited the adhesion of SRBC and leukocytes to endothelial cells, increased microvascular flow velocities, and reduced mortality in SCD mice under hypoxic conditions.[67] Its use as a therapeutic agent is challenged by its exceptionally short half-life in the circulation.

Recombinant human P-selectin glycoprotein ligand-1 immunoglobulin (rPSGL-Ig) chimera is produced in modified Chinese hamster ovary cells,[138] blocks adhesion to P-selectin, and in preclinical studies retarded inflammation, thrombosis, and hemostasis. It must be administered parenterally. In a phase 2 clinical trial of acute myocardial infarction outcome, rPSGL-Ig chimera did not meet its primary end point.[139] It is no longer in active development.

PERSPECTIVE

The foregoing discussion includes different conclusions regarding the importance of P-selectin and E-selectin in the adhesion that leads to abnormal sickle cell blood flow and different approaches to antiadhesion-based therapy. Although the reasons for these differences have not been examined systematically, biological and pharmacologic variations may be less likely than variations in experimental design to account for these differences. Such disparities include the agonists and conditions used to activate endothelial cells and the pathophysiologic severity of the types of sickle cell mice used. For instance, endothelial cell activation has been accomplished with a variety of agonists and conditions, including TNF-α,[61] hypoxia/reoxygenation,[36] platelet-activating factor,[140] and PAR-1 agonist peptide.[66] There also has been great variance in the pathophysiologic severity of the sickle cell mice used, which has included C57BL mice that had undergone transplantation with bone marrow from the pathophysiologically severe Paszty or Berk mice,[60,61] SAD and NY sickle cell mice that have less severe pathophysiology,[141] and a chimeric sickle mouse system in which host Paszty mice, C57BL control mice, or P-selectin knockout mice were transfused with SRBC from Paszty mice.[60,66,72] Until such time that these experimental systems have been rigorously vetted, it might be judicious to consider the experimental systems as provisos in divergent conclusions.

SUMMARY

The development of novel therapeutic approaches to SCD remains an unmet need. In this regard, in addition to antisickling therapies (via fetal hemoglobin induction or other approaches), it has become clear that targeting phenomena downstream from the Gordian knot of deoxyhemoglobin-S polymerization has a definite role in ameliorating the clinical severity of the disease, decreasing morbidity, and improving the quality of life. Targeting impaired microvascular blood flow by decreasing SRBC adhesion has been shown to improve flow in vitro, in experimental animals, and in human patients. P-selectin as the initiator of SRBC and white blood cell adhesion to the endothelium is an attractive target. It is encouraging to see a multitude of antiselectin therapies in clinical trials. An important consideration for drugs being developed is the ease of administration and patient adherence of a particular drug (oral vs parenteral) and the intended application of new agents (prophylaxis vs treatment of acute pain crises). The next few years are likely to provide important information on these issues.

REFERENCES

1. McEver RP. Adhesive interactions of leukocytes, platelets, and the vessel wall during hemostasis and inflammation. Thromb Haemost 2001;86:746–56.
2. McEver RP. Selectins: lectins that initiate cell adhesion under flow. Curr Opin Cell Biol 2002;14:581–6.
3. Vandendries ER, Furie BC, Furie B. Role of P-selectin and PSGL-1 in coagulation and thrombosis. Thromb Haemost 2004;92:459–66.
4. Ley K, Laudanna C, Cybulsky MI, et al. Getting to the site of inflammation: the leukocyte adhesion cascade updated. Nat Rev Immunol 2007;7:678–89.
5. Klug PP, Lessin LS, Radice P. Rheological aspects of sickle cell disease. Arch Intern Med 1974;133:577–90.
6. Thomas AN, Pattison C, Serjeant GR. Causes of death in sickle-cell disease in Jamaica. Br Med J (Clin Res Ed) 1982;285:633–5.
7. Powars D, Chan LS, Schroeder WA. The variable expression of sickle cell disease is genetically determined. Semin Hematol 1990;27:360–76.
8. Francis RB Jr, Johnson CS. Vascular occlusion in sickle cell disease: current concepts and unanswered questions. Blood 1991;77:1405–14.
9. Chien S. The Benjamin W. Zweifach Award Lecture. Blood cell deformability and interactions: from molecules to micromechanics and microcirculation. Microvasc Res 1992;44:243–54.
10. Francis RB. Large-vessel occlusion in sickle cell disease: pathogenesis, clinical consequences, and therapeutic implications. Med Hypotheses 1991;35: 88–95.
11. Hillery CA, Panepinto JA. Pathophysiology of stroke in sickle cell disease. Microcirculation 2004;11:195–208.
12. Embury SH, Hebbel RP, Mohandas N, et al. Pathogenesis of vasoocclusion. In: Embury SH, Hebbel RP, Mohandas N, et al, editors. Sickle cell disease: basic principles and clinical practice. New York: Raven Press; 1994. p. 311–26.
13. Embury SH. The not-so-simple process of sickle cell vasoocclusion. Microcirculation 2004;11:101–13.
14. Ballas SK, Mohandas N. Sickle red cell microrheology and sickle blood rheology. Microcirculation 2004;11:209–25.
15. Platt OS, Brambilla DJ, Rosse WF, et al. Mortality in sickle cell disease: life expectancy and risk factors for early death. N Engl J Med 1994;330: 1639–44.
16. Powars DR, Chan LS, Hiti A, et al. Outcome of sickle cell anemia: a 4-decade observational study of 1056 patients. Medicine (Baltimore) 2005;84:363–76.
17. van Tuijn CF, van Beers EJ, Schnog JJ, et al. Pain rate and social circumstances rather than cumulative organ damage determine the quality of life in adults with sickle cell disease. Am J Hematol 2010;85:532–5.
18. Platt OS, Thorington BD, Brambilla DJ, et al. Pain in sickle cell disease: rates and risk factors. N Engl J Med 1991;325:11–6.
19. Rodgers GP, Schechter AN, Noguchi CT, et al. Periodic microcirculatory flow in patients with sickle-cell disease. N Engl J Med 1984;311:1534–8.
20. Lipowsky HH, Sheikh NU, Katz DM. Intravital microscopy of capillary microdynamics in sickle cell disease. J Clin Invest 1987;80:117–27.

21. Cheung AT, Chen PC, Larkin EC, et al. Microvascular abnormalities in sickle cell disease: a computer-assisted intravital microscopy study. Blood 2002;99: 3999–4005.
22. Rodgers GP, Schechter AN, Noguchi CT, et al. Microcirculatory adaptations in sickle cell anemia: reactive hyperemia response. Am J Physiol 1990;258:H113–20.
23. Francis RB Jr, Hebbel RP. Hemostasis. In: Embury SH, Hebbel RP, Mohandas N, et al, editors. Sickle cell disease: basic principles and clinical practice. New York: Raven Press; 1994. p. 299–310.
24. Tomer A, Harker LA, Kasey S, et al. Thrombogenesis in sickle cell disease. J Lab Clin Med 2001;137:398–407.
25. Ataga KI, Orringer EP. Hypercoagulability in sickle cell disease: a curious paradox. Am J Med 2003;115:721–8.
26. Nur E, Biemond BJ, Otten HM, et al. Oxidative stress in sickle cell disease; pathophysiology and potential implications for disease management. Am J Hematol 2011;86:484–9.
27. Hebbel RP, Osarogiagbon R, Kaul D. The endothelial biology of sickle cell disease: inflammation and a chronic vasculopathy. Microcirculation 2004;11:129–51.
28. Okpala I. Leukocyte adhesion and the pathophysiology of sickle cell disease. Curr Opin Hematol 2006;13:40–4.
29. Kato GJ, Gladwin MT, Steinberg MH. Deconstructing sickle cell disease: reappraisal of the role of hemolysis in the development of clinical subphenotypes. Blood Rev 2007;21:37–47.
30. Hebbel RP. Adhesive interactions of sickle erythrocytes with endothelium. J Clin Invest 1997;99:2561–4.
31. Conran N, Costa FF. Hemoglobin disorders and endothelial cell interactions. Clin Biochem 2009;42:1824–38.
32. Lei H, Karniadakis GE. Quantifying the rheological and hemodynamic characteristics of sickle cell anemia. Biophys J 2012;102:185–94.
33. Kaul D. Sickle cell disease. In: Tuma RF, Durán WN, Ley K, editors. Handbook of physiology: microcirculation. Amsterdam: Academic Press; 2008. p. 769–93.
34. Ferrone FA. Polymerization and sickle cell disease: a molecular view. Microcirculation 2004;11:115–28.
35. Wallace KL, Linden J. Adenosine A2A receptors induced on iNKT and NK cells reduce pulmonary inflammation and injury in mice with sickle cell disease. Blood 2010;116:5010–20.
36. Kaul DK, Hebbel RP. Hypoxia/reoxygenation causes inflammatory response in transgenic sickle mice but not in normal mice. J Clin Invest 2000;106:411–20.
37. Horne MK. Sickle cell anemia as a rheologic disease. Am J Med 1981;70: 288–98.
38. Hebbel RP, Vercellotti GM. The endothelial biology of sickle cell disease. J Lab Clin Med 1997;129:288–93.
39. Coates TD. So what if blood is thicker than water? Blood 2011;117:745–6.
40. Alexy T, Pais E, Armstrong JK, et al. Rheologic behavior of sickle and normal red blood cell mixtures in sickle plasma: implications for transfusion therapy. Transfusion 2006;46:912–8.
41. Hulbert ML, McKinstry RC, Lacey JL, et al. Silent cerebral infarcts occur despite regular blood transfusion therapy after first strokes in children with sickle cell disease. Blood 2011;117:772–9.
42. Schmalzer EA, Lee JO, Brown AK, et al. Viscosity of mixtures of sickle and normal red cells at varying hematocrit levels: implications for transfusion. Transfusion 1987;27:228–33.

43. Detterich J, Alexy T, Rabai M, et al. Low-shear red blood cell oxygen transport effectiveness is adversely affected by transfusion and further worsened by deoxygenation in sickle cell disease patients on chronic transfusion therapy. Transfusion 2013;53(2):297–305.

44. Usami S, Chien S, Bertles JF. Deformability of sickle cells as studied by microsieving. J Lab Clin Med 1975;86:274–9.

45. Lipowsky HH, Usami S, Chien S. Human SS red cell rheologic behavior in the microcirculation of cremaster muscle. Blood Cells 1982;8:113–26.

46. Nash GB, Johnson CS, Meiselman HJ. Influence of oxygen tension on the viscoelastic behavior of red blood cells in sickle cell disease. Blood 1986; 67:110–8.

47. Itoh T, Chien S, Usami S. Effects of hemoglobin concentration on deformability of individual sickle cells after deoxygenation. Blood 1995;85:2245–53.

48. Hoover R, Rubin R, Wise G, et al. Adhesion of normal sickle erythrocytes to endothelial monolayer cultures. Blood 1979;54:872–6.

49. Hebbel RP, Yamada O, Moldow CF, et al. Abnormal adherence of sickle erythrocytes to cultured vascular endothelium. Possible mechanism for microvascular occlusion in sickle cell disease. J Clin Invest 1980;65:154–60.

50. Hebbel RP, Boogaerts MA, Eaton JW, et al. Erythrocyte adherence to endothelium in sickle-cell anemia. N Engl J Med 1980;302:992–5.

51. Kaul DK, Fabry ME, Nagel RL. Erythrocytic and vascular factors influencing the microcirculatory behavior of blood in sickle cell anemia. Ann N Y Acad Sci 1989; 565:316–26.

52. Kaul DK, Fabry ME, Nagel RL. Microvascular sites and characteristics of sickle cell adhesion to vascular endothelium in shear flow conditions: pathophysiological implications. Proc Natl Acad Sci U S A 1989;86:3356–60.

53. Kaul DK, Tsai HM, Liu XD, et al. Monoclonal antibodies to alphaVbeta3 (7E3 and LM609) inhibit sickle red blood cell-endothelium interactions induced by platelet-activating factor. Blood 2000;95:368–74.

54. Kaul DK, Liu X, Nagel RL. Ameliorating effects of fluorocarbon emulsion on sickle red blood cell-induced obstruction in an ex vivo vasculature. Blood 2001;98:3128–31.

55. Kutlar A, Ataga KI, McMahon L, et al. A potent oral P-selectin blocking agent improves microcirculatory blood flow and a marker of endothelial cell injury in patients with sickle cell disease. Am J Hematol 2012;87:536–9.

56. Matsui NM, Borsig L, Rosen SD, et al. P-selectin mediates the adhesion of sickle erythrocytes to the endothelium. Blood 2001;98:1955–62.

57. Wood K, Russell J, Hebbel RP, et al. Differential expression of E- and P-selectin in the microvasculature of sickle cell transgenic mice. Microcirculation 2004;11: 377–85.

58. Solovey A, Lin Y, Browne P, et al. Circulating activated endothelial cells in sickle cell anemia. N Engl J Med 1997;337:1584–9.

59. Embury SH, Mohandas N, Paszty C, et al. In vivo blood flow abnormalities in the transgenic knockout sickle cell mouse. J Clin Invest 1999;103:915–20.

60. Paszty C, Brion CM, Manci E, et al. Transgenic knockout mice with exclusively human sickle hemoglobin and sickle cell disease. Science 1997;278:876–8.

61. Turhan A, Weiss LA, Mohandas N, et al. Primary role for adherent leukocytes in sickle cell vascular occlusion: a new paradigm. Proc Natl Acad Sci U S A 2002; 99:3047–51.

62. Frenette PS. Sickle cell vasoocclusion: heterotypic, multicellular aggregations driven by leukocyte adhesion. Microcirculation 2004;11:167–77.

63. French JA, Kenny D, Scott JP, et al. Mechanisms of stroke in sickle cell disease: sickle erythrocytes decrease cerebral blood flow in rats after nitric oxide synthase inhibition. Blood 1997;89:4591–9.

64. Lutty GA, Taomoto M, Cao J, et al. Inhibition of TNF-alpha-induced sickle RBC retention in retina by a VLA-4 antagonist. Invest Ophthalmol Vis Sci 2001;42:1349–55.

65. Lutty GA, Otsuji T, Taomoto M, et al. Mechanisms for sickle red blood cell retention in choroid. Curr Eye Res 2002;25:163–71.

66. Embury SH, Matsui NM, Ramanujam S, et al. The contribution of endothelial cell P-selectin to the microvascular flow of mouse sickle erythrocytes in vivo. Blood 2004;104:3378–85.

67. Gutsaeva DR, Parkerson JB, Yerigenahally SD, et al. Inhibition of cell adhesion by anti-P-selectin aptamer: a new potential therapeutic agent for sickle cell disease. Blood 2011;117:727–35.

68. Lawrence MB, Springer TA. Leukocytes roll on a selectin at physiologic flow rates: distinction from and prerequisite for adhesion through integrins. Cell 1991;65:859–73.

69. Springer TA. Traffic signals for lymphocyte recirculation and leukocyte emigration: the multistep paradigm. Cell 1994;76:301–14.

70. Lasky LA. Selectin-carbohydrate interactions and the initiation of the inflammatory response. Annu Rev Biochem 1995;64:113–39.

71. Robinson SD, Frenette PS, Rayburn H, et al. Multiple, targeted deficiencies in selectins reveal a predominant role for P-selectin in leukocyte recruitment. Proc Natl Acad Sci U S A 1999;96:11452–7.

72. Mayadas TN, Johnson RC, Rayburn H, et al. Leukocyte rolling and extravasation are severely compromised in P selectin-deficient mice. Cell 1993;74:541–54.

73. Konstantopoulos K, McIntire LV. Effects of fluid dynamic forces on vascular cell adhesion. J Clin Invest 1996;98:2661–5.

74. McEver RP. Selectins. Curr Opin Immunol 1994;6:75–84.

75. Kansas GS. Selectins and their ligands: current concepts and controversies. Blood 1996;88:3259–87.

76. Sako D, Comess KM, Barone KM, et al. A sulfated peptide segment at the amino terminus of PSGL-1 is critical for P-selectin binding. Cell 1995;83:323–31.

77. Furie B, Furie BC. The molecular basis of platelet and endothelial cell interaction with neutrophils and monocytes: role of P-selectin and the P-selectin ligand, PSGL-1. Thromb Haemost 1995;74:224–7.

78. Finger EB, Puri KD, Alon R, et al. Adhesion through L-selectin requires a threshold hydrodynamic shear. Nature 1996;379:266–9.

79. Lawrence MB, Kansas GS, Kunkel EJ, et al. Threshold levels of fluid shear promote leukocyte adhesion through selectins (CD62L, P,E). J Cell Biol 1997;136: 717–27.

80. Bullard DC. P- and E-selectin. In: Ley K, editor. Adhesion molecules: function and inhibition. Basel (Switzerland): Birkhäuser Verlag AG; 2007. p. 71–95.

81. Stenberg PE, McEver RP, Shuman MA, et al. A platelet alpha-granule membrane protein (GMP-140) is expressed on the plasma membrane after activation. J Cell Biol 1985;101:880–6.

82. McEver RP. Regulation of expression of E-selectin and P-selectin. In: Vestweber D, editor. The selectins: initiators of leukocyte endothelial adhesion. Amsterdam: Harwood; 1997. p. 31–47.

83. Belcher JD, Nguyen J, Chen C, et al. Plasma hemoglobin and heme trigger Weibel Palade body exocytosis and vaso-occlusion in transgenic sickle mice. Blood 2011;118:896A.

84. Silverstein RL. The vascular endothelium. In: Gallin JI, Snyderman R, editors. Inflammation: basic principles and clinical correlates. Philadelphia: Lippincott Williams & Wilkins; 1999. p. 207–25.

85. Takano M, Meneshian A, Sheikh E, et al. Rapid upregulation of endothelial P-selectin expression via reactive oxygen species generation. Am J Physiol Heart Circ Physiol 2002;283:H2054–61.

86. Pinsky DJ, Naka Y, Liao H, et al. Hypoxia-induced exocytosis of endothelial cell Weibel-Palade bodies. A mechanism for rapid neutrophil recruitment after cardiac preservation. J Clin Invest 1996;97:493–500.

87. Hahne M, Jager U, Isenmann S, et al. Five tumor necrosis factor-inducible cell adhesion mechanisms on the surface of mouse endothelioma cells mediate the binding of leukocytes. J Cell Biol 1993;121:655–64.

88. Harlan JM. Introduction: anti-adhesion therapy in sickle cell disease. Blood 2000;95:365–7.

89. Hebbel RP. Clinical implications of basic research: blockade of adhesion of sickle cells to endothelium by monoclonal antibodies. N Engl J Med 2000; 342:1910–2.

90. Matsui NM, Varki A, Embury SH. Heparin inhibits the flow adhesion of sickle red blood cells to P-selectin. Blood 2002;100:3790–6.

91. Koenig A, Norgard-Sumnicht K, Linhardt R, et al. Differential interactions of heparin and heparan sulfate glycosaminoglycans with the selectins. Implications for the use of unfractionated and low molecular weight heparins as therapeutic agents. J Clin Invest 1998;101:877–89.

92. Coughlin SR. Thrombin signalling and protease-activated receptors. Nature 2000;407:258–64.

93. Embury SH, Baran CE, Hefner CA, et al. The nature of P-selectin ligands on sickle cells. Blood 2004;104(Suppl 1):107a [abstract# 363].

94. Telen MJ. Red blood cell surface adhesion molecules: their possible roles in normal human physiology and disease. Semin Hematol 2000;37:130–42.

95. Johnson C, Telen M. Adhesion molecules and hydroxyurea in the pathophysiology of sickle cell disease. Haematologica 2008;93:481–6.

96. Yao L, Setiadi H, Xia L, et al. Divergent inducible expression of P-selectin and E-selectin in mice and primates. Blood 1999;94:3820–8.

97. Khew-Goodall Y, Butcher CM, Litwin MS, et al. Chronic expression of P-selectin on endothelial cells stimulated by the T-cell cytokine, interleukin-3. Blood 1996; 87:1432–8.

98. Yao L, Pan J, Setiadi H, et al. Interleukin 4 or oncostatin M induces a prolonged increase in P-selectin mRNA and protein in human endothelial cells. J Exp Med 1996;184:81–92.

99. Subramaniam M, Koedam JA, Wagner DD. Divergent fates of P- and E-selectins after their expression on the plasma membrane. Mol Biol Cell 1993;4:791–801.

100. Sultana C, Shen Y, Rattan V, et al. Interaction of sickle erythrocytes with endothelial cells in the presence of endothelial cell conditioned medium induces oxidant stress leading to transendothelial migration of monocytes. Blood 1998;92:3924–35.

101. Marui N, Offermann MK, Swerlick R, et al. Vascular cell adhesion molecule-1 (VCAM-1) gene transcription and expression are regulated through an antioxidant-sensitive mechanism in human vascular endothelial cells. J Clin Invest 1993;92:1866–74.

102. Ulbrich H, Eriksson EE, Lindbom L. Leukocyte and endothelial cell adhesion molecules as targets for therapeutic interventions in inflammatory disease. Trends Pharmacol Sci 2003;24:640–7.

103. Ludwig RJ, Schon MP, Boehncke WH. P-selectin: a common therapeutic target for cardiovascular disorders, inflammation and tumour metastasis. Expert Opin Ther Targets 2007;11:1103–17.

104. Hebbel RP, Vercellotti G, Nath KA. A systems biology consideration of the vasculopathy of sickle cell anemia: the need for multi-modality chemo-prophylaxis. Cardiovasc Hematol Disord Drug Targets 2009;9:271–92.

105. Morris CR, Kato GJ, Poljakovic M, et al. Dysregulated arginine metabolism, hemolysis-associated pulmonary hypertension, and mortality in sickle cell disease. JAMA 2005;294:81–90.

106. Niihara Y, Matsui NM, Shen YM, et al. L-glutamine therapy reduces endothelial adhesion of sickle red blood cells to human umbilical vein endothelial cells. BMC Blood Disord 2005;5:4.

107. Adam SS, Hoppe C. Potential role for statins in sickle cell disease. Pediatr Blood Cancer 2013;60:550–7.

108. Head CA, Swerdlow P, McDade WA, et al. Beneficial effects of nitric oxide breathing in adult patients with sickle cell crisis. Am J Hematol 2010;85:800–2.

109. Rinder HM, Bonan JL, Rinder CS, et al. Dynamics of leukocyte-platelet adhesion in whole blood. Blood 1991;78:1730–7.

110. de Bruijne-Admiraal LG, Modderman PW, Von dem Borne AE, et al. P-selectin mediates Ca(2+)-dependent adhesion of activated platelets to many different types of leukocytes: detection by flow cytometry. Blood 1992;80:134–42.

111. Ott I, Neumann FJ, Gawaz M, et al. Increased neutrophil-platelet adhesion in patients with unstable angina. Circulation 1996;94:1239–46.

112. Michelson AD, Barnard MR, Krueger LA, et al. Circulating monocyte-platelet aggregates are a more sensitive marker of in vivo platelet activation than platelet surface P-selectin: studies in baboons, human coronary intervention, and human acute myocardial infarction. Circulation 2001;104:1533–7.

113. Polanowska-Grabowska R, Wallace K, Field JJ, et al. P-selectin-mediated platelet-neutrophil aggregate formation activates neutrophils in mouse and human sickle cell disease. Arterioscler Thromb Vasc Biol 2010;30:2392–9.

114. Skinner MP, Lucas CM, Burns GF, et al. GMP-140 binding to neutrophils is inhibited by sulfated glycans. J Biol Chem 1991;266:5371–4.

115. Vermeire E, Hearnshaw H, Van Royen P, et al. Patient adherence to treatment: three decades of research. A comprehensive review. J Clin Pharm Ther 2001;26:331–42.

116. Osterberg L, Blaschke T. Adherence to medication. N Engl J Med 2005;353:487–97.

117. Fallowfield L, Atkins L, Catt S, et al. Patients' preference for administration of endocrine treatments by injection or tablets: results from a study of women with breast cancer. Ann Oncol 2006;17:205–10.

118. DiBonaventura MD, Wagner JS, Girman CJ, et al. Multinational internet-based survey of patient preference for newer oral or injectable Type 2 diabetes medication. Patient Prefer Adherence 2010;4:397–406.

119. Barthel SR, Gavino JD, Descheny L, et al. Targeting selectins and selectin ligands in inflammation and cancer. Expert Opin Ther Targets 2007;11:1473–91.

120. Chang J, Patton JT, Sarkar A, et al. GMI-1070, a novel pan-selectin antagonist, reverses acute vascular occlusions in sickle cell mice. Blood 2010;116:1779–86.

121. Wun T, De Castro LM, Styles L, et al. Effects of GMI-1070, a pan-selectin inhibitor, on leukocyte adhesion in sickle cell disease: results from a phase 1/2 study. Blood 2010;116:120, 262A.

122. Wagner MC, Eckman JR, Wick TM. Histamine increases sickle erythrocyte adherence to endothelium. Br J Haematol 2005;132:512–22.

123. Smith CM, Hebbel RP, Tukey DP, et al. Pluronic F-68 reduces the endothelial adherence and improves the rheology of liganded sickle erythrocytes. Blood 1987;69:1631–6.
124. Armstrong JK, Meiselman HJ, Fisher TC. Inhibition of red blood cell-induced platelet aggregation in whole blood by a nonionic surfactant, poloxamer 188 (RheothRx injection). Thromb Res 1995;79:437–50.
125. Cheung AT, Chan MS, Ramanujam S, et al. Effects of poloxamer 188 treatment on sickle cell vaso-occlusive crisis: computer-assisted intravital microscopy study. J Investig Med 2004;52:402–6.
126. Orringer EP, Casella JF, Ataga KI, et al. Purified poloxamer 188 for treatment of acute vaso-occlusive crisis of sickle cell disease: a randomized controlled trial. JAMA 2001;286:2099–106.
127. Nelson RM, Cecconi O, Roberts WG, et al. Heparin oligosaccharides bind L- and P-selectin and inhibit acute inflammation. Blood 1993;82:3253–8.
128. Baughman RA, Kapoor SC, Agarwal RK, et al. Oral delivery of anticoagulant doses of heparin. A randomized, double-blind, controlled study in humans. Circulation 1998;98:1610–5.
129. Arbit E, Goldberg M, Gomez-Orellana I, et al. Oral heparin: status review. Thromb J 2006;4:6.
130. Qari MH, Aljaouni SK, Alardawi MS, et al. Reduction of painful vaso-occlusive crisis of sickle cell anaemia by tinzaparin in a double-blind randomized trial. Thromb Haemost 2007;98:392–6.
131. Maffrand JP, Herbert JM, Bernat A, et al. Experimental and clinical pharmacology of pentosan polysulfate. Semin Thromb Hemost 1991;17(Suppl 2):186–98.
132. Höpfner M, Alban S, Schumacher G, et al. Selectin-blocking semisynthetic sulfated polysaccharides as promising anti-inflammatory agents. J Pharm Pharmacol 2003;55:697–706.
133. FDA. Elmiron: FDA safety information and adverse event reporting system. 2013:1. Available at: http://www.fda.gov/Safety/MedWatch/SafetyInformation/Safety-RelatedDrugLabelingChanges/ucm125235.htm.
134. Simon M, McClanahan RH, Shah JF, et al. Metabolism of [^{3}H]pentosan polysulfate sodium (PPS) in healthy human volunteers. Xenobiotica 2005;35:775–84.
135. Kaila N, Xu GY, Camphausen RT, et al. Identification and structural determination of a potent P-selectin inhibitor. Bioorg Med Chem 2001;9:801–86.
136. Bedard PW, Clerin V, Sushkova N, et al. Characterization of the novel P-selectin inhibitor PSI-697 [2-(4-chlorobenzyl)-3-hydroxy-7,8,9,10-tetrahydrobenzo[h] quinoline-4-carboxylic acid] in vitro and in rodent models of vascular inflammation and thrombosis. J Pharmacol Exp Ther 2008;324:497–506.
137. Meier TR, Myers DD Jr, Wrobleski SK, et al. Prophylactic P-selectin inhibition with PSI-421 promotes resolution of venous thrombosis without anticoagulation. Thromb Haemost 2008;99:343–51.
138. Kumar A, Villani MP, Patel UK, et al. Recombinant soluble form of PSGL-1 accelerates thrombolysis and prevents reocclusion in a porcine model. Circulation 1999;99:1363–9.
139. Romano SJ. Selectin antagonists: therapeutic potential in asthma and COPD. Treat Respir Med 2005;4:85–94.
140. Kaul DK, Tsai HM, Nagel RL, et al. Platelet-activating factor enhances adhesion of sickle erythrocytes to vascular endothelium: the role of vascular integrin $a_v b_3$ and von Willebrand factor. In: Beuzard Y, Lubin B, Rosa J, editors. Sickle cell

disease and thalassaemias: new trends in therapy. Paris: INSERM; 1995. p. 497–500.

141. Nagel RL. A knockout of a transgenic mouse—animal models of sickle cell anemia. N Engl J Med 1998;339:194–5.

Cellular Adhesion and the Endothelium

E-Selectin, L-Selectin, and Pan-Selectin Inhibitors

Marilyn J. Telen, MD

KEYWORDS

- Adhesion • Sickle cell disease • Endothelium • Selectins • Integrins

KEY POINTS

- Adhesion of sickle red blood cells (RBCs) and leukocytes to endothelium, as well as to each other, is critical to the process of vasoocclusion in sickle cell disease (SCD).
- Selectins mediate rapidly reversible adhesive interactions, leading to rolling and tethering of cells under conditions of shear stress. This type of transient slowing or immobilization can lead to integrin activation and firm integrin-mediated adhesion.
- Both in vitro and in vivo preclinical studies support the hypothesis that E-selectin-mediated interactions have a critical role in vasoocclusion in SCD.
- Early-phase clinical studies suggest that an investigational drug, GMI-1070, which is a pan-selectin inhibitor with most activity against E-selectin, may be an effective intervention capable of shortening time to resolution of vasoocclusion in SCD.

INTRODUCTION

Sickle cell disease is characterized by episodic, acutely painful vasoocclusive episodes. The pathophysiology of vasoocclusion is thought to involve a wide variety of adhesive interactions involving erythrocytes (RBCs), the endothelium, and leukocytes, including neutrophils, monocytes, and lymphocytes. Platelets likely also contribute to the vasoocclusive process that characterizes SCD (**Fig. 1**).

All hematopoietic cells, as well as endothelial cells, express multiple adhesion molecules, and many of these have been demonstrated in a variety of in vitro, in vivo, and ex vivo model systems to play a role in adhesive interactions that occur as a result of the presence of sickle RBCs (SS RBCs). Because such adhesive events are believed to be critical to the vasoocclusive process, they are a particularly attractive therapeutic

Disclosure Statement: Dr M.J. Telen has received research funding from GlycoMimetics, Inc (Gaithersburg, MD, USA) and Dilaforette, A.B (Solna, Sweden) and honoraria from Pfizer, Inc (New York, NY, USA) and Biogen Idec, Inc (Cambridge, MA, USA).
Division of Hematology, Department of Medicine and Duke Comprehensive Sickle Cell Center, Duke University Medical Center, Box 2615, Durham, NC 27710, USA
E-mail address: marilyn.telen@duke.edu

Hematol Oncol Clin N Am 28 (2014) 341–354
http://dx.doi.org/10.1016/j.hoc.2013.11.010
0889-8588/14/$ – see front matter © 2014 Elsevier Inc. All rights reserved.

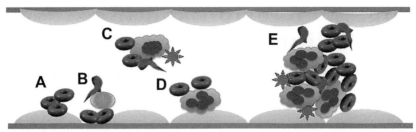

Fig. 1. Interactions between blood cells and the endothelium in sickle cell disease. (*A*) Red cells containing primarily HbS (SS RBCs) adhere directly to the endothelium, a process that initially involves tethering via endothelial P-selectin and then results in firm adhesion via red cell ICAM-4 (LW blood group antigen protein) and endothelial αVβ3 integrin. (*B*) SS RBCs can activate endothelial cells, causing them to retract as well as to upregulate adhesion molecule expression. Retraction exposes subendothelial matrix, which contains both thrombospondin and laminin, for which RBCs express specific receptors. The laminin receptor is BCAM/Lu, the protein that bears Lutheran blood group antigens. Mature SS RBCs bind to thrombospondin via CD47; CD36 expressed by reticulocytes can also bind to thrombospondin. (*C*) SS RBCs can interact with leukocytes during low shear stress conditions and directly activate their ability to adhere to endothelial cells. Monocytes in the circulation can form circulating aggregates with both RBCs and platelets. (*D*) Neutrophils can roll and tether to endothelial cells via P- and E-selectins, after which they bind more firmly to endothelial integrins. Adherent neutrophils "capture" SS RBCs. (*E*) Adherent neutrophils and SS RBCs, or circulating multicellular aggregates, can form large adherent cellular masses that grow to obstruct or nearly obstruct postcapillary venules. Slow blood flow promotes sickling of already deoxygenated SS RBCs.

target by which to address the cause of greater than 90% of health care required by patients with SCD. Most patients with SCD experience at least one such acutely painful episode annually, and many experience multiple events each year. Each event typically requires parenteral opioid therapy, often during a hospital stay of many days. However, identifying the most important adhesion receptors to target with potentially therapeutic drugs has been challenging.

SELECTINS AND SELECTIN-MEDIATED ADHESION

Among the adhesion receptors expressed by both hematopoietic and endothelial cells are the 3 known types of selectins: P-selectin, E-selectin, and L-selectin. Selectin ligands comprise a variety of sialylated and fucosylated carbohydrates containing an epitope common to both sialyl-Lewis a (sialyl-Le[a]) and sialyl-Lewis X (sialyl-Le[x]).[1–3] Selectins contribute to a wide variety of physiologically important processes, including interactions of hematopoietic stem cells with the bone marrow microenvironment, homing of lymphocytes to high endothelial venules, migration of leukocytes to areas of inflammation,[4] and metastasis of cancer cells.[5]

In general, selectins mediate rapid on-off interactions, whereas integrins, another class of ubiquitous adhesion receptors, mediate high-affinity, stable adhesion. Selectins are therefore thought to provide the initial interaction between hematopoietic cells in motion and other cells, which may be stationary (such as endothelial cells) or also in motion, such as other circulating blood cells.[6] Shear stress may be critical to the activation of at least some selectin-mediated events, which then lead to "tethering," or short-lived adhesion of one cell to another. In interactions involving endothelial cells, "rolling" is then observed,[6] consisting of repeated short-lived interactions of hematopoietic cells in motion with the stationary surface of the endothelium. Ulti-mately, these transient interactions are followed by firmer cell-cell adhesion provided by other adhesion receptors and ligands. Thus, selectins are responsible for rolling of circulating cells on endothelial surfaces, while integrins and some other adhesion receptors are responsible for more permanent capture of such cells.

Structural Characteristics of Selectins

The 3 species of selectin compose a family of adhesion receptors with similar struc-tures but variable size and ligand specificity (**Fig. 2**). The region responsible for binding carbohydrate ligands is at the N-terminus and is a lectin domain largely dependent on calcium for its activity. Further toward the membrane is the epidermal growth factor (EGF) domain, which is linked to consensus repeats. The number of consensus re-peats is unique to each selectin, ranging from 2 in L-selectin to 6 in E-selectin and 9 in P-selectin. The rest of the molecules consist of a transmembrane domain and short cytoplasmic domain. All 3 selectin molecules share about 60% homology in their lectin and EGF domains.[3]

E-Selectin

E-selectin, also known as CD62E, endothelial-leukocyte adhesion molecule 1, or leukocyte-endothelial cell adhesion molecule 2, is encoded by the *SELE* gene, which is on chromosome 1 near the gene encoding L-selectin. E-selectin is primarily expressed by activated endothelial cells. It is poorly expressed by resting endothelial cells; it is also expressed in skin and bone marrow. In general, E-selectin is expressed after inflammatory stimuli induce expression of *SELE*; thus, E-selectin expression re-quires de novo protein synthesis and takes 3 to 5 hours to appear after stimulation, peaking up to 12 hours after exposure to an appropriate cytokine. Exposure to shear

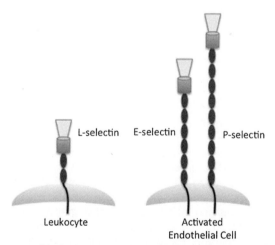

L-selectin   E-selectin   P-selectin

Leukocyte   Activated Endothelial Cell

Fig. 2. Selectins expressed by leukocytes and endothelial cells. Leukocytes constitutively ex-press L-selectin, which can undergo cleavage from the cell when activation occurs. Endothe-lial cells increase expression of both E- and P-selectins when activated. The most N-terminal extracellular domain of all selectins is a lectin domain (▽) responsible for binding to sialyl Lewis structures. This lectin domain extends from an epidermal growth factor (■) domain, which is itself attached to a series of consensus repeats, ranging from 2 in L-selectin to 9 in P-selectin. The consensus repeats are linked to a transmembrane domain and a short C-terminal cytoplasmic domain.

stress also affects E-selectin expression, with high shear stress increasing E-selectin expression.[7]

Both polymorphonuclear and mononuclear leukocytes express E-selectin ligands and use them in their interactions with the endothelium during inflammation.

L-Selectin

L-selectin (CD62L) is a constitutively expressed selectin, present on subsets of T lymphocytes, including both naive and central memory T cells. L-selectin is also expressed by neutrophils and monocytes. Thus, it can play a broad role in leukocyte trafficking. Expression of L-selectin by lymphocytes and neutrophils is regulated by the action of endometalloproteases that cleave L-selectin from the cell surface when cells are activated.[3] Loss of L-selectin is normally accompanied by increased expression of other leukocyte adhesion receptors. As L-selectin is cleaved from leukocyte surfaces, the level of plasma-soluble L-selectin (sL-selectin) increases. Soluble L-selectin may play a role in downregulation of leukocyte adhesion, as it retains biological activity and thus may block leukocyte adhesion generally. Ligand binding to cell surface L-selectin has been shown to set off a signaling cascade involving src-tyrosine kinase p56^{lck}, Ras, mitogen-activating protein kinase, and Rac2, leading to increased synthesis of O_2^-.[8] On the endothelial side, L-selectin-mediated adhesion depends on activation of the endothelium, as endothelial cells express little ligand without activation.

Characteristics of P-selectin are discussed in an article by Kutlar and Embury elsewhere in this issue.

PRECLINICAL STUDIES OF THE ROLE OF E- AND L-SELECTINS IN SCD

Both P-selectin and E-selectin have been shown to contribute to adhesive events in in vitro models of SCD. They seem to play critical roles in vasoocclusion in animal models of SCD, and reagents that block P-selectin- and E selectin-mediated interactions have been demonstrated to prevent or ameliorate vasoocclusion in experimental models.[7,9–11] The role of L-selectin in SCD is less clear.

L-Selectin in Sickle Cell Disease

Several studies have shown that neutrophils are activated in SCD, even at steady state. Although neutrophil activation in SCD is widely recognized, expression of L-selectin by neutrophils in SCD has been variably described as both increased and decreased. Lard and colleagues[12] found a significant decrease in L-selectin expression by neutrophils in steady state SCD, as well as increased levels of plasma sL-selectin. This observation is consistent with the view that neutrophils decrease expression of cell-surface L-selectin in response to activation. These investigators also found that this decrease was significantly more pronounced during vasoocclusive episodes.[12] Other neutrophil markers were also consistent with neutrophil activation. However, Okpala and colleagues[13] described SCD neutrophils and lymphocytes as having increased L-selectin expression compared with HbAA controls and reported that monocyte L-selectin expression increased during vasoocclusion. This group also suggested that subjects with higher leukocyte L-selectin and integrin expression levels had more severe disease complications. A study of silent cerebral infarcts in children with SCD has shown a small but statistically significant increase in plasma-soluble L-selectin levels.[14] However, another study of L-selectin gene polymorphisms and L-selectin levels showed no relationship among gene polymorphisms, L-selectin levels, and SCD complications.[15]

Hydroxyurea (HU) has been postulated to exert its effects partially through its ability to decrease neutrophilia in SCD, and several studies have attempted to determine if it also has an effect on neutrophil activation and concomitantly on neutrophil expression of L-selectin. Saleh and colleagues[16] found that institution of HU therapy had no effect on sL-selectin levels. However, Benkerrou and colleagues[17] have reported that HU corrected the dysregulated expression of L-selectin, which they found otherwise to be decreased without exogenous activation, and that HU also increased neutrophil production of H_2O_2 after stimulation, which had been decreased in SCD neutrophils from subjects not exposed to HU.

When hypoxia/reperfusion injury is produced in sickle mice, an exaggerated inflammatory response is elicited.[9] Neutrophils also seem to have an important direct role in vasoocclusion, as shown by the studies of Turhan and colleagues.[18] They demonstrated that SS RBCs bind readily to leukocytes when the latter are adherent to endothelial cells in sickle mice. However, the role of L-selectin, if any, in this process is unclear. When sickle mice were deficient in both P- and E-selectins, they had many fewer leukocytes adhering to the vascular walls and were protected from vasoocclusion precipitated by the proinflammatory cytokine tumor necrosis factor α (TNFα),[18] as further discussed later. However, these and other in vivo studies did not report investigation of the role of L-selectin.

E-Selectin in Sickle Cell Disease

Endothelial P-selectin has been shown to bind circulating SS RBCs and contribute to vasoocclusion,[9] whereas E-selectin seems to have a critical role to play in vasoocclusion by mediating rolling and initial adhesion of leukocytes to endothelium. Once adherent, leukocytes then "capture" SS RBCs, causing a growing blockade of small vessels (**Fig. 3**).

Zennadi and colleagues[11] have explored the relationship between the abnormal SS RBC and leukocyte activation. They have shown that, in vitro, coincubation of SS RBCs and mononuclear leukocytes (a mixture of lymphocytes and monocytes) activates the leukocytes, which then show increased adhesion to nonactivated cultured

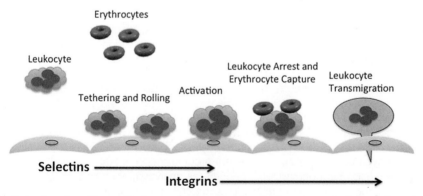

Fig. 3. Leukocyte rolling, adhesion, and transmigration. In the presence of shear stress, leukocytes form quickly reversible bonds with selectins, causing them to appear to be "rolling" along the surface of the endothelium. Selectins also mediate short-term tethering, which induces further slowing of leukocyte passage relative to the other blood elements. As these "on-off" events occur, both the leukocytes and endothelial cells become activated, which ultimately can lead to expression of activated integrins, which then mediate firm adhesion. After establishment of integrin-mediated adhesion, leukocytes may then migrate into the tissues by passing either through intercellular junctions or through the endothelial cells themselves. Adherent leukocytes have also been shown to "capture" slow-flowing SS RBCs.

endothelial cells.[11] Significant inhibition of leukocyte adhesion to endothelium was observed when the cultured human umbilical vein endothelial cells used in these studies were preincubated with monoclonal antibodies reactive with E-selectin. However, antibodies to P-selectin did not inhibit leukocyte adhesion in this model. Zennadi and colleagues also showed that the SS RBC adhesion receptors critical for this stimulation of leukocyte adhesion seem to be ICAM-4 (LW protein) and CD44. More recently, this group has shown that contact with SS RBCs can also induce neutrophil adhesion.[19]

Blood cells from patients with SCD can also directly activate endothelial cells, causing upregulation of expression of VCAM-1, E-selectin, and ICAM-1.[20] In studies by Brown and colleagues,[20] this effect seemed to depend on TNFα and interleukin (IL)-1 produced by leukocytes. In an earlier and in some respects complementary study, Sultana and colleagues[21] demonstrated the effect of SS RBCs on endothelial cells. They showed that interaction of SS RBCs with cultured human umbilical vein endothelial cells resulted in markedly increased indicators of cellular oxidant stress; interaction with normal RBCs did not have a similar effect. In addition, endothelial cell expression of several adhesion receptors, including E-selectin, were upregulated when endothelial cells were exposed to SS RBCs, and transendothelial migration of monocytes was also increased. Shiu and colleagues[22] also showed that perfusion of cultured endothelial cells with SS RBCs caused increased gene expression of ICAM-1 and a more modest increase in VCAM-1 expression.

Mononuclear leukocytes from patients with SCD have also been described as having the capability of activating endothelial cells, although cell-cell contact was not required. Belcher and colleagues[23] showed that SCD monocytes, but not normal monocytes, caused TNFα- and IL-1β-dependent activation of endothelial cells, which then led to nuclear translocation of nuclear factor-kB. However, Safaya and colleagues[24] were unable to demonstrate that isolated monocytes from patients with SCD upregulated endothelial cell expression of L-selectin, E-selectin, VCAM-1, and ICAM-1 more than did normal monocytes.

In Vivo Studies in Animal Models of Sickle Cell Disease

In studies of the cremasteric vasculature of sickle mice, Hidalgo and colleagues[25] in 2009 showed that inactivation of E-selectin led to protection from vasoocclusion in sickle mice, as well as protection from transfusion-related acute lung injury, also in a mouse model. However, in at least one similar model, only a P-selectin antibody, and not an E-selectin antibody, blocked the exaggerated hypoxia/reperfusion inflammatory response of sickle mice and enhanced blood flow in the affected vessels.[9]

Additional studies were performed by Chang and colleagues,[10] in which they studied the contribution of E-selectin as well as the activity of a small molecule selectin inhibitor, GMI-1070. GMI-1070 is a small carbohydrate molecule designed to mimic the bioactive domain of sLe$_x$ and present a conformation suitable for binding to the carbohydrate-binding domain of E-selectin, as analyzed by nuclear magnetic resonance techniques. The investigators first used enzyme-linked immunosorbent assays in which selectin chimeras were bound to the wells of the plates. They demonstrated that GMI-1070 bound to all 3 types of selectins, although its ability to bind E-selectin was about 100-fold higher than its ability to bind to L- and P-selectins in that assay. The IC_{50} for E-selectin was 4.3 μM, whereas it was 423 μM and 337 μM for P-selectin and L-selectin, respectively.

They then used a flow chamber assay, in which human umbilical vein endothelial cells were cultured with TNFα to induce E-selectin expression or IL-4 and histamine to induce P-selectin expression.[10] They found that adhesion of neutrophils was inhibited more readily by GMI-1070 when E-selectin expression was induced by TNFα than when P-selectin expression was induced by IL-4 and histamine.

The same authors then studied the activity of GMI-1070 in a mouse model of vasoocclusion.[10] They treated mice with SCD that had undergone transplantation (C57BL/6 male mice, lethally irradiated and transplanted with Berkeley sickle cell mouse nucleated bone marrow cells), with both intraperitoneal injection of TNFα to induce cell adhesion and vasoocclusion and antibodies against P- and E-selectins (combined), GMI-1070, or control. Intravital microscopy of cremasteric muscle vessels was used to observe and measure cell adhesion and blood flow. They compared the ability of GMI-1070 and anti-P- and anti-E-selectin antibodies to affect leukocyte rolling and adhesion, as well as to abrogate vasoocclusion.[10] Although they found that GMI-1070 slightly increased the percentage of rolling leukocytes, it also increased leukocyte rolling velocity and decreased the percentage of adherent leukocytes. The combined use of anti-P- and anti-E-selectin antibodies was even more effective in reducing leukocyte adhesion. GMI-1070 reduced the capture of SS RBCs by adherent leukocytes and improved blood flow in this model. The improvement in blood flow was equivalent when the effects of GMI-1070 and the combination of anti-P- and anti-E-selectin antibodies were compared. In addition, the investigators also studied the effect of GMI-1070 administered nearly 2 hours after the inflammatory stimulus and after the vasoocclusive process was established. In that setting, GMI-1070 also greatly increased blood flow and increased mouse survival. These studies confirmed the importance of both P- and E-selectins in vasoocclusion and the therapeutic potential of a compound such as GMI-1070, which could reduce E-selectin-mediated adhesion.

THERAPEUTIC APPROACHES TO E-SELECTIN-MEDIATED ADHESION IN HUMAN SCD

Given evidence for a contribution from at least P- and E-selectins to the vasoocclusive process, the development of a pan-selectin antagonist rather than a reagent that inhibits only one selectin makes sense in the context of SCD. It may be that only such agents can prevent the initiation or propagation of vasoocclusion and reduce the inflammation secondary to the response to hypoxia/reperfusion injury.

Clinical Studies Focusing on Selectins in Human Disease

At this writing, 99 studies involving selectins as targets are listed in clinicaltrials.gov, and these focus on the roles of selectins in a variety of human diseases. Most have targeted P-selectin, whereas only a few have used agents that inhibit E- or L-selectin or have pan-selectin inhibitory activity (**Table 1**). Among drugs targeting selectins, trials of only 2 potential drugs have commenced for SCD. The first of these to be studied has been GMI-1070, the pan-selectin inhibitor that decreases both E- and P-selectin-dependent leukocyte adhesion. In animal models, it not only decreased vasoocclusion (as described earlier) but also ameliorated other conditions requiring leukocyte adhesion, including delayed-type hypersensitivity responses and cardiac ischemia/reperfusion injury.[26]

GMI-1070 Phase 1 Studies

GMI-1070 was first studied in healthy volunteers.[27] A total of 72 subjects were randomized to GMI-1070 or placebo in 2 blinded studies. In the first, a dose-escalation study was performed, with single intravenous doses of 2, 5, 10, 20, and 40 mg/kg. In the first part of the second study, each subject received 5, 10, or 20 mg/kg every 8 hours for 13 doses (4 days); in the second part of the study, subjects received

Table 1
Clinical studies of E-, L-, and pan-selectin inhibitors in human disease

Investigational Agent	Type of Study	Disease Target	Identifier
Aselizumab (anti-L-selectin antibody)	Phase 2	Trauma	na
Bimosiamose (inhaled)	Phase 2	Chronic obstructive pulmonary disease	NCT01108913, NCT00962481
Bimosiamose cream	Phase 2	Psoriasis	NCT00823693
E-selectin protein, administered as a nasal spray	Phase 1	Stroke prevention	NCT00012454
GI-270384X (oral ICAM-1 and E-selectin inhibitor)	Phase 1	Ulcerative colitis	NCT00457171
GMI-1070 (pan-selectin inhibitor)	Phase 1	Sickle cell disease	NCT00911495
GMI-1070 (pan-selectin inhibitor)	Phase 2	Sickle cell disease vasoocclusive crisis	NCT01119833
YSPSL (rPSGL-Ig, pan-selectin inhibitor)	Phase 1/2	Solid organ transplant (prevention of delayed graft function)	NCT00298181, NCT00298168

a loading dose regimen of 40 mg/kg followed by 20 mg/kg every 8 hours for 6 doses (2 days). No serious adverse events (SAEs) were associated with the drug, and all adverse events (AEs) that were observed were rated as mild or moderate. These included one apparently drug-related pruritic rash that necessitated discontinuation of drug treatment. There were also no dose-related AEs noted. In the multiple dose regimen, the drug half-life was estimated at 8 hours. Based on these studies, a phase 1/2 trial was conducted in patients with SCD.

The phase 1/phase 2 study evaluated GMI-1070 in adults with stable SCD, to assess safety, pharmacokinetics, and microvascular effects of intravenous GMI-1070 in the outpatient setting. This study (entitled "Phase 1/Phase 2 Study of the Safety, Pharmacokinetics, and Microvascular Effect of Titrating Doses of Intravenous GMI-1070, a Pan-Selectin Inhibitor, in Adults With Sickle Cell Disease," NCT00911495) was performed in 2009–2010 and enrolled 15 subjects, 4 of whom were taking HU.[28] GMI-1070 was administered intravenously (IV) at 20 mg/kg loading dose, followed by a single dose of 10 mg/kg 10 hours later. Subjects had the genotypes SS or Sβ^0 thalassemia and were between 18 and 45 years of age. They were in steady state, with stable disease and no vasoocclusive crises during the previous 3 months.

This phase1/2 study showed the drug to be cleared by the kidneys, with renal clearance averaging 18.0 ± 7.93 mL/min and accounting for essentially all drug elimination; the elimination half-life of GMI-1070 averaged 7.73 ± 2.45 hours.[28] AEs were minimal, with 4 subjects reporting headache within 24 hours of dosing. No unexpected SAEs occurred. Most clinical laboratory results remained unaffected by the drug. However, the drug had a pronounced effect on neutrophil count, which increased significantly when measured 24 and 48 hours after drug administration[29]; mean baseline white blood cell (WBC) count was $10 \times 10^3/mm^3$, and baseline absolute neutrophil count (ANC) was $5.4 \times 10^3/mm^3$. The mean WBC count increased to 10.4, 11.6, 10.2, and $8.7 \times 10^3/mm^3$ at 8, 24, and 48 hours and 7 days, respectively. The baseline ANC increased to 5.5, 7.5, 5.6, and $4.2 \times 10^3/mm^3$ at the same time points. The change in ANC was statistically significant at 24 and 48 hours, while no changes were observed in monocyte and lymphocyte counts. However, despite sometimes quite marked elevations in ANC, no AEs were associated with this change. There was no apparent relationship between drug clearance rate and degree of leukocytosis, HU use, or AEs.

The lack of AEs despite marked elevations in ANC may have been related to the reduced leukocyte adhesion found in vitro in these patients.[29] Using intravital microscopy of the bulbar conjunctivae, no significant changes in microvascular blood flow were identified, although there was a slight change toward improvement right after drug administration. In ex vivo measurement of neutrophil adhesion, adhesion to matrix proteins was also reduced at 4 and 8 hours after infusion; however, these changes also did not reach statistical significance.

In a companion study, Simon and colleagues[30] showed that GMI-1070 significantly inhibited in vitro activation of the β2 integrin Mac-1 by soluble recombinant human E-selectin/Fc chimera on isolated neutrophils. In the same study, the investigators also studied neutrophils from subjects with sickle cell who received GMI-1070 in the study described earlier and found that activation markers of neutrophils were decreased 4 and 8 hours after drug administration. They also found that the amount of platelet-monocyte aggregates were reduced after drug administration.

Additional evidence regarding the effect of GMI-1070 was gained from yet another study by Simon and colleagues.[31] When adhesion of neutrophils was tested in a microfluidic flow chamber in which E-selectin and ICAM-1 were immobilized to present substrates for rolling and adhesion, GMI-1070 was able to reduce neutrophil arrest and also reduced neutrophil activation. This study also suggested that different concentrations of GMI-1070 had somewhat different effects; at low concentrations, GMI-1070 blocked the capacity of E-selectin to activate CD18 and mediate arrest. However, higher concentrations of GMI-1070 were required to increase the rolling velocity on a substrate of E-selectin during fluid shear stress.

GMI-1070 Phase 2 Study

A phase 2 study of the use of GMI-1070 during vasoocclusive episodes has completed enrollment. This study was entitled "A Phase 2 Randomized, Double-Blind, Placebo-Controlled Study of the Efficacy, Safety, and Pharmacokinetics of GMI-1070, A Pan-Selectin Inhibitor, In Subjects Hospitalized For Sickle Cell Vaso-Occlusive Crisis" (NCT01119833). Seventy-six patients aged 12 to 60 years, with Hb SS or Sβ^0 thalassemia, admitted with vasoocclusive crisis, were randomly assigned to receive either GMI-1070 or a placebo IV, in addition to usual care for vasoocclusion. GMI-1070 or placebo was given twice daily until patients met criteria for resolution of vasoocclusive crisis, had no improvement at 5 days, or had completed 7 days of therapy. Follow-up studies were then done 1 month after discharge.

Although the results of this study have not yet been released in detail, a press release from the company has indicated that patients treated with GMI-1070 experienced a wide range of improved outcomes compared with patients receiving placebo. Those receiving active drug had a reduction in the duration of vasoocclusive crisis as well as shorter hospital stays. In addition, active drug was associated with reduced requirement for narcotics. AE rates were said to be comparable between the treatment and placebo arms.

The second antiselectin to be studied in SCD is SelG1, a humanized monoclonal antibody to P-selectin. This "Study to Assess Safety and Impact of SelG1 With or Without Hydroxyurea Therapy in Sickle Cell Disease Patients With Pain Crises (SUSTAIN)" (clinicaltrials.gov NCT01895361) is being conducted by Selexys Pharmaceuticals. This phase I clinical study commenced in 2011 and is designed to study the pharmacokinetics of 2 dose levels of this compound in patients with SCD, as well as to determine the safety of monthly administration of this compound, potentially to reduce the frequency of vasoocclusive crises. Further information about studies of P-selectin inhibitors of various types is provided in an article by Kutlar and Embury elsewhere in this volume.

L- AND E-SELECTIN TARGETED THERAPY: A BROADER PICTURE

Neutrophils are the primary defense against bacterial infection and are the first cells recruited during an innate immune response to the site of infection.[32] The selectin family of adhesion molecules mediates some of the critical early steps of leukocyte tethering and rolling in postcapillary venules, the site at which neutrophils adhere and from which they then migrate into areas of infection and inflammation. This same site is also thought to be most important in SCD vasoocclusion. Although neutrophils are important components of host defenses, they are also critical to the pathophysiology not only of SCD but also of diabetic retinopathy, acute lung injury due to several causes, renal microvasculopathy, stroke, and acute coronary artery syndrome.[33] Thus, it is clear that, in many situations and sites, interfering with E- and L-selectin function may have both beneficial as well as deleterious effects.

In addition, selectins support other critical physiologic cell-cell interactions, including the homing of lymphocytes to high endothelial venules,[4] the proliferation of hematopoietic stem cells,[34] and the antitumor effect of central memory T cells.[35] However, selectins can also directly mediate adhesion via sialyl Lewis ligands expressed by cancer cells, leading to tumor metastasis; all 3 types of selectins seem to be able to facilitate this process.[36] Thus, interfering with those interactions have been proposed as an approach to cancer therapy.[5,35] Partial deficiency of E-selectin-ligand1 reduces atherosclerotic plaque instability in mice, whereas complete deficiency is an embryonic lethal trait.[37] Thus, although therapies targeting selectin-mediated adhesion may be effective in modulating the severity of vasoocclusion and may also become relevant to cancer therapy, it also remains to be seen to what degree and for what duration one can safely afford to interfere with selectin function while avoiding untoward side effects of such therapy.

Nevertheless, selectin inhibitors are being explored in many disease settings (see **Table 1**). Such inhibitors have been especially attractive in the search for ways to treat inflammatory conditions, including most notably ischemia/reperfusion injury.[38] For example, E-selectin-deficient mice are protected from the consequences of experimentally induced renal ischemia, and a function-blocking monoclonal antibody to E-selectin produces a similar benefit in wild-type mice.[39]

Bimosiamose, an E- and P-Selectin Inhibitor

The synthetic pan-selectin antagonist, bimosiamose, inhibits both E- and P-selectins and decreases lymphocyte adhesion under flowing conditions. It has been studied in several disease settings, including reactive airway disease and ischemia/reperfusion injury in several organs.[40–45] In yet another setting, the compound resulted in improvements in disease activity in both an animal model of psoriasis as well as in affected patients.[46] Another selectin inhibitor, efomycine M, blocks L-selectin-mediated leukocyte adhesion and also was effective in murine models of psoriasis[47] but has not been reported as having been tested in humans.

GI270384X—Inhibition of E-Selectin Expression

Another drug, GI270384X, inhibits cytokine-induced ICAM-1 and E-selectin expression and has been studied in experimental inflammatory colitis.[48] In vitro, this drug reduced TNFα-induced neutrophil adhesion to cultured endothelial cells. In mice, the drug reduced expression of ICAM-1 but not E-selectin and reduced leukocyte recruitment to the inflamed colon. However, a phase 1 study of this drug (NCT00457171) was terminated in 2009, and results have not been reported.

Aselizumab—L-Selectin Inhibition

A humanized monoclonal antibody (aselizumab) targeting L-selectin specifically has also been studied. However, it resulted in both increased infections and no significant effects on clinical course in patients who had experienced severe trauma.[49]

YSPSL (rPSGL-Ig)—A Pan-Selectin Inhibitor Targeting P- and E-Selectins

Other pan-selectin inhibitors that have been used in clinical trials predominantly target P-selectin, although some have measurable activity against other selectins as well. For example, YSPSL (rPSGL-Ig) predominantly targets P-selectin but also inhibits E- and L-selectins. In animal models, it has been shown to reduce cytokine production as well as to decrease the tissue damage associated with ischemia reperfusion. It has also led to improved renal function posttransplant.[50] Thus, 4 trials listed at clinicaltrials.gov involve YSPSL in a transplant setting to decrease delayed graft function and prevent ischemia/reperfusion injury.

SUMMARY

The current state of understanding of the pathophysiologic mechanisms of vasoocclusion in SCD has led to great interest in the development of therapies designed to reduce erythrocyte and leukocyte adhesion to endothelial cells, as well as red cell-leukocyte interactions and inflammation generally. Considerable evidence points to E-selectin as an especially attractive target in this regard, and phase 1 and 2 studies have been performed that support this avenue of research. Although only 1 new drug has yet been developed to target E-selectin, and phase 3 studies remain to be conducted, results to date are promising in regards to both safety and efficacy. This avenue of investigation is therefore likely to attract continued interest among both translational and clinical investigators, as well as pharmaceutical companies.

REFERENCES

1. Berg E, Robinson MK, Mansson O, et al. A carbohydrate domain common to both sialyl Lea and sialyl Lex is recognized by the endothelial cell leukocyte adhesion molecule ELAM-1. J Biol Chem 1991;266(23):14869–72.
2. Tedder T, Steeber D, Chen A, et al. The selectins: vascular adhesion molecules. FASEB J 1995;9(10):866–73.
3. Smith CW. Adhesion molecules and receptors. J Allergy Clin Immunol 2008; 121(Suppl 2):S375–9.
4. Tedder TF, Steeber DA, Pizcueta P. L-selectin-deficient mice have impaired leukocyte recruitment into inflammatory sites. J Exp Med 1995;181(6):2259–64.
5. St Hill CA. Interactions between endothelial selectins and cancer cells regulate metastasis. Front Biosci 2011;17:3233–51.
6. McEver RP, Zhu C. Rolling cell adhesion. Annu Rev Cell Dev Biol 2010;26: 363–96.
7. Chase S, Magnani J, Simon S. E-selectin ligands as mechanosensitive receptors on neutrophils in health and disease. Ann Biomed Eng 2012;40(4):849–59.
8. Brenner B, Gulbins E, Schlottmann K, et al. L-selectin activates the Ras pathway via the tyrosine kinase p56lck. Proc Natl Acad Sci U S A 1996;24(26):15376–81.

9. Kaul DK, Hebbel RP. Hypoxia/reoxygenation causes inflammatory response in transgenic sickle mice but not in normal mice. J Clin Invest 2000;106(3):411–20.

10. Chang J, Patton JT, Sarkar A, et al. GMI-1070, a novel pan-selectin antagonist, reverses acute vascular occlusions in sickle cell mice. Blood 2010;116(10): 1779–86.

11. Zennadi R, Chien A, Xu K, et al. Sickle red cells induce adhesion of lymphocytes and monocytes to endothelium. Blood 2008;112(8):3474–83.

12. Lard LR, Mul FP, de Haas M, et al. Neutrophil activation in sickle cell disease. J Leukoc Biol 1999;66(3):411–5.

13. Okpala I, Daniel Y, Haynes R, et al. Relationship between the clinical manifestations of sickle cell disease and the expression of adhesion molecules on white blood cells. Eur J Haematol 2002;69(3):135–44.

14. Faulcon LM, Fu Z, Dulloor P, et al. Thrombospondin-1 and L-selectin are associated with silent cerebral infarct in children with sickle cell anaemia. Br J Haematol 2013;162(3):421–4.

15. Ugochukwu CC, Okpala I, Pantelidis P, et al. L-selectin gene polymorphisms and complications of sickle cell disease. Int J Lab Hematol 2008;30(4):312–6.

16. Saleh AW, Hillen HF, Duits AJ. Levels of endothelial, neutrophil and platelet-specific factors in sickle cell anemia patients during hydroxyurea therapy. Acta Haematol 1999;102(1):31–7.

17. Benkerrou M, Delarche C, Brahimi L, et al. Hydroxyurea corrects the dysregulated L-selectin expression and increased H(2)O(2) production of polymorphonuclear neutrophils from patients with sickle cell anemia. Blood 2002;99(7):2297–303.

18. Turhan A, Weiss LA, Mohandas N, et al. Primary role for adherent leukocytes in sickle cell vascular occlusion: a new paradigm. Proc Natl Acad Sci U S A 2002; 99(5):3047–51.

19. Boateng LA, Zennadi R, Telen MJ. Sickle red blood cell induced adhesion of neutrophils to endothelial cells and biologic correlates of leukocyte activation. Blood 2011;118:1055.

20. Brown MD, Wick TM, Eckman JR. Activation of vascular endothelial cell adhesion molecule expression by sickle blood cells. Pediatr Pathol Mol Med 2001; 20(1):47–72.

21. Sultana C, Shen Y, Rattan V, et al. Interaction of sickle erythrocytes with endothelial cells in the presence of endothelial cell conditioned medium induces oxidant stress leading to transendothelial migration of monocytes. Blood 1998;92(10): 3924–35.

22. Shiu YT, Udden MM, McIntire LV. Perfusion with sickle erythrocytes up-regulates ICAM-1 and VCAM-1 gene expression in cultured human endothelial cells. Blood 2000;95(10):3232–41.

23. Belcher JD, Marker PH, Weber JP, et al. Activated monocytes in sickle cell disease: potential role in the activation of vascular endothelium and vaso-occlusion. Blood 2000;96(7):2451–9.

24. Safaya S, Steinberg MH, Klings ES. Monocytes from sickle cell disease patients induce differential pulmonary endothelial gene expression via activation of NF-kappaB signaling pathway. Mol Immunol 2012;50(1–2):117–23.

25. Hidalgo A, Chang J, Jang JE, et al. Heterotypic interactions enabled by polarized neutrophil microdomains mediate thromboinflammatory injury. Nat Med 2009;15(4):384–91.

26. Magnani JL, Sarkar A, Li Y, et al. GMI-1070: a small pan-selectin antagonist that inhibits leukocyte adhesion and migration in multiple disease models in vivo. Blood (ASH Annual Meeting Abstracts) 2007;110(11):2410.

27. Xie YL, Seufert R, Magnani JL, et al. Safety, tolerability and pharmacokinetics of GMI-1070, a pan-selectin inhibitor for treatment of vaso-occlusive crisis: single and multiple dose studies in healthy volunteers. Blood (ASH Annual Meeting Abstracts) 2009;114:1526.
28. Styles L, Wun T, De Castro LM, et al. GMI-1070, a pan-selectin inhibitor: safety and PK in a phase 1/2 study in adults with sickle cell disease. Blood (ASH Annual Meeting Abstracts) 2010;116(21):1632.
29. Wun T, De Castro LM, Styles L, et al. Effects of GMI-1070, a pan-selectin inhibitor, on leukocyte adhesion in sickle cell disease: results from a phase 1/2 study. ASH Annual Meeting Abstracts 2010;116(21):262.
30. Simon SI, Chase S, Larkin SK, et al. Effects of selectin antagonist GMI-1070 on the activation state of leukocytes in sickle cell patients not in crisis. Blood (ASH Annual Meeting Abstracts) 2010;116(21):2672.
31. Simon SI, Chase S, Thackray H, et al. Inhibition of E-selectin inflammatory function by the glycomimetic GMI-1070. Blood (ASH Annual Meeting Abstracts) 2011;118(21):851.
32. Hickey MJ, Kubes P. Intravascular immunity: the host–pathogen encounter in blood vessels. Nat Rev Immunol 2009;9:364–75.
33. Segel GB, Halterman MW, Lichtman MA. The paradox of the neutrophil's role in tissue injury. J Leukoc Biol 2011;89(3):359–72.
34. Winkler IG, Barbier V, Nowlan B, et al. Vascular niche E-selectin regulates hematopoietic stem cell dormancy, self renewal and chemoresistance. Nat Med 2012;18(11):1651–7.
35. Stark FC, Gurnani K, Sad S, et al. Lack of functional selectin ligand interactions compromises long term tumor protection by CD8+ T cells. PloS one 2012;7(2): e32211.
36. Läubli H, Borsig L. Selectins promote tumor metastasis. Semin Cancer Biol 2010;20(3):169–77.
37. Luo W, Wang H, Guo C, et al. Haploinsufficiency of E-selectin ligand-1 is associated with reduced atherosclerotic plaque macrophage content while complete deficiency leads to early embryonic lethality in mice. Atherosclerosis 2012; 224(2):363–7.
38. Rossi B, Constantin G. Anti-selectin therapy for the treatment of inflammatory diseases. Inflamm Allergy Drug Targets 2008;7(2):85–93.
39. Singbartl K, Ley K. Protection from ischemia-reperfusion induced severe acute renal failure by blocking E-selectin. Crit Care Med 2000;28(7):2507–14.
40. Jayle C, Milinkevitch S, Favreau F, et al. Protective role of selectin ligand inhibition in a large animal model of kidney ischemia-reperfusion injury. Kidney Int 2006;69(10):1749–55.
41. Kirsten A, Watz H, Kretschmar G, et al. Efficacy of the pan-selectin antagonist bimosiamose on ozone-induced airway inflammation in healthy subjects–a double blind, randomized, placebo-controlled, cross-over clinical trial. Pulm Pharmacol Ther 2011;24(5):555–8.
42. Langer R, Wang M, Stepkowski SM, et al. Selectin inhibitor bimosiamose prolongs survival of kidney allografts by reduction in intragraft production of cytokines and chemokines. J Am Soc Nephrol 2004;15(11):2893–901.
43. Nemoto T, Burne MJ, Daniels F, et al. Small molecule selectin ligand inhibition improves outcome in ischemic acute renal failure. Kidney Int 2001;60(6):2205–14.
44. Palma-Vargas JM, Toledo-Pereyra L, Dean RE, et al. Small-molecule selectin inhibitor protects against liver inflammatory response after ischemia and reperfusion. J Am Coll Surg 1997;185(4):365–72.

45. Watz H, Bock D, Meyer M, et al. Inhaled pan-selectin antagonist bimosiamose attenuates airway inflammation in COPD. Pulm Pharmacol Ther 2013;26(2): 265–70.
46. Friedrich M, Bock D, Philipp S, et al. Pan-selectin antagonism improves psoriasis manifestation in mice and man. Arch Dermatol Res 2006;297(8):345–51.
47. Schon MP, Krahn T, Schon M, et al. Efomycine M, a new specific inhibitor of selectin, impairs leukocyte adhesion and alleviates cutaneous inflammation. Nat Med 2002;8(4):366–72.
48. Panés J, Aceituno M, Gil F, et al. Efficacy of an inhibitor of adhesion molecule expression (GI270384X) in the treatment of experimental colitis. Am J Physiol Gastrointest Liver Physiol 2007;293(4):G739–48.
49. Seekamp A, van Griensven M, Dhondt E, et al. The effect of anti-L-selectin (aselizumab) in multiple traumatized patients–results of a phase II clinical trial. Crit Care Med 2004;32(10):2021–8.
50. Gaber AO, Mulgaonkar S, Kahan BD, et al. YSPSL (rPSGL-Ig) for improvement of early renal allograft function: a double-blind, placebo-controlled, multi-center phase IIa study. Clin Transplant 2011;25(4):523–33.

Role of the Hemostatic System on Sickle Cell Disease Pathophysiology and Potential Therapeutics

Zahra Pakbaz, MD[a], Ted Wun, MD[a,b,*]

KEYWORDS

- Sickle cell • Thromboembolism • Hypercoagulable • Anti-platelets • Anticoagulants

KEY POINTS

- Although the pathogenesis of sickle cell disease (SCD) lies in disordered hemoglobin structure and function, downstream effects of sickle hemoglobin include changes in the hemostatic system that overall result in a prothrombotic phenotype.
- These changes include thrombin activation, decreased levels of anticoagulants, impaired fibrinolysis, and platelet activation.
- Limited studies to date suggest that biomarkers of activation can be affected by currently available antithrombotic drugs, and provocative data from pilot studies indicate there may be improvement in clinically important outcomes.
- Therefore, clinical trials with antithrombotic therapies are justified with both SCD-related complications (vaso-occlusive crisis, pain) and thrombotic complications as outcome events of interest.

INTRODUCTION

Sickle cell disease (SCD) is the result of homozygous or compound heterozygous inheritance of mutation in the β-globin gene. The resulting substitution of the hydrophilic amino acid glutamic acid at the sixth position by the hydrophobic amino acid valine, leads to the production of hemoglobin S (HbS). HbS polymerizes when deoxygenated and this polymerization is associated with cell dehydration and increased red cell density.[1–3] The dense, rigid, and sickling red cells lead to vaso-occlusion and impaired blood flow,[2,4] and is thought to underlie acute (painful episodes, acute chest

Z. Pakbaz has no conflict of interest. T. Wun receives grant funding from Glycomimetics, Inc.
[a] Division of Hematology Oncology, Davis School of Medicine, 4501 X Street, Suite 3016, Sacramento, CA 95817, USA; [b] UC Davis Clinical and Translational Sciences Center, VA Northern California Health Care System, Sacramento, CA, USA
* Corresponding author. Division of Hematology Oncology, UC Davis Comprehensive Cancer Center, 4501 X Street, Suite 3016, Sacramento, CA 95817.
E-mail address: ted.wun@ucdmc.ucdavis.edu

Hematol Oncol Clin N Am 28 (2014) 355–374
http://dx.doi.org/10.1016/j.hoc.2013.11.011
0889-8588/14/$ – see front matter Published by Elsevier Inc.

syndrome) and chronic (avascular necrosis, renal insufficiency) complications of the disease. Also, intracellular polymerization ultimately damages the red cell membrane and leads to chronic and episodic extravascular and intravascular hemolytic anemia, hemolysis-linked nitric oxide (NO) dysregulation, and endothelial dysfunction,[5] resulting in leg ulcer, pulmonary arterial hypertension (PAH), priapism, and stroke.[6]

Several investigators have reported increased thromboembolic events and alteration in hemostatic system in SCD both under steady state and during acute events. This suggests that perturbation in the hemostatic system may contribute to SCD pathophysiology. Changes that have been described include increased expression of tissue factor (TF) on blood monocytes[7–9] and endothelial cells,[10,11] abnormal exposure of phosphatidylserine on the red cell surface,[12,13] and increased microparticles, which both promote activation of the coagulation cascade,[14–16] and high incidence of antiphospholipid antibodies.[17,18] In fact, SCD meets the requirements of the Virchow triad (slow flow, activated procoagulant proteins, and vascular injury); therefore, it should not be surprising that sickle disease is accompanied by thrombosis. Clinical manifestations of the prothrombotic state of patients with SCD include venous thromboembolism (VTE), in situ thrombosis, and stroke.[2,19–22]

In this section, we highlight the existing evidence for contribution of hemostatic system perturbation to SCD pathophysiology. We will also review the data showing increased risk of thromboembolic events, particularly newer information on the incidence of VTE. Finally, the potential role of platelet inhibitors and anticoagulants in SCD will be briefly reviewed.

EVIDENCE FOR INCREASED THROMBOEMBOLIC EVENTS IN SCD

Stroke has an overall prevalence of 3.75% in patients with SCD and 11% in patients younger than 20 years with sickle cell anemia (HbSS), and is most often caused by large vessel arterial obstruction with superimposed thrombosis.[20,23] New and old thrombi in the pulmonary vasculature are prevalent in autopsy series.[21,24,25] The analysis of a large discharge database in Pennsylvania from 2001 to 2006 found that the incidence of pulmonary embolism was 50-fold to 100-fold higher in the SCD population (0.22%–0.52%) than in the general Pennsylvania population (0.0039%–0.0058%).[26] A retrospective study of reported discharge diagnoses showed that patients with SCD younger than 40 years were more likely to be diagnosed with pulmonary embolism compared with African Americans without SCD (0.44% vs 0.12%); however, the prevalence of deep vein thrombosis was similar between the 2 groups.[19] In contrast, in a retrospective study of 404 patients with SCD cared for at the Sickle Cell Center for Adults at Johns Hopkins between August 2008 and January 2012, 25% of the patients had a history of VTE (18.8% non–catheter related), with a median age at diagnosis of 30 years. Sickle cell variant genotypes, such as HbSC or HbSβ+ thalassemia, were associated with increased risk of non–catheter-related VTE compared with HbSS. A history of non–catheter-related VTE was an independent risk factor for death in adults with SCD.[27]

SCD also appears to be a significant risk factor for pregnancy-related VTE, with an odds ratio of 6.7.[28,29] A retrospective study showed that patients with SCD had more antenatal complications than those with sickle cell trait, without affecting the fetal outcome.[30] Sickle cell trait is generally benign, but one study suggested that sickle cell trait increases the risk of VTE in pregnancy compared with race-matched controls, with an odds ratio of about 2.5. Although in another study of pregnancy, sickle cell trait was associated with pulmonary embolism (PE) rather than deep vein thrombosis.[31] In a recent larger study, investigators could not detect a statistically significant difference in peripartum VTE or PE incidence between women with and without sickle cell trait in a large hospital cohort study.[32]

EVIDENCE OF HEMOSTASIS SYSTEM ALTERATION IN SCD

The pathophysiology of hypercoagulability in SCD is multifactorial and is a result of alteration in almost every component of the hemostasis system (**Table 1**). These alterations in platelets, and procoagulant, anticoagulant, and fibrinolytic systems are overall prothrombotic.

Activation of the Coagulation Cascade

Many investigators have shown biomarker evidence for ongoing activation of the coagulation cascade both during steady state (clinically well) and during vaso-occlusive crisis (VOC). These markers denote an ongoing hypercoagulable state in SCD. Thrombin generation is increased in SCD, evidenced by increased prothrombin fragment 1.2 (F1.2), thrombin-antithrombin complexes, plasma fibrinogen products, D-dimer, and decreased factor V.[33–35] Also, Factor VII and activated Factor VII are decreased in SCD compared with non-SCD individuals, most likely due to accelerated FVII turnover by increased TF activity.[36,37] High levels of thrombin-antithrombin complex, prothrombin fragment F1.2, and D-dimer are associated with an activated vascular endothelium in patients with SCD with PAH (defined by echocardiographic criteria), and this correlates with the rate of hemolysis in these patients.[38] However, in a cohort of patients with SCD with mild pulmonary hypertension, there was no association between the hypercoagulable state of SCD and the early phase of PAH.[39]

Alterations in proximal intrinsic pathway proteins have been reported as well. In a small study of homozygous SS disease, plasma prekallikrein levels were decreased during steady state with a further reduction during VOC.[40] In a concomitant study, there was additional 50% decrease in kininogen during VOC compared with low levels of kininogen at baseline. High molecular weight kinonogen (HMWK) was not directly evaluated, but plasma kallikrein almost exclusively digests HMWK; therefore, contact activation is the likely cause of the decrease in plasma kininogen levels.[41] The levels of Factor XII, HMWK, and prekallikrein are slightly decreased in children with homozygous SS disease in steady state.[42] Because components of the contact system are mediators of inflammation, including pain and local vasodilatation, activation

Table 1	
Hemostatic alterations in patients with sickle cell disease	
Increased Levels	**Decreased Levels**
Platelet activation	Factor V
Platelet aggregation	Factor XII
Phosphatidylserine-rich platelets	Factor IX
Thrombin-antithrombin complexes	Protein C
Prothrombin fragment F 1.2	Protein S
Plasmin-antiplasmin complexes	
Fibrinogen and fibrin-fibrinogen complex	
Fibrinopeptide A	
D-dimer	
Plasminogen activator inhibitor	

Data from De Franceschi L, Cappellini MD, Olivieri O. Thrombosis and sickle cell disease. Semin Thromb Hemost 2011;37(3):228.

of this system might play a role in inflammatory pathway perturbations as wells as coagulation pathway abnormalities that contribute to SCD pathophysiology.

Reduction in Physiologic Anticoagulant Level

Decreases in anticoagulant proteins of hemostasis system would further promote a hypercoagulable state and have been reported in SCD. Onyemelukwe and Jibril[43] described significantly lower level of plasma antithrombin III (AT-III, now called anti-thrombin or AT) in patients with SCD compared with healthy non-SCD controls. The anticoagulants protein C and S are low in patients with SCD in steady state (crisis free), and tend to decrease to even lower levels during crisis episodes.[35,44,45] In a survey of patients with SCD in steady state from Turkey, protein C and AT were significantly lower compared with non-SCD controls.[46] Also, significantly decreased levels of proteins C and S were reported in patients with SCD who developed thrombotic strokes compared with neurologically healthy children with SCD.[47] However, the association with stroke was not seen in the report by Liesner and colleagues,[48] despite demonstrating a reduction in proteins C and S and increased thrombin generation (denoted by increased thrombin-antithrombin complexes and prothrombin fragment 1 + 2) in the steady state, which was only partially reversed by transfusion.[48] Plasma levels of the serine protease inhibitor, heparin cofactor II (HCII), are also decreased in SCD.[49] In total, these findings suggest a possible alteration in either anticoagulant synthesis related to liver disease or chronic consumption due to increased thrombin production.

Impaired Fibrinolysis

The thrombophilia in SCD is also associated with abnormalities in the fibrinolytic system, characterized by increased plasma levels of plasminogen activator inhibitor (PAI)-1 in both steady state and during sickle acute events compared with the healthy population.[50,51] This may be a result of increased synthesis of PAI-1 by damaged endothelial cells and activated platelets,[52] and might participate in the pathogenesis of VOC in SCD. Elevations in plasma plasmin-antiplasmin complexes (PAP)[33] were also observed in patients with SCD in the noncrisis, steady state. The frequency of pain episodes in patients with SCD correlated with the extent of fibrinolytic activity (assessed by D-dimer levels) in the noncrisis steady state, suggesting that D-dimer levels may predict the frequency of pain crises.[33]

Activated Platelets

Platelet abnormalities (function, number, and survival) both in baseline crisis-free state and acute events were some of the earliest hemostatic changes documented in SCD.[53–60] Several biomarkers have been measured to document the functional abnormalities. Urinary thromboxane-A2 and prostaglandin metabolites are increased, and platelet trombospondin-1 level is decreased in SCD.[61,62] These findings suggested ongoing platelet activation. Increased platelet activation markers, such as P-selectin (CD62), CD63, activated glycoprotein (GP) IIb/IIIa, plasma soluble factors (PF)-3, PF4, β-thromboglobulin, and platelet-derived soluble CD40 ligand (sCD40L) were reported in patients with SCD using cytofluorimetric approaches.[33,59,63,64] Also, platelet adherence to fibrinogen was found to be increased through modulation of intracellular signaling pathways associated with increased αIIβ3-integrin activation.[65] Platelet aggregation in adults has been found to be increased, perhaps because of an increase in the number of megathrombocytes in the peripheral circulation[60,66,67] or as a result of increase in levels of platelet agonists, such as thrombin, adenosine diphosphate, or epinephrine. In contrast to adults, platelet aggregation in children was normal or reduced, perhaps because of better preservation of splenic function or fewer circulating megathrombocytes.[53,55,57] Increased phosphatidylserine-rich platelets have also been described in patients with SCD, which might accelerate the activation of the coagulation system.[33]

Platelet number and survival are also abnormal in both steady state and acute events. In steady state there is moderate thrombocytosis in older children and adults with sickle cell anemia.[66] The number of circulating megathrombocytes, which are young and metabolically active platelets, is also increased. These findings have been attributed to the functional asplenia exhibited by these patients.[67] Although studies performed during steady state suggest normal platelet survival,[54,68] decrease in platelet lifespan has been reported in VOC.[54,69,70] Platelet and megathrombocyte counts may decrease markedly, especially when the crisis is severe.[56] These decreases are followed by marked rebound increases in platelet and megathrombocyte counts, with levels peaking 10 to 14 days after the onset of the crisis.[54,70]

All of these findings suggest that both shortened platelet survival and enhanced platelet consumption occur during VOCs, possibly because platelets are being deposited at sites of vascular injury or vascular occlusion. It has been demonstrated that labeled platelets accumulate at the putative sites of vaso-occlusion.[69]

PATHOPHYSIOLOGY OF HEMOSTASIS SYSTEM ACTIVATION IN SCD

As shown previously, in SCD there is a chronic increase in plasma markers of thrombin generation, decrease in natural anticoagulants, and inhibited fibrinolytic system, and some data show these changes are accentuated during a VOC. Although the role of genetic predisposition for thrombophilia in SCD (separate from the sickle cell mutation itself) is still under investigation, several other factors have been identified as contributors to the altered hemostatic system in SCD. Although some of these play major roles in the pathophysiology of SCD, such as altered red blood cell (RBC) membrane, inflammation due to vaso-occlusion/reperfusion oxidative stress, hemolysis resulting in cell-free hemoglobin, abnormal bioavailability of NO, and endothelial dysfunction, the role of others remains under investigation. These include activated circulating endothelial cells, monocytes, microparticles, and platelets. All of these factors have potential to activate the coagulation cascade by increased TF expression on endothelial cells, monocytes, and circulating microparticles derived from RBCs, monocytes, endothelial cells, and platelets.[9,71] Possible mechanisms for increased TF expression in SCD are (1) increased cell-free heme from hemolysis inducing TF expression on vascular endothelial cells[72]; (2) ischemia-reperfusion (hypoxia and inflammation), in fact, in an experimental mouse model, 3 hours of exposure to a hypoxic environment and subsequent return to 18 hours of ambient air resulted in an increase in pulmonary vein TF expression, suggesting that ischemia-reperfusion injury in patients with SCD may play a role in activation of procoagulant proteins[71]; and (3) platelet activation and exposure of CD40 ligand.[63]

Role of RBC Membrane

There has been extensive research on the abnormal RBC membrane and its role in pathophysiology of SCD, which is beyond the scope of this review. In summary, abnormal phosphatidylserine (PS) exposure of the sickle cell RBC membrane[12] alters the adhesive properties of sickle RBCs,[73] leading to an increase in capillary transit time and stasis, enhancing the potential for the activation of coagulation factors and cellular elements in the microvasculature and postcapillary venules. Additionally, the exposed PS functions as a docking site for procoagulant proteins.[74–76] The number of PS-positive sickle RBCs significantly correlates with plasma levels of prothrombin fragment 1.2, D-dimer, and PAP complexes,[75,76] and may contribute to increased risk of stroke in SCD.[77] These PS-positive RBCs are a signal for apoptosis[78,79] and lead to TF-positive microparticle generation. Antiphospholipid antibodies against PS are also markedly elevated in homozygous SCD and correlate strongly with plasma D-dimer, suggesting a role for antiphospholipid antibodies in coagulation activation in SCD.[35] The mechanism may be inhibition of protein S binding to β_2-glycoprotein-1,[80] resulting in inactivation of protein S by circulating C4b-binding protein. In addition, RBCs with increased PS exposure may bind directly to protein S, contributing to reduction in free protein S.[81,82]

Role of Hemolysis-Free Hemoglobin-NO-Spleen Axis

Physiologically, endothelial-derived NO is protected from the scavenging effects of intracellular hemoglobin by the erythrocyte membrane barrier and the cell-free zone that forms along endothelium in laminar flowing blood.[83–86] Also, haptoglobin, CD163, hemoxygenase, and biliverdin reductase detoxify cell-free hemoglobin after hemolysis. However, during intravascular hemolysis, the haptoglobin-hemoxygenase-biliverdin reductase system is overwhelmed. Consequently, the cell-free hemoglobin is accumulated in plasma and interacts with NO, generating reactive oxygen species. In addition, arginase I, which is released from the RBC during hemolysis, metabolizes arginine, which is the substrate for NO synthesis.[87]

NO not only regulates the vascular tone and inhibits endothelial adhesion molecule expression, but also has potent antithrombotic effects. NO inhibits platelet activation via cycle guanosine monophosphate-dependent signaling.[88–91] Nitric oxide may also inhibit TF expression.[92–94]

In addition to scavenging NO, cell-free hemoglobin can inhibit ADAMTS13 activity affecting von Willebrand factor (vWF) cleavage in patients with thrombotic thrombocytopenic purpura.[95] In fact, ADAMTS13 activity and ADAMTS13-to-vWF antigen ratio is decreased in patients with SCD compared with healthy controls.[96–98] This would decrease the proteolysis of vWF and could lead to the accumulation of ultra-large adhesive vWF on the vascular endothelium surface and thrombosis. This mechanism may be a novel mechanism contributing to the complex microvascular pathophysiology of SCD. As mentioned earlier, free heme can also induce endothelial TF expression.

The spleen clears senescent, oxidized, and phosphatidylserine-exposing red cells from the circulation and thus limits intravascular cell microvesiculation, hemolysis, and phosphatidylserine exposure.[99–101] Increase in the plasma concentration of cell free hemoglobin and red cell microparticles after splenectomy could increase NO scavenging, vascular injury, and thrombosis. Interestingly, because priapism may also be a complication of hemolytic anemia and low NO bioavailability,[102–104] an increase in intravascular cell free plasma hemoglobin and red cell microparticles after splenectomy could also explain the observed development of priapism after splenectomy.[105,106] It is also well established that splenectomy in other patient populations is associated with increased risk of VTE.[107]

The Microparticles

Microparticles (MPs) are small membrane vesicles released from cells when activated or during apoptosis. MPs in the blood can originate from platelets, erythrocytes, leukocytes, and endothelial cells.[108] In healthy individuals, circulating MPs are mainly derived from platelets and to a lesser extent leukocyte and endothelial cells.[109] Elevated numbers of circulating microparticles have been reported in patients suffering from a variety of diseases with vascular involvement and hypercoagulability, including SCD.[110–115] The exact mechanism by which circulating microparticles trigger coagulation in SCD remains unclear. Most circulating microparticles in SCD originate from erythrocytes and platelets and by exposure of phosphatidylserine facilitate coagulation cascade complex formation.

Additionally, increased exposure of TF has been demonstrated on monocyte-derived microparticles.[110] TF-positive microparticles derived from RBCs, platelets, endothelial cells, and monocytes are elevated in patients with SCD both in steady state and during acute events compared with healthy controls,[110] suggesting their possible role in the sickle cell prothrombotic state.[48] The high levels of erythroid and platelet-derived microparticles in sickle cell patients may further increase during acute vaso-occlusive events, although this has not been a consistent finding.[59]

The erythroid-derived microparticles are able to activate the coagulation system independent of the TF and their level correlates with markers of hemolysis, von Willebrand factor, D-dimer and F1+2 levels,[14] pain crisis, and elevated tricuspid regurgitant jet velocity measured by echocardiogram.[15] Their ability to activate the coagulation system through factor XIIa[16] could explain this third pathway. The increase in thrombin generation seems to primarily be caused by erythroid-derived microparticles and hydroxyurea is associated with decreased circulating microparticles compared with untreated patients.[116]

GENETIC PREDISPOSITION FOR THROMBOPHILIA IN SCD

Genetic modifiers with functional effects on the hemostatic system have been studied in patients with SCD. Many of the thrombophilic mutations described to date are not prevalent in people of African descent.[117,118] However, in some populations, patients with SCD might be carrying thrombophilic mutations more than the general population. Studies of human platelet alloantigen (HPA) polymorphism showed a possible prothrombotic role in these patients. Few investigators have studied the role of genetic modifiers of vascular endothelium as well.

Thrombophilic Mutations

Many studies reported the low frequency of thrombophilic mutations (Factor V Leiden [FVL], MTHFR C677T, and prothrombin G20210A) and the lack of association between these mutations and risk of thromboembolism in African American, sub-Saharan African, West Indies, Maghrib, Brazilian, Jamaican, and eastern Saudi Arabian patients with SCD, likely because of the low frequency of these genes in the related general population.[119–127] However, despite the moderate prevalence of FVL mutation (2.97%–5.50%) among the general population of Iran,[128] the prevalence of FVL mutation is higher (14.30%) among Iranian patients with SCD[129] with a significant association between this mutation and SCD (odds ratio = 6.5). Also, a study from Brazil suggests that MTHFR C677T might be a risk factor for vascular complications in SCD.[123] Also, 3 studies of inherited risk factors of venous thromboembolism in patients with SCD from southern Mediterranean countries[130–132] report high prevalence of thrombophilic mutations in patients with SCD and their association with thromboembolic events. Among Lebanese sickle/β^0-thalassemia patients, a high prevalence of the thrombophilic mutations of FVL (42%), homozygous and heterozygous MTHFR C677T (59%), and prothrombin G20210A (8%) has been reported.[130] In this report, patients with sickle/β-thalassemia were 5.24-fold and 4.39-fold more likely to have FVL mutation as compared with the healthy controls and patients with thalassemia intermedia, respectively. Also, the presence of extensive large vessel thrombosis in a patient with sickle/β^0-thalassemia from Lebanon who was homozygous for FVL and heterozygous for MTHFRC677T has been reported.[131] In another case report, a patient with SCD from Israel with recurrent cerebrovascular accident and deep venous thrombosis, was found to be heterozygous for FVL and MTHFR C677T.[132] Therefore, the prevalence of thrombophilic mutations in the non-African SCD population may be of clinical relevance.

Human Platelet Alloantigen Polymorphism

Polymorphisms in HPA genes may determine platelet reactivity and have been associated with variable risk of thrombotic events, mostly arterial.[133] Studies on polymorphisms of HPA show a possible prothrombotic role in different thrombotic disorders and in patients with SCD with cerebrovascular events.[133–137] In a case-control study, Al-Subaie and colleagues[137] reported that the HPA-3 variant, which has an isoleucine-to-serine substitution close to the C-terminus of the GPIIb heavy chain, is an independent risk factor for acute vaso-occlusive events in SCD.

Genetic modifiers affecting vascular endothelium in patients with SCD have been evaluated in a few studies; however, the mechanism by which they affect the vascular endothelium needs to be investigated further and in larger patient populations.

THERAPEUTIC IMPLICATIONS OF HEMOSTATIC SYSTEM ACTIVATION IN SCD

Although hemostatic activation is somewhat downstream in the SCD pathophysiological cascade, it is plausible that a therapy targeted at decreasing platelet and coagulation activation might ameliorate or prevent sickle cell–related complications. This is analogous to the use of platelet inhibitors in atherosclerotic vascular disease and anticoagulants in venous thromboembolism. The underlying pathogenesis is not targeted; nonetheless, blocking downstream effects does decrease the incidence and severity of complications. In addition, emerging data suggesting increased venous thromboembolism in patients with SCD[26,27,138] provides further rationale for treatment with either platelet inhibitors or anticoagulants. Finally, platelet inhibitors and anticoagulants are widely used and studied, and their safety profiles are well known in diverse populations. All of this makes study of these agents attractive in SCD.

Trials of Platelet Inhibitors in SCD

To date, there are only 3 studies in humans evaluating the therapeutic effect of aspirin in SCD (**Table 2**). These studies were conducted in the 1980s and results are limited by the study design. When hemoglobin was incubated with aspirin in vitro, the acetyl group was incorporated into hemoglobin and led to increased oxygen affinity.[139] Subsequently, Osamo and colleagues[140] investigated the therapeutic effect of aspirin in 100 patients aged 11 to 20 years with homozygous SCD. In this study, half of patients were randomized to receive a total daily dose of 1200 mg soluble aspirin for 6 weeks, whereas the other half received placebo in addition to usual care. Hemoglobin levels and oxygen saturation increased in the aspirin arm with increased red cell survival in the 3 patients whose red cell survival was measured. There were no comparative values for the placebo arm. There were no serious hemorrhagic events in the treatment group. Pain was not formally assessed. However, in a double-blind placebo-controlled crossover study of a lower dose of aspirin (3–6 mg/kg) for a longer period of time (21 months) in 49 children aged 2 to 17 years with HbSS, HbSC, or HbSO-Arab, there was no difference in the number of painful episodes, number of total days in pain, duration of pain crisis, or pain severity during crisis between the aspirin-treated and placebo-treated periods using pain assessment forms completed by their parents. Irrespective of the treatment, there was a marked decrease in the number of pain

Table 2
Studies of platelet inhibition in sickle cell disease

Author	Genotypes	Study Type (n)	Therapy	Overall Result
Chaplin et al,[143] 1980	HbSS	Nonrandomized crossover (3)	Aspirin and diypyridamole	Decrease in pain frequency, platelet count, and fibrinogen
Osamo et al,[140] 1981	HbSS	Randomized (100)	Aspirin	Increase in oxygen affinity, Hb, and red cell life span Pain not formally assessed
Greenberg et al,[141] 1983	HbSS/SO-Arab/SC	Randomized (49)	Aspirin vs placebo	No decrease in pain frequency
Semple et al,[69] 1984	HbSS/Sβ thalassemia	Randomized (9)	Ticlopidine vs placebo	No change in pain, but decrease in platelet activation biomarkers
Cabannes et al,[144] 1984	HbSS	Randomized (140)	Ticlopidine vs placebo	Reduction in frequency and duration of vaso-occlusive crisis
Zago et al,[142] 1984	HbSS/Sβ thalassemia	Randomized (29)	Aspirin vs placebo	No change in pain episodes or laboratory values
Wun et al,[138] 2013	HbSS/Sβ thalassemia/SC	Randomized Phase 2 (62)	Prasugrel vs placebo	Decrease in platelet activation and trend to decreased pain frequency and rate

Data from Ataga KI, Key NS. Hypercoagulability in sickle cell disease: new approaches to an old problem. Hematology Am Soc Hematol Educ Program 2007;94.

crises after the first 6 months of study.[141] Similarly, a single-blind crossover study of 29 patients aged 4 to 31 years receiving 17 to 45 mg/kg per day of aspirin for 5 months followed by no aspirin for the next 5 months,[142] did not find a difference in the painful events.

The data for use of dipyridamole in SCD is sparse. Chaplin and colleagues[143] treated 3 patients with aspirin 650 mg by mouth twice a day and dipyridamole (a phosphodiesterase inhibitor) 50 mg by mouth twice daily for acute pain crisis and compared the frequency and severity of pain for the 2 years on therapy to the next 2 years off the therapy. The severity of pain and the total number of hospitalizations for pain decreased. During the study there was no evidence of increased bleeding.

Therapeutic effect of thienopyridines has also been studied in SCD. Semple and colleagues[69] assessed platelet survival and activation in 9 asymptomatic patients with SCD who were randomized to placebo for 28 days followed by ticlopidine 250 mg by mouth twice daily for next 28 days. Ticlopidine did not prolong platelet survival (measured by radiolabeled platelets) but 40% reduction in collagen and ADP-induced maximal platelet aggregation was observed in this double-blind placebo-controlled trial. One patient had a painful episode during the therapy, but this study was not powered to determine a difference in pain. Cabannes and colleagues[144] randomized 140 patients with SCD to ticlopidine 500 to 750 mg daily for 6 months or placebo to study the efficacy of ticlopidine in the prevention of acute pain crisis. Frequency of crisis, crisis duration, and crisis severity decreased in the ticlopidine arm compared with the placebo arm. More recently, Wun and colleagues[138] studied the third-generation thienopyridine, prasugrel, in a randomized, double-blind adaptive Phase 2 study in adults with all genotypes of SCD. Patients were randomized to prasugrel 5 mg daily (n = 41) or placebo (n = 21) for 30 days. Platelet function was significantly inhibited in prasugrel-treated compared with placebo-treated patients with SCD. Biomarkers of in vivo platelet activation, including platelet surface P-selectin and plasma soluble P-selectin, were significantly reduced in patients with SCD treated with prasugrel compared with placebo. Mean pain rate (percentage of days with pain) and intensity decreased in the prasugrel arm but did not reach statistical significance. Prasugrel was well tolerated and not associated with serious hemorrhagic events. Despite the small size and short duration of this study, there was a decrease in platelet activation biomarkers and a trend toward decreased pain. An international Phase 3 study of prasugrel in children with SCD is currently enrolling.

Anticoagulant Therapy for Sickle Cell Disease

Anticoagulants might be used in SCD for the primary or secondary prevention of VTE, to treat or prevent complications of SCD, or both. For the primary or secondary prevention of VTE, there is no evidence that the use of anticoagulant medications should be any different than in other medically ill patients with regard to indications, dose, intensity, or duration of therapy. This is because of the lack of SCD-specific studies addressing the management of VTE in this population. Special considerations include the possibility that filling defects on CT angiogram for diagnosis of pulmonary embolism may represent in situ sickling rather than a classic fibrin-rich clot, and the lack of utility of D-dimer in diagnostic algorithms for VTE due to persistent elevations in many patients. In addition, if one considers SCD to be a potent and persistent hypercoagulable state, then there is a stronger argument for extended secondary prophylaxis after a first unprovoked event. This would be concordant with current American College of Chest Physician guidelines that suggest extended anticoagulation after unprovoked events for all patients when there is a low risk of bleeding.

There have been a handful of studies examining chronic anticoagulation in SCD; most have been small and uncontrolled (**Table 3**). A series of 12 patients treated with warfarin was reported by Salvaggio and colleagues[145] in 1963. Each patient served as his or her own control. Although no formal statistics were performed, the frequency of pain episodes did not seem to improve and there were 7 episodes of bleeding, 1 nearly fatal. The investigators concluded that warfarin was not beneficial in SCD.

Schnog and colleagues[146] performed a randomized, double blind, placebo-controlled, crossover pilot study to assess the efficacy and safety of low adjusted-dose acenocoumarol. Treatment was either acenocoumarol or placebo for 14 weeks, after which treatment was discontinued for a period of 5 weeks. Patients were then crossed over. Efficacy was assessed by comparing the frequency of VOC, incident bleeding, and biomarkers of coagulation activation between acenocoumarol and placebo treatment of each patient. Twenty-two patients (14 homozygous [HbSS] and 8 compound heterozygous sickle-C [HbSC]; aged 20–59 years) completed the entire

Table 3
Studies of anticoagulation in sickle cell disease

Author	Genotypes	Study Type (n)	Therapy	Overall Results
Salvaggio et al,[145] 1963	HbSS	Nonrandomized (12)	Warfarin	Slight decrease in frequency of pain episodes
Chaplin et al,[143] 1980	HbSS	Nonrandomized (4)	Heparin	Reduced frequency of pain episodes
Wolters et al,[149] 1995	HbSS/SC	Nonrandomized (7)	Acenocoumarol	Reduction in biomarker of thrombin activation
Schnog et al,[146] 2001	HbSS/SC	Randomized (22)	Acenocoumarol vs placebo	Decreased markers of thrombin activation but no effect on pain
Qari et al,[148] 2007	HbSS	Randomized (253)	Tinzaprain vs placebo	Reduction in the duration and severity of vaso-occlusive crisis

Data from Ataga KI, Key NS. Hypercoagulability in sickle cell disease: new approaches to an old problem. Hematology Am Soc Hematol Educ Program 2007;94.

study. Acenocoumarol treatment did not result in a significant reduction of VOC events. There was a marked reduction of the hypercoagulable state, as denoted by biomarkers (decreased plasma levels of prothrombin F1.2 fragments [$P = .002$], thrombin-antithrombin complexes [$P = .003$], and D-dimer fragments [$P = .001$]) without the major bleeding. Even though no clinical benefit (pertaining to the frequency of painful crises) was detected in this pilot study, the investigators concluded the value of low adjusted-dose acenocoumarol for preventing specific events (such as strokes) and as a long-term treatment of patients with SCD should be a subject of further study.

Anticoagulation also has been studied in the acute VOC setting. Ahmed and colleagues[147] measured plasma D-dimer in 37 adult patients with SCD who were hospitalized for VOC. D-dimer level of patients who were on low-dose warfarin was compared with those patients who were not on any anticoagulation treatment. Patients were on warfarin either for VTE or catheter prophylaxis; this was not a randomized study. Overall median D-dimer level in 65 samples was 2.7 µg fibrinogen equivalent units (FEU)/mL (0.34–4.00). Patients who were on low-dose warfarin had a median D-dimer level of 0.81 µg FEU/mL (0.34–1.80) compared with 3.1 µg FEU/mL (0.94–4.00) in those patients who were not on anticoagulation treatment. Using analysis of variance to model D-dimer levels, only warfarin was significantly correlated with low D-dimer levels after controlling for other variables. They concluded that patients with SCD during a vaso-occlusive painful crisis have an elevated D-dimer level and that low-dose anticoagulation treatment is associated with a significant reduction in the D-dimer levels. There was no assessment of clinically important outcomes.

A randomized double-blind clinical trial was performed to test the safety and efficacy of a low molecular weight heparin, tinzaparin, for the management of VOC.[148] A total of 253 patients with acute painful crisis, but with no other complications of SCD, were randomized to tinzaparin at 175 IU/kg, subcutaneous once daily, along with supportive care, including morphine analgesia; in the comparator group, 126 patients received placebo and the same supportive care. The maximal treatment period was 7 days. Tinzaparin-treated patients had significantly fewer total hospital days (mean of 7.08 vs 12.06 days), crisis duration (mean of 2.57 vs 4.35 days), and days of severest pain score (mean of 1.28 vs 1.74) compared with placebo-treated patients. There were 2 minor bleeding events in the tinzaparin arm. As noted, heparin in the setting of SCD may inhibit P-selectin–mediated red cell adhesion in addition to anticoagulant effects. These provocative findings should be confirmed in future studies, especially as one could argue that low molecular weight heparin at prophylactic doses should be routine in hospitalized patients with SCD.

SUMMARY

Although the pathogenesis of SCD lies in disordered hemoglobin structure and function, downstream effects of sickle hemoglobin include changes in hemostatic system that overall result in a prothrombotic phenotype. These changes include thrombin activation, decreased levels of anticoagulants, impaired fibrinolysis, and platelet activation. Limited studies to date suggest that biomarkers of activation can be affected by currently available antithrombotic drugs, and provocative data from pilot studies indicate there may be improvement in clinically important outcomes. Therefore, clinical trials with antithrombotic therapies are justified, with both SCD-related complications (VOC, pain) and thrombotic complications as outcome events of interest.

REFERENCES

1. Eaton WA, Hofrichter J. Sickle cell hemoglobin polymerization. Adv Protein Chem 1990;40:63–279.
2. Steinberg MH. Management of sickle cell disease. N Engl J Med 1999;340(13): 1021–30.
3. Ballas SK, Smith ED. Red blood cell changes during the evolution of the sickle cell painful crisis. Blood 1992;79(8):2154–63.
4. Solovey AA, Solovey AN, Harkness J, et al. Modulation of endothelial cell activation in sickle cell disease: a pilot study. Blood 2001;97(7):1937–41.
5. Kato GJ, Gladwin MT, Steinberg MH. Deconstructing sickle cell disease: reappraisal of the role of hemolysis in the development of clinical subphenotypes. Blood Rev 2007;21(1):37–47.
6. Ohene-Frempong KS, Steinberg MH. Clinical aspects of sickle cell anemia in adults and children. In: Steinberg BF, Forget BG, Higgs DR, et al, editors. Disorders of hemoglobin: genetics, pathophysiology, and clinical management. Cambridge (United Kingdom): Cambridge University Press; 2001. p. 611–70.
7. Belcher JD, Marker PH, Weber JP, et al. Activated monocytes in sickle cell disease: potential role in the activation of vascular endothelium and vaso-occlusion. Blood 2000;96(7):2451–9.
8. Setty BN, Key NS, Rao AK, et al. Tissue factor-positive monocytes in children with sickle cell disease: correlation with biomarkers of haemolysis. Br J Haematol 2012;157(3):370–80.
9. Key NS, Slungaard A, Dandelet L, et al. Whole blood tissue factor procoagulant activity is elevated in patients with sickle cell disease. Blood 1998;91(11): 4216–23.
10. Solovey A, Gui L, Key NS, et al. Tissue factor expression by endothelial cells in sickle cell anemia. J Clin Invest 1998;101(9):1899–904.
11. Setty BN, Betal SG, Zhang J, et al. Heme induces endothelial tissue factor expression: potential role in hemostatic activation in patients with hemolytic anemia. J Thromb Haemost 2008;6(12):2202–9.

12. Kuypers FA, Lewis RA, Hua M, et al. Detection of altered membrane phospholipid asymmetry in subpopulations of human red blood cells using fluorescently labeled annexin V. Blood 1996;87(3):1179–87.

13. Wood BL, Gibson DF, Tait JF. Increased erythrocyte phosphatidylserine exposure in sickle cell disease: flow-cytometric measurement and clinical associations. Blood 1996;88(5):1873–80.

14. van Beers EJ, Schaap MC, Berckmans RJ, et al. Circulating erythrocyte-derived microparticles are associated with coagulation activation in sickle cell disease. Haematologica 2009;94(11):1513–9.

15. Tantawy AA, Adly AA, Ismail EA, et al. Circulating platelet and erythrocyte microparticles in young children and adolescents with sickle cell disease: relation to cardiovascular complications. Platelets 2013;24(8):605–14.

16. Van Der Meijden PE, Van Schilfgaarde M, Van Oerle R, et al. Platelet- and erythrocyte-derived microparticles trigger thrombin generation via factor XIIa. J Thromb Haemost 2012;10(7):1355–62.

17. Westerman MP, Unger L, Kucuk O, et al. Phase changes in membrane lipids in sickle red cell shed-vesicles and sickle red cells. Am J Hematol 1998;58(3): 177–82.

18. Kucuk O, Gilman-Sachs A, Beaman K, et al. Antiphospholipid antibodies in sickle cell disease. Am J Hematol 1993;42(4):380–3.

19. Stein PD, Beemath A, Meyers FA, et al. Deep venous thrombosis and pulmonary embolism in hospitalized patients with sickle cell disease. Am J Med 2006; 119(10):897.e7–11.

20. Prengler M, Pavlakis SG, Prohovnik I, et al. Sickle cell disease: the neurological complications. Ann Neurol 2002;51(5):543–52.

21. Adedeji MO, Cespedes J, Allen K, et al. Pulmonary thrombotic arteriopathy in patients with sickle cell disease. Arch Pathol Lab Med 2001;125(11):1436–41.

22. Haque AK, Gokhale S, Rampy BA, et al. Pulmonary hypertension in sickle cell hemoglobinopathy: a clinicopathologic study of 20 cases. Hum Pathol 2002; 33(10):1037–43.

23. Ohene-Frempong K, Weiner SJ, Sleeper LA, et al. Cerebrovascular accidents in sickle cell disease: rates and risk factors. Blood 1998;91(1):288–94.

24. Graham JK, Mosunjac M, Hanzlick RL, et al. Sickle cell lung disease and sudden death: a retrospective/prospective study of 21 autopsy cases and literature review. Am J Forensic Med Pathol 2007;28(2):168–72.

25. Manci EA, Culberson DE, Yang YM, et al. Causes of death in sickle cell disease: an autopsy study. Br J Haematol 2003;123(2):359–65.

26. Novelli EM, Huynh C, Gladwin MT, et al. Pulmonary embolism in sickle cell disease: a case-control study. J Thromb Haemost 2012;10(5):760–6.

27. Naik RP, Streiff MB, Haywood C Jr, et al. Venous thromboembolism in adults with sickle cell disease: a serious and under-recognized complication. Am J Med 2013;126(5):443–9.

28. Villers MS, Jamison MG, De Castro LM, et al. Morbidity associated with sickle cell disease in pregnancy. Am J Obstet Gynecol 2008;199(2):125.e1–5.

29. James AH, Jamison MG, Brancazio LR, et al. Venous thromboembolism during pregnancy and the postpartum period: incidence, risk factors, and mortality. Am J Obstet Gynecol 2006;194(5):1311–5.

30. Zia S, Rafique M. Comparison of pregnancy outcomes in women with sickle cell disease and trait. J Pak Med Assoc 2013;63(6):743–6.

31. Austin H, Key NS, Benson JM, et al. Sickle cell trait and the risk of venous thromboembolism among blacks. Blood 2007;110(3):908–12.

32. Pintova S, Cohen HW, Billett HH. Sickle cell trait: is there an increased VTE risk in pregnancy and the postpartum? PLoS One 2013;8(5):e64141.

33. Tomer A, Harker LA, Kasey S, et al. Thrombogenesis in sickle cell disease. J Lab Clin Med 2001;137(6):398–407.

34. Peters M, Plaat BE, Ten Cate H, et al. Enhanced thrombin generation in children with sickle cell disease. Thromb Haemost 1994;71(2):169–72.

35. Westerman MP, Green D, Gilman-Sachs A, et al. Antiphospholipid antibodies, proteins C and S, and coagulation changes in sickle cell disease. J Lab Clin Med 1999;134(4):352–62.

36. Kurantsin-Mills J, Ofosu FA, Safa TK, et al. Plasma factor VII and thrombin-antithrombin III levels indicate increased tissue factor activity in sickle cell patients. Br J Haematol 1992;81(4):539–44.

37. Hagger D, Wolff S, Owen J, et al. Changes in coagulation and fibrinolysis in patients with sickle cell disease compared with healthy black controls. Blood Coagul Fibrinolysis 1995;6(2):93–9.

38. Ataga KI, Moore CG, Hillery CA, et al. Coagulation activation and inflammation in sickle cell disease-associated pulmonary hypertension. Haematologica 2008; 93(1):20–6.

39. van Beers EJ, Spronk HM, Ten Cate H, et al. No association of the hypercoagulable state with sickle cell disease related pulmonary hypertension. Haematologica 2008;93(5):e42–4.

40. Miller R, Verma P, Adams R. Studies of the kallikrein-kinin system in patients with sickle cell disease. J Natl Med Assoc 1983;75(6):551–6.

41. Verma P, Adams R, Miller R. Reduced plasma kininogen concentration during sickle cell crisis. Res Commun Chem Pathol Pharmacol 1983;41(2):313–22.

42. Gordon E, Klein B, Berman B, et al. Reduction of contact factors in sickle cell disease. J Pediatr 1985;106(3):427–30.

43. Onyemelukwe GC, Jibril HB. Anti-thrombin III deficiency in Nigerian children with sickle cell disease. Possible role in the cerebral syndrome. Trop Geogr Med 1992;44(1–2):37–41.

44. Wright JG, Malia R, Cooper P, et al. Protein C and protein S in homozygous sickle cell disease: does hepatic dysfunction contribute to low levels? Br J Haematol 1997;98(3):627–31.

45. el-Hazmi MA, Warsy AS, Bahakim H. Blood proteins C and S in sickle cell disease. Acta Haematol 1993;90(3):114–9.

46. Bayazit AK, Kilinc Y. Natural coagulation inhibitors (protein C, protein S, antithrombin) in patients with sickle cell anemia in a steady state. Pediatr Int 2001;43(6):592–6.

47. Tam DA. Protein C and protein S activity in sickle cell disease and stroke. J Child Neurol 1997;12(1):19–21.

48. Liesner R, Mackie I, Cookson J, et al. Prothrombotic changes in children with sickle cell disease: relationships to cerebrovascular disease and transfusion. Br J Haematol 1998;103(4):1037–44.

49. Porter JB, Young L, Mackie IJ, et al. Sickle cell disorders and chronic intravascular haemolysis are associated with low plasma heparin cofactor II. Br J Haematol 1993;83(3):459–65.

50. Nsiri B, Gritli N, Mazigh C, et al. Fibrinolytic response to venous occlusion in patients with homozygous sickle cell disease. Hematol Cell Ther 1997;39(5): 229–32.

51. Nsiri B, Gritli N, Bayoudh F, et al. Abnormalities of coagulation and fibrinolysis in homozygous sickle cell disease. Hematol Cell Ther 1996;38(3):279–84.

52. Yamamoto K, Saito H. A pathological role of increased expression of plasminogen activator inhibitor-1 in human or animal disorders. Int J Hematol 1998; 68(4):371–85.

53. Stuart MJ, Stockman JA, Oski FA. Abnormalities of platelet aggregation in the vaso-occlusive crisis of sickle-cell anemia. J Pediatr 1974;85(5):629–32.

54. Haut MJ, Cowan DH, Harris JW. Platelet function and survival in sickle cell disease. J Lab Clin Med 1973;82(1):44–53.

55. Gruppo RA, Glueck HI, Granger SM, et al. Platelet function in sickle cell anemia. Thromb Res 1977;10(3):235.

56. Freedman ML, Karpatkin S. Elevated platelet count and megathrombocyte number in sickle cell anemia. Blood 1975;46(4):579–82.

57. Mehta P, Mehta J. Abnormalities of platelet aggregation in sickle cell disease. J Pediatr 1980;96(2):209–13.

58. Papadimitriou CA, Travlou A, Kalos A, et al. Study of platelet function in patients with sickle cell anemia during steady state and vaso-occlusive crisis. Acta Haematol 1993;89(4):180–3.

59. Wun T, Paglieroni T, Rangaswami A, et al. Platelet activation in patients with sickle cell disease. Br J Haematol 1998;100(4):741–9.

60. Westwick J, Watson-Williams EJ, Krishnamurthi S, et al. Platelet activation during steady state sickle cell disease. Am J Med 1983;14(1):17–36.

61. Browne PV, Mosher DF, Steinberg MH, et al. Disturbance of plasma and platelet thrombospondin levels in sickle cell disease. Am J Hematol 1996;51(4): 296–301.

62. Foulon I, Bachir D, Galacteros F, et al. Increased in vivo production of thromboxane in patients with sickle cell disease is accompanied by an impairment of platelet functions to the thromboxane A2 agonist U46619. Arterioscler Thromb 1993;13(3):421–6.

63. Lee SP, Ataga KI, Orringer EP, et al. Biologically active CD40 ligand is elevated in sickle cell anemia: potential role for platelet-mediated inflammation. Arterioscler Thromb Vasc Biol 2006;26(7):1626–31.

64. Famodu AA, Oduwa D. Platelet count and platelet factor 3 (PF-3) availability in sickle cell disease. Br J Biomed Sci 1995;52(4):323–4.

65. Proenca-Ferreira R, Franco-Penteado CF, Traina F, et al. Increased adhesive properties of platelets in sickle cell disease: roles for alphaIIb beta3-mediated ligand binding, diminished cAMP signalling and increased phosphodiesterase 3A activity. Br J Haematol 2010;149(2):280–8.

66. Francis RB Jr. Platelets, coagulation, and fibrinolysis in sickle cell disease: their possible role in vascular occlusion. Blood Coagul Fibrinolysis 1991;2(2):341–53.

67. Kenny MW, George AJ, Stuart J. Platelet hyperactivity in sickle-cell disease: a consequence of hyposplenism. J Clin Pathol 1980;33(7):622–5.

68. Mehta P. Significance of plasma beta-thromboglobulin values in patients with sickle cell disease. J Pediatr 1980;97(6):941–4.

69. Semple MJ, Al-Hasani SF, Kioy P, et al. A double-blind trial of ticlopidine in sickle cell disease. Thromb Haemost 1984;51(3):303–6.

70. Alkjaersig N, Fletcher A, Joist H, et al. Hemostatic alterations accompanying sickle cell pain crises. J Lab Clin Med 1976;88(3):440–9.

71. Solovey A, Kollander R, Shet A, et al. Endothelial cell expression of tissue factor in sickle mice is augmented by hypoxia/reoxygenation and inhibited by lovastatin. Blood 2004;104(3):840–6.

72. Ataga KI. Hypercoagulability and thrombotic complications in hemolytic anemias. Haematologica 2009;94(11):1481–4.

73. Setty BN, Kulkarni S, Stuart MJ. Role of erythrocyte phosphatidylserine in sickle red cell-endothelial adhesion. Blood 2002;99(5):1564–71.

74. Zwaal RF, Schroit AJ. Pathophysiologic implications of membrane phospholipid asymmetry in blood cells. Blood 1997;89(4):1121–32.

75. Setty BN, Kulkarni S, Dampier CD, et al. Fetal hemoglobin in sickle cell anemia: relationship to erythrocyte adhesion markers and adhesion. Blood 2001;97(9): 2568–73.

76. Setty BN, Rao AK, Stuart MJ. Thrombophilia in sickle cell disease: the red cell connection. Blood 2001;98(12):3228–33.

77. Styles L, de Jong K, Vichinsky E, et al. Increased RBC phosphatidylserine exposure in sickle cell disease patients at risk for stroke by transcranial Doppler screening. Blood 1997;(90):604.

78. Fadok VA, Voelker DR, Campbell PA, et al. Exposure of phosphatidylserine on the surface of apoptotic lymphocytes triggers specific recognition and removal by macrophages. J Immunol 1992;148(7):2207–16.

79. Martin SJ, Reutelingsperger CP, McGahon AJ, et al. Early redistribution of plasma membrane phosphatidylserine is a general feature of apoptosis regardless of the initiating stimulus: inhibition by overexpression of Bcl-2 and Abl. J Exp Med 1995;182(5):1545–56.

80. Stuart MJ, Setty BN. Hemostatic alterations in sickle cell disease: relationships to disease pathophysiology. Pediatr Pathol Mol Med 2001;20(1):27–46.

81. Kuypers FA, Larkin SK, Emeis JJ, et al. Interaction of an annexin V homodimer (Diannexin) with phosphatidylserine on cell surfaces and consequent antithrombotic activity. Thromb Haemost 2007;97(3):478–86.

82. Lane PA, O'Connell JL, Marlar RA. Erythrocyte membrane vesicles and irreversibly sickled cells bind protein S. Am J Hematol 1994;47(4):295–300.

83. Schechter AN, Gladwin MT. Hemoglobin and the paracrine and endocrine functions of nitric oxide. N Engl J Med 2003;348(15):1483–5.

84. Huang KT, Han TH, Hyduke DR, et al. Modulation of nitric oxide bioavailability by erythrocytes. Proc Natl Acad Sci U S A 2001;98(20):11771–6.

85. Vaughn MW, Huang KT, Kuo L, et al. Erythrocytes possess an intrinsic barrier to nitric oxide consumption. J Biol Chem 2000;275(4):2342–8.

86. Butler AR, Megson IL, Wright PG. Diffusion of nitric oxide and scavenging by blood in the vasculature. Biochim Biophys Acta 1998;1425(1):168–76.

87. Morris CR, Kato GJ, Poljakovic M, et al. Dysregulated arginine metabolism, hemolysis-associated pulmonary hypertension, and mortality in sickle cell disease. JAMA 2005;294(1):81–90.

88. Villagra J, Shiva S, Hunter LA, et al. Platelet activation in patients with sickle disease, hemolysis-associated pulmonary hypertension, and nitric oxide scavenging by cell-free hemoglobin. Blood 2007;110(6):2166–72.

89. Kermarrec N, Zunic P, Beloucif S, et al. Impact of inhaled nitric oxide on platelet aggregation and fibrinolysis in rats with endotoxic lung injury. Role of cyclic guanosine 5'-monophosphate. Am J Respir Crit Care Med 1998; 158(3):833–9.

90. Radomski MW, Palmer RM, Moncada S. The role of nitric oxide and cGMP in platelet adhesion to vascular endothelium. Biochem Biophys Res Commun 1987;148(3):1482–9.

91. Radomski MW, Palmer RM, Moncada S. Endogenous nitric oxide inhibits human platelet adhesion to vascular endothelium. Lancet 1987;2(8567): 1057–8.

92. Gerlach M, Keh D, Bezold G, et al. Nitric oxide inhibits tissue factor synthesis, expression and activity in human monocytes by prior formation of peroxynitrite. Intensive Care Med 1998;24(11):1199–208.

93. Fiorucci S, Santucci L, Cirino G, et al. IL-1 beta converting enzyme is a target for nitric oxide-releasing aspirin: new insights in the antiinflammatory mechanism of nitric oxide-releasing nonsteroidal antiinflammatory drugs. J Immunol 2000; 165(9):5245–54.

94. Dusse LM, Cooper AJ, Lwaleed BA. Tissue factor and nitric oxide: a controversial relationship! J Thromb Thrombolysis 2007;23(2):129–33.

95. Studt JD, Kremer Hovinga JA, Antoine G, et al. Fatal congenital thrombotic thrombocytopenic purpura with apparent ADAMTS13 inhibitor: in vitro inhibition of ADAMTS13 activity by hemoglobin. Blood 2005;105(2):542–4.

96. Schnog JJ, Kremer Hovinga JA, Krieg S, et al. ADAMTS13 activity in sickle cell disease. Am J Hematol 2006;81(7):492–8.

97. Krishnan S, Siegel J, Pullen G Jr, et al. Increased von Willebrand factor antigen and high molecular weight multimers in sickle cell disease associated with nocturnal hypoxemia. Thromb Res 2008;122(4):455–8.

98. Zhou Z, Han H, Cruz MA, et al. Haemoglobin blocks von Willebrand factor proteolysis by ADAMTS-13: a mechanism associated with sickle cell disease. Thromb Haemost 2009;101(6):1070–7.

99. Kuypers FA, de Jong K. The role of phosphatidylserine in recognition and removal of erythrocytes. Cell Mol Biol (Noisy-le-grand) 2004;50(2): 147–58.

100. Connor J, Pak CC, Schroit AJ. Exposure of phosphatidylserine in the outer leaflet of human red blood cells. Relationship to cell density, cell age, and clearance by mononuclear cells. J Biol Chem 1994;269(4):2399–404.

101. Schwartz RS, Tanaka Y, Fidler IJ, et al. Increased adherence of sickled and phosphatidylserine-enriched human erythrocytes to cultured human peripheral blood monocytes. J Clin Invest 1985;75(6):1965–72.

102. Kato GJ, McGowan V, Machado RF, et al. Lactate dehydrogenase as a biomarker of hemolysis-associated nitric oxide resistance, priapism, leg ulceration, pulmonary hypertension, and death in patients with sickle cell disease. Blood 2006;107(6):2279–85.

103. Nolan VG, Adewoye A, Baldwin C, et al. Sickle cell leg ulcers: associations with haemolysis and SNPs in Klotho, TEK and genes of the TGF-beta/BMP pathway. Br J Haematol 2006;133(5):570–8.

104. Nolan VG, Wyszynski DF, Farrer LA, et al. Hemolysis-associated priapism in sickle cell disease. Blood 2005;106(9):3264–7.

105. Jackson N, Franklin IM, Hughes MA. Recurrent priapism following splenectomy for thalassaemia intermedia. Br J Surg 1986;73(8):678.

106. Macchia P, Massei F, Nardi M, et al. Thalassemia intermedia and recurrent priapism following splenectomy. Haematologica 1990;75(5):486–7.

107. Boyle S, White RH, Brunson A, et al. Splenectomy and the incidence of venous thromboembolism and sepsis in patients with immune thrombocytopenia. Blood 2013;121(23):4782–90.

108. Lovren F, Verma S. Evolving role of microparticles in the pathophysiology of endothelial dysfunction. Clin Chem 2013;59(8):1166–74.

109. Tushuizen ME, Diamant M, Sturk A, et al. Cell-derived microparticles in the pathogenesis of cardiovascular disease: friend or foe? Arterioscler Thromb Vasc Biol 2011;31(1):4–9.

110. Shet AS, Aras O, Gupta K, et al. Sickle blood contains tissue factor-positive microparticles derived from endothelial cells and monocytes. Blood 2003;102(7): 2678–83.
111. Nieuwland R, Berckmans RJ, Rotteveel-Eijkman RC, et al. Cell-derived microparticles generated in patients during cardiopulmonary bypass are highly procoagulant. Circulation 1997;96(10):3534–41.
112. Nieuwland R, Berckmans RJ, McGregor S, et al. Cellular origin and procoagulant properties of microparticles in meningococcal sepsis. Blood 2000;95(3): 930–5.
113. Joop K, Berckmans RJ, Nieuwland R, et al. Microparticles from patients with multiple organ dysfunction syndrome and sepsis support coagulation through multiple mechanisms. Thromb Haemost 2001;85(5):810–20.
114. Berckmans RJ, Nieuwland R, Tak PP, et al. Cell-derived microparticles in synovial fluid from inflamed arthritic joints support coagulation exclusively via a factor VII-dependent mechanism. Arthritis Rheum 2002;46(11):2857–66.
115. Lok CA, Nieuwland R, Sturk A, et al. Microparticle-associated P-selectin reflects platelet activation in preeclampsia. Platelets 2007;18(1):68–72.
116. Gerotziafas GT, Van Dreden P, Chaari M, et al. The acceleration of the propagation phase of thrombin generation in patients with steady-state sickle cell disease is associated with circulating erythrocyte-derived microparticles. Thromb Haemost 2012;107(6):1044–52.
117. Patel RK, Arya R. Tests for hereditary thrombophilia are of limited value in the black population. Stroke 2003;34(12):e236.
118. Mack R, Chowdary D, Streck D, et al. Inherited thrombophilia genes in minorities. Genet Test 1999;3(4):371–3.
119. Helley D, Besmond C, Ducrocq R, et al. Polymorphism in exon 10 of the human coagulation factor V gene in a population at risk for sickle cell disease. Hum Genet 1997;100(2):245–8.
120. Kahn MJ, Scher C, Rozans M, et al. Leiden is not responsible for stroke in patients with sickling disorders and is uncommon in African Americans with sickle cell disease. Am J Hematol 1997;54(1):12–5.
121. Kahn JE, Veyssier-Belot C, Renier JL, et al. Recurrent thromboembolism in a patient with beta-thalassemia major associated with double heterozygosity for factor V R506Q and prothrombin G20210A mutations. Blood Coagul Fibrinolysis 2002;13(5):461–3.
122. Wright JG, Cooper P, Malia RG, et al. Activated protein C resistance in homozygous sickle cell disease. Br J Haematol 1997;96(4):854–6.
123. Moreira Neto F, Lourenco DM, Noguti MA, et al. The clinical impact of MTHFR polymorphism on the vascular complications of sickle cell disease. Braz J Med Biol Res 2006;39(10):1291–5.
124. Andrade FL, Annichino-Bizzacchi JM, Saad ST, et al. Prothrombin mutant, factor V Leiden, and thermolabile variant of methylenetetrahydrofolate reductase among patients with sickle cell disease in Brazil. Am J Hematol 1998;59(1):46–50.
125. Kordes U, Janka-Schaub G, Schneppenheim R, et al. Leiden mutation in sickle cell anaemia. Br J Haematol 2002;116(1):236.
126. Fawaz NA, Bashawery L, Al-Sheikh I, et al. Factor V-Leiden, prothrombin G20210A, and MTHFR C677T mutations among patients with sickle cell disease in Eastern Saudi Arabia. Am J Hematol 2004;76(3):307–9.
127. Zimmerman SA, Ware RE. Inherited DNA mutations contributing to thrombotic complications in patients with sickle cell disease. Am J Hematol 1998;59(4): 267–72.

128. Zeinali S, Duca F, Zarbakhsh B, et al. Thrombophilic mutations in Iran. Thromb Haemost 2000;83(2):351–2.
129. Rahimi Z, Vaisi-Raygani A, Nagel RL, et al. Thrombophilic mutations among Southern Iranian patients with sickle cell disease: high prevalence of factor V Leiden. J Thromb Thrombolysis 2008;25(3):288–92.
130. Isma'eel H, Arnaout MS, Shamseddeen W, et al. Screening for inherited thrombophilia might be warranted among Eastern Mediterranean sickle-beta-0 thalassemia patients. J Thromb Thrombolysis 2006;22(2):121–3.
131. Otrock ZK, Mahfouz RA, Taher AT. Should we screen Eastern Mediterranean sickle beta-thalassemia patients for inherited thrombophilia? J Thromb Haemost 2005;3(3):599–600.
132. Koren A, Zalman L, Levin C, et al. Venous thromboembolism, factor V Leiden, and methylenetetrahydrofolate reductase in a sickle cell anemia patient. Pediatr Hematol Oncol 1999;16(5):469–72.
133. Bray PF. Platelet glycoprotein polymorphisms as risk factors for thrombosis. Curr Opin Hematol 2000;7(5):284–9.
134. Furihata K, Nugent DJ, Kunicki TJ. Influence of platelet collagen receptor polymorphisms on risk for arterial thrombosis. Arch Pathol Lab Med 2002;126(3):305–9.
135. Deckmyn H, Ulrichts H, Van De Walle G, et al. Platelet antigens and their function. Vox Sang 2004;87(Suppl 2):105–11.
136. Castro V, Alberto FL, Costa RN, et al. Polymorphism of the human platelet antigen-5 system is a risk factor for occlusive vascular complications in patients with sickle cell anemia. Vox Sang 2004;87(2):118–23.
137. Al-Subaie AM, Fawaz NA, Mahdi N, et al. Human platelet alloantigens (HPA) 1, HPA2, HPA3, HPA4, and HPA5 polymorphisms in sickle cell anemia patients with vaso-occlusive crisis. Eur J Haematol 2009;83(6):579–85.
138. Wun T, Soulieres D, Frelinger AL, et al. A double-blind, randomized, multicenter phase 2 study of prasugrel versus placebo in adult patients with sickle cell disease. J Hematol Oncol 2013;6:17.
139. Clotz I, Tam J. Acetylation of sickle cell hemoglobin by aspirin. Proc Natl Acad Sci U S A 1973;70(5):1313–5.
140. Osamo NO, Photiades DP, Famodu AA. Therapeutic effect of aspirin in sickle cell anaemia. Acta Haematol 1981;66(2):102–7.
141. Greenberg J, Ohene-Frempong K, Halus J, et al. Trial of low doses of aspirin as prophylaxis in sickle cell disease. J Pediatr 1983;102(5):781–4.
142. Zago MA, Costa FF, Ismael SJ, et al. Treatment of sickle cell diseases with aspirin. Acta Haematol 1984;72(1):61–4.
143. Chaplin H Jr, Alkjaersig N, Fletcher AP, et al. Aspirin-dipyridamole prophylaxis of sickle cell disease pain crises. Thromb Haemost 1980;43(3):218–21.
144. Cabannes R, Lonsdorfer J, Castaigne JP, et al. Clinical and biological double-blind-study of ticlopidine in preventive treatment of sickle-cell disease crises. Agents Actions Suppl 1984;15:199–212.
145. Salvaggio JE, Arnold CA, Banov CH. Long-term anti-coagulation in sickle-cell disease. A clinical study. N Engl J Med 1963;269:182–6.
146. Schnog JB, Kater AP, Mac Gillavry MR, et al. Low adjusted-dose acenocoumarol therapy in sickle cell disease: a pilot study. Am J Hematol 2001;68(3):179–83.
147. Ahmed S, Siddiqui AK, Iqbal U, et al. Effect of low-dose warfarin on D-dimer levels during sickle cell vaso-occlusive crisis: a brief report. Eur J Haematol 2004;72(3):213–6.

148. Qari MH, Aljaouni SK, Alardawi MS, et al. Reduction of painful vaso-occlusive crisis of sickle cell anaemia by tinzaparin in a double-blind randomized trial. Thromb Haemost 2007;98(2):392–6.

149. Wolters HJ, Ten Cate H, Thomas LL, et al. Low-intensity oral anticoagulation in sickle-cell disease reverses the prethrombotic state: promises for treatment? Br J Haematol 1995;90(3):715–7.

Modulators of Erythropoiesis

Emerging Therapies for Hemoglobinopathies and Disorders of Red Cell Production

Laura Breda, PhD[a,*], Stefano Rivella, PhD[a,b]

KEYWORDS

- Steady state • Stress and ineffective erythropoiesis • Hemoglobinopathies • JAK2
- Transforming growth factor β • ACE-011 • ACE-536 • LY-2157299

KEY POINTS

- Increased proliferation of erythroid progenitors is a feature common to many pathologic conditions associated with anemia or an excessive production of red cells.
- Chronic stress erythropoiesis (associated with ineffective erythropoiesis and anemia or erythrocytosis) leads to severe comorbidities that aggravate the patient's condition.
- In the context of tumorigenesis, the level of JAK2 activity or activin seems to correlate directly with disease progression.
- Development of drugs that target Epo-dependent or Epo-independent pathways, like JAK2 or activin signaling, can be beneficial in hemoglobinopathies and other erythroid disorders.

JAK2 AND DISORDERS ASSOCIATED WITH CHRONIC STRESS ERYTHROPOIESIS

Erythropoiesis is a tightly regulated process that includes cytokine signaling and cell-cell interactions in the specialized niche called erythroblastic islands.[1–3] Because of the essential role of erythrocytes in oxygen delivery, erythropoiesis can effectively respond and adapt quickly to changes in tissue oxygen tension. This situation is mediated primarily by erythropoietin (EPO).[4–6] EPO signals through the EPO receptor (EPOR).[7–9] One of the main factors activated by EPO/EPOR interaction is the cytoplasmic kinase JAK2.[10–12] Through autophosphorylation and crossphosphorylation events, JAK2 activates STAT5 and parallel signaling pathways.[13,14] STAT5 migrates to the nucleus activating genes necessary for proliferation, differentiation, and survival of erythroid progenitors. The crucial role of EPO, EPOR, JAK2, and STAT5 has been shown by knocking out these factors in mice. Absence of each one of these molecules

a Department of Pediatrics, Hematology-Oncology, Weill Cornell Medical College, 1300 York Avenue, New York, NY 10021, USA; b Department of Cell and Developmental Biology, Weill Cornell Medical College, 1300 York Avenue, New York, NY 10021, USA
* Corresponding author.
E-mail address: lab2002@med.cornell.edu

Hematol Oncol Clin N Am 28 (2014) 375–386
http://dx.doi.org/10.1016/j.hoc.2013.12.001
0889-8588/14/$ – see front matter © 2014 Elsevier Inc. All rights reserved.

resulted in a lethal anemia during fetal development.[12] In particular, phosphorylation of STAT5 is essential for basal erythropoiesis and for its acceleration during hypoxic stress (stress erythropoiesis).[15] Some of the conditions in which the JAK2/STA5 pathway is chronically activated and erythropoiesis is accelerated are polycythemia vera and β-thalassemia.[3,16,17]

The most recurrent mutation in JAK2, JAK2 V617F, is associated with myeloprolif-erative neoplasms (MPNs). This mutation is associated with constitutive phosphoryla-tion of JAK2 and EPO hypersensitivity.[18–23] JAK2 inhibitors such as ruxolitinib, LY2784544, and SAR302503 are currently being tested or used to treat myelofibrosis, essential thrombocythemia, and polycythemia vera.[24–26] In particular, polycythemia vera, one of the MPNs, is characterized by increased production of erythroid progen-itors, erythrocytes, and splenomegaly.[16,27–29]

In β-thalassemia, hypoxia leads to high levels of EPO in circulation and, in turn, increased erythroid proliferation.[16,27–29] Thus, even in absence of JAK2 mutations, the activity of JAK2 is enhanced, leading to increased proliferation and decreased differentiation of erythroid progenitors (chronic stress erythropoiesis, **Fig. 1**A). This sit-uation causes a net increase in the number of erythroid progenitors, leading to extra-medullary hematopoiesis and splenomegaly.[16,27–29] Splenomegaly, in turn, increases sequestration of red blood cells (RBC), exacerbating the anemia and ineffective eryth-ropoiesis (IE).[16,27–33]

POTENTIAL USE OF JAK2 INHIBITORS IN β-THALASSEMIA

IE is the hallmark of a group of anemias characterized by cell death associated with increased proliferation and decreased differentiation of erythroblasts, leading to an expansion in the number of erythroid progenitors, but with suboptimal or ab-sent production of normal RBC.[16] The discovery that JAK2 plays an important role in the progression and exacerbation of IE suggests that drugs inhibiting the activity of JAK2 could mitigate IE (see **Fig. 1**B) and reverse splenomegaly. In pre-clinical studies, it has been shown that a JAK2 inhibitor (200mg/Kg/d dose) dramat-ically decreased the spleen size and modulated the IE.[16,27–33] Based on these observations, use of JAK2 inhibitors could be used to reverse splenomegaly, thereby avoiding the need for splenectomy. Ideally, this treatment could also be helpful in reducing the rate of blood transfusions. leading to improved management of anemia and iron overload.[16,27–33]

ACTIVINS, MEMBERS OF THE TRANSFORMING GROWTH FACTOR β FAMILY SIGNALING

Activins are soluble ligands, which, along with bone morphogenetic proteins (BMPs) and growth and differentiation factors (GDFs), belong to a large group of proteins called the transforming growth factor β (TGF-β) family. The most well-characterized activins are homodimeric or heterodimeric structures composed of 2 similar β-chains, A or B. Inhibins, on the other hand, are heterodimers composed of α-chains and β-chains (from activins) and antagonize activins and BMP signaling. Generally, ligands of TGF-β family are synthesized from a common precursor with a prodomain that can determine the activity and localization of a ligand.[34]

The TGF-β family signal through 7 different type I and 5 different type II transmem-brane serine/threonine kinase receptors.[35] Type I receptors (activin receptorlike ki-nases) ALK2, ALK4, and ALK7 (also indicated as ACVR1, ACVR1B, and ACVR1C, respectively) and activin receptor IIA (ActRIIA) and ActRIIB (also indicated as ACVR2A, ACVR2B) are typically the mediators of activin effect.[36] ActRIIs are shared by some of the BMPs and GDFs.[37] Activin signaling is carried out through formation

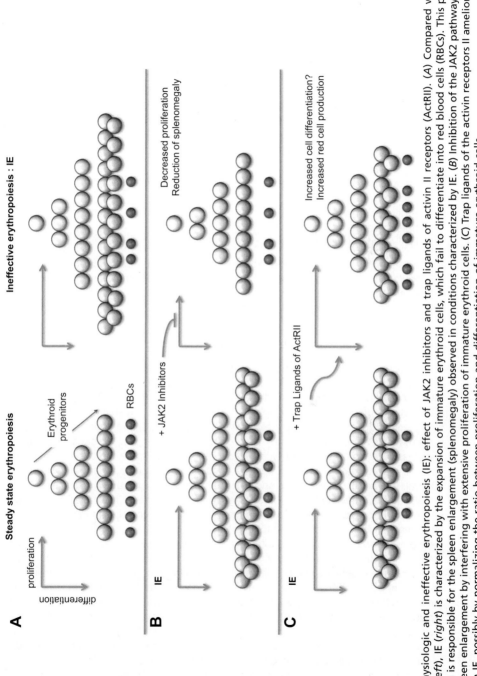

Fig. 1. Physiologic and ineffective erythropoiesis (IE): effect of JAK2 inhibitors and trap ligands of activin II receptors (ActRII). (*A*) Compared with normal (*left*), IE (*right*) is characterized by the expansion of immature erythroid cells, which fail to differentiate into red blood cells (RBCs). This phenomenon is responsible for the spleen enlargement (splenomegaly) observed in conditions characterized by IE. (*B*) Inhibition of the JAK2 pathway reduces spleen enlargement by interfering with extensive proliferation of immature erythroid cells. (*C*) Trap ligands of the activin receptors II ameliorate anemia in IE, possibly by normalizing the ratio between proliferation and differentiation of immature erythroid cells.

of a ternary complex between the ligand, the type II and the type I receptors, which phosphorylates SMAD proteins.[35,36] SMADs multimerize, and these complexes translocate to the nucleus and regulate gene expression in concert with other transcription factors. Follistatin (FST) and FST-related protein (FRP) bind extracellularly to activins and other related TGF-β ligands, controlling their signaling and availability.[38–40] FST inhibits activin by hiding one-third of its residues as well as type I and II receptor binding sites.[38–40] Mice with a disrupted FST gene have musculoskeletal and skin abnormalities, whereas mice with the gene encoding FRP (FST-related gene or FLRG) deleted show dysregulated glucose metabolism and fat homeostasis.[41]

Activins are expressed in various tissues and have a broad range of activities that regulate:

- Gonadal function
- Hormonal homeostasis
- Growth and differentiation of musculoskeletal tissues
- Growth and metastasis of cancer cells
- Proliferation and differentiation of embryonic/hematopoietic stem and erythropoietic cells
- Higher brain function

Activin activities are involved in the cause and pathogenesis of several diseases.[42] Dysregulation of activin signaling has been associated with many malignant disorders as well as diseases affected by anemia. For these conditions, the inhibition of activin signaling represents an interesting therapeutic approach.[42]

CANCER-RELATED ANEMIA AND INEFFECTIVE ERYTHROPOIESIS

Anemia is a condition that affects hematologic malignancies like multiple myeloma and myelodysplastic syndromes (MDS). MDS encompass a heterogeneous group of closely related clonal hematopoietic disorders characterized by a marrow with impaired maturation (dysmyelopoiesis) and peripheral blood cytopenias, resulting from ineffective blood cell production[43] and develop when a clonal mutation predominates in the bone marrow, suppressing healthy stem cells. Anemia can also be caused by myelosuppressive chemotherapy. Anemia is also observed in some tumors in absence of chemotherapy treatment and it can be considered a prognostic factor of reduced survival. IE also leads to anemia and it is the hallmark of a group of diseases such as β-thalassemia. Individuals with these anemias have markedly increased EPO levels, which result in massive erythroid expansion in the hypercellular marrow.[44,45] When abnormalities in the red cells lead to their intramedullary demise, erythropoiesis is ineffective and leads to enhanced intestinal iron absorption, and resultant tissue iron loading and toxicity. The thalassemia syndromes (both α-thalassemia and β-thalassemia) are the most frequent conditions associated with IE and result from diminished production of α-globin or β-globin chains, respectively, the 2 subunits of the hemoglobin A (adult) molecule.[27,46–48] As a result of IE, patients develop several comorbidities, including iron overload and bone abnormalities. Another group of conditions characterized by IE are congenital and acquired sideroblastic anemias. In these conditions, the bone marrow produces sideroblasts, characterized by granules of iron accumulated in perinuclear mitochondria, forming a ring around the erythroblast nucleus. These ringed sideroblasts fail to differentiate into healthy erythrocytes.[49] Acquired sideroblastic anemias may be caused either by a genetic disorder or indirectly as part of the MDS.[50] Other erythroid disorders that might benefit from ameliorating the IE are congenital dyserythropoietic anemias, chronic pernicious anemia, and hereditary spherocytosis.[51]

Individuals affected by thalassemia and MDS receive blood transfusion to compensate for the anemia, but with time, several comorbidities develop, including iron overload, bone abnormalities, and, in patients with MDS, progression to acute myeloid leukemia. Although improved transfusion and iron chelation treatments over the past 2 decades or so have reduced morbidity and improved the life expectancy of patients, they do not provide a definitive cure and lack the ability to correct IE. Therefore, alternative pharmacologic therapies that target the direct recovery of terminal erythroid differentiation are urgently needed.

The use of EPO and its derivatives, also referred to as erythropoiesis stimulating agents (ESAs), to treat cancer-related anemia can be controversial, because it has been speculated that it might aggravate tumor progression.[52] In addition, ESAs have been used for diseases characterized by anemia caused by IE but with limited benefits.[53] Therefore, new pharmacologic treatments with different mechanisms of action are needed. In this perspective, the use of molecules that can target EPO-unrelated pathways, like activin signaling, might be potential candidates to ameliorate anemia.

EFFECT OF ACTIVIN SIGNALING IN BONE

In vitro and in vivo data on activin signaling are discordant. Mice injected with activin A show increase of bone formation and bone strength, although in rats, similar results were reproduced using inhibin A.[54] In perimenopausal and postmenopausal women, follicle-stimulating hormone (FSH) seems to indirectly exert its anabolic effect on bone through an ovarian mediator (possibly inhibin A).[55] Withdrawal of inhibin A could be related to bone loss observed in perimenopause and postmenopause. FST has been shown to have an opposite effect,[56] indicating that FST and inhibins do not operate as analogue in the bone context. In relationship to metastatic bone progression, increased levels of circulating activin A seem to be a prognostic factor. Patients who have breast and prostatic cancer with bone metastasis present higher levels of activin A than nonmetastatic patients.[57] A similar observation was made for patients with multiple myeloma, in whom high activin levels correlate with extensive bone involvement and lower survival rate.[58] Moreover, in vitro studies have shown that multiple myeloma cells stimulate stromal cells to produce activin, which in turn leads to inhibition of osteoblast differentiation in vitro.[59]

EFFECT OF ACTIVIN SIGNALING IN CANCER

In vivo studies showed that lack of inhibin in transgenic mice causes gonadal and adrenal tumorigenesis, indicating that these activin repressors are important tumor repressors in these tissues.[60] Overexpression of FST in these mice does not reduce tumor incidence but modulates tumor progression and reduces the tumor cachexia-like syndrome associated with high levels of activin.[61] As for the liver, FST adenoviral-induced overexpression causes hyperproliferation of hepatocytes.[62] The opposite effect is observed when overexpression of FST is induced in small cell lung cancer cells, which seem to produce a reduction of experimental metastases in various organs in NOD-SCID (nonobese diabetic/severe combined immunodeficiency) mice.[41] Compared with transgenic activin-deficient mice, FST-deficient mice die before birth because of compromised development of growth, skin, muscle, and skeletal development. Therefore, FST operates on many signaling pathway in addition to the activin-related ones. The function of FST and activin in different tissues can differ vastly, and therefore, their levels as indicators of tumor development, progression, and metastases might be challenging, although certainly impactful.[42]

EFFECT OF ACTIVIN SIGNALING IN HEMATOPOIESIS AND ERYTHROPOIESIS

Members of the TGF-β family are also key regulators of human hematopoiesis, modulating various cellular responses, such as proliferation, differentiation, migration, and apoptosis. Activin expression can be detected in bone marrow cells, including erythroid cells. Recombinant activin induces cellular shrinking and nuclear condensation of CD34+ cells during in vitro differentiation. This process is reverted by addition of FRP, BMP2, and BMP4.[63,64]

Activin A and BMP2 and BMP4, alone or in combination, have been shown to have a role in the regulation of erythropoiesis in various models.[65,66]

The biological function of activin A, BMP2, and BMP4 was assessed measuring clonogenic potential in colony forming cell assay of human CD34+ cells isolated from either mobilized peripheral blood or bone marrow.[63] Activin was found to increase the number of both late erythroid burst-forming unit (BFU-E) and erythroid colony-forming unit (CFU-E). This observation was confirmed in vivo through injection of activin in anemic (phlebotomized) and normal mice.[67] On the other hand, BMP2 was found to increase the number of early BFU-E. Cells treated with activin A showed a significant decrease in nuclear size, a phenomenon associated with maturation of erythroid cells. Compared with activin A alone, addition of BMP4 induces an inhibitory effect in the number of late BFU-E and CFU-E and increases nuclear size.[68-70] This finding suggests that BMP4 facilitates differentiation of the erythroid progenitors before they lose their ability to form colonies and their nuclear size starts shrinking. BMP2 antagonizes the effect of activin A on nuclear size reduction.[63,64] Therefore, BMP molecules may have a different effect on the activin A–mediated biological activities.

In hematopoiesis, FST has an inhibitory effect on activin.[64] Both FST and FRP also neutralize GDF11 and myostatin.[71] Both repressors interfere with the ability of activin to induce nuclear size reduction and increase counts of early BFU and CFU, and also inhibit BMP2-induced early BFU proliferation. Bone morphogenetic stromal cells are among the tissues that produce at steady state the highest levels of FLRG transcripts.[72] They also produce activin and FST.[72] Among hematopoietic lineages, monocytes have the highest level of expression of FLRG.[72] Expression of FLRG in erythroid cells is mostly observed in immature cells, whereas FST is expressed at highest levels in most mature erythroid cells.[63,64,72] The expression of both FST and FLRG transcripts are induced by activin A as well as TGF-β, indicating that these 2 repressors participate in a negative feedback loop that regulates activin signaling. Additional regulation of activin and TGF-β ligand signaling pathways occurs intracellularly via the SMAD inhibitory proteins 6 and 7.[73,74] These proteins induce ubiquitin-dependent degradation of SMAD2, 3, and 4.[73-75]

THERAPEUTIC INTERVENTIONS THAT TARGET ACTIVIN SIGNALING

Several strategies have been developed to hinder the dysregulation of activin signaling. These strategies include the use of:

- Small molecules that inhibit type 1 receptors
- Antibodies that inhibit the interaction between activins and their receptors
- Activin mutant proteins that bind to ActIIRA but block subsequent ternary interaction with receptor type 1, ALK4
- Chimeric polypeptides that sequester activin but not GDF8 or 11
- Ligand traps that act in a similar fashion to FST/FSRG

Currently, the approaches with highest clinical impact are those based on small molecules that inhibit type 1 receptors or ligand trap soluble molecules that sequester ligands of ActRIIA and B, like ACE-011 and ACE-536.

SMALL MOLECULES TARGETING TYPE 1 RECEPTORS

These molecules have been developed mainly to target ALK5, the type 1 receptor of TGF-β, with specific focus on cancer treatment. Most molecules developed have shown broader range of affinity and target not only ALK5 but also ALK4 and 7.[42] Therefore, they are considered inhibitors of activin and TGF-β as well. Because of the broader mechanism of action, they are still evaluated, and their use in clinical trial is subject to further screening. Among these molecules, molecule LY-2157299, a potent inhibitor of ALK 5, has now been used in 5 different clinical trials, which include phase 1-2 cancer and metastatic cancer as well MDS studies.[42]

Zhou and colleagues[74] showed that SMAD7 expression (an inhibitor of the SMAD pathway activated by TGF-β) is significantly reduced in bone marrow-derived CD34$^+$ cells isolated from patients with low-grade MDS compared with healthy individuals. This downregulation induces more sensibility to TGF-β stimulation.[74] Therefore, the pathways associated with TGF-β are hyperactivated, likely affecting cell differentiation and proliferation. This situation is mostly mediated through ALK5. When LY-2157299 is given to a mouse model of MDS, this ameliorates RBC synthesis, with increased hematocrit and hemoglobin levels.[74] MDS bone marrow cells show poor hematopoietic colony formation. Treatment of mononuclear cells isolated from patients with low-grade MDS with the ALK5 inhibitor increased both erythroid and myeloid colony numbers, which points to a high therapeutic potential of ALK5 inhibition by LY-2157299 in patients with MDS who do not have increased blast counts.[74]

PRECLINICAL AND CLINICAL STUDIES WITH ACE-011/RAP-011

ACE-011 is a receptor fusion protein that functions as a soluble trap that sequesters ligands of ActRIIA. It is a truncated form of the extracellular domain of human ActRIIA combined with the Fc of the human immunoglobulin IgG1. In the mouse ortholog, RAP-011, the extracellular domain of the human ActRIIA is combined with the Fc of the mouse immunoglobulin IgG2a.

Several studies have shown beneficial effects of RAP-011 in mouse models of various conditions. RAP-011 was able to ameliorate anemia induced by chemotherapy treatment of mice with paclitaxel.[76] RBC levels were also increased after treatment of normal mice with the drug.

Reduction of osteolytic lesions and number of multiple myeloma tumor cells, in addition to strengthening of the bones, was observed in a humanized mouse model of multiple myeloma.[59] RAP-011 also reduced osteolytic lesions and metastatic progression in a breast cancer mouse model, prolonging mouse survival.[77]

Two clinical studies[78,79] in healthy volunteers have shown that in postmenopausal women, a single administration (intravenous or subcutaneous, up to 3 mg/kg) of ACE-011

- Reduces FSH serum levels
- Increases levels of bone formation biomarkers like bone-specific alkaline phosphatase
- Increases RBC, hematocrit, and hemoglobin levels (leaving white cells and platelet counts unchanged) in a dose-dependent manner and in a fashion that differs from the mechanism of action of ESAs.

The half-life of the drug is 24 to 32 days. The increase of RBC count suggests that 1 or more ligands of ActRIIA might act as a negative regulator in normal erythropoiesis.

Iancu-Rubin and colleagues[80] investigated the mechanisms behind the beneficial effect of ACE-011 on RBC production in vitro. Although they could not detect a direct effect on erythroid differentiation of human CD34+ cells, they found that ACE-011 attenuates the inhibitory effect of bone marrow conditioned media on cell differentiation. Therefore, the effect of the drug could be attributed to an indirect modulation of the microenvironment in which CD34+ cells differentiate rather than a direct action on the erythroid precursors.

Because of its ability to ameliorate anemia, ACE-011 has been used in clinical trials for patients with multiple myeloma (NCT00747123, completed, and NCT01562405, currently recruiting patients). In addition, the drug is under investigation in several ongoing trials that are recruiting patients for:

- The treatment of anemia in low-risk or intermediate-1-risk MDS or nonproliferative chronic myelomonocytic leukemia (NCT01736683)
- Testing safety and efficacy in adults with transfusion-dependent Diamond-Blackfan anemia (NTC01464164)
- Testing safety and tolerability in adults with β-thalassemia (NTC01571635)

PRECLINICAL AND CLINICAL STUDIES WITH ACE-536/RAP-536

As mentioned earlier, several members of the TGF-β superfamily are involved in regulating erythropoiesis. ACE-536 (and its mouse ortholog RAP-536) is a modified activin type IIB receptor (Act-RIIB) fusion protein that does not inhibit activin A–induced signaling, but inhibits signaling induced by other members of the TGF-β superfamily. Although EPO increases proliferation of erythroid progenitors, RAP-536 promotes maturation of terminally differentiating erythroblasts. In thalassemic mice ($Hbb^{th1/th1}$), RAP-536 ameliorates hematologic parameters as well as comorbidities that develop as a consequence of the erythroid hyperplasia.[81]

In NUP98-HOXD13 (NHD13) MDS mice, RAP-536 corrects IE and normalizes myeloid/erythroid ratio, retarding progression to leukemia.[81,82] In both mouse models, RAP-536 rescued disease phenotypes by promoting terminal erythroid differentiation, thereby enhancing effective erythropoiesis. Cell cycle analyses of bone and splenic erythroblasts isolated from mice treated with RAP-536 showed decrease in S-phase and increase in G1/2 phases compared with placebo-treated animals. At 72 hours after treatment with RAP-536, a decrease of basophilic and increase of orthochromatic and polychromatic erythroblasts and reticulocytes is observed, with a resultant increase in hemoglobin compared with placebo-treated wild type mice. Altogether, these observations suggest that the mechanism of action of these trap ligands works through acceleration of the differentiation of the erythroid precursors, normalizing the ratio between proliferation and differentiation of the erythroid precursors under conditions of IE (see **Fig. 1**C). In addition, these preclinical data have provided a rationale for clinical studies of the human ortholog ACE-536, which is in 2 European phase 2 clinical trials, for the treatment of β-thalassemia intermedia (NCT01749540) and MDS (NCT01749514).

SUMMARY

Use of new compound such as inhibitors of JAK2 or TGF-β-like molecules might soon revolutionize the treatment of β-thalassemia and related disorders. However, this situation requires careful optimization, noting the potential for off-target immune suppression for JAK2 inhibitors and the lack of mechanistic insights for the use of the ligand trap soluble molecules that sequester ligands of ActRIIA and B.

REFERENCES

1. Chasis JA. Erythroblastic islands: specialized microenvironmental niches for erythropoiesis. Curr Opin Hematol 2006;13:137–41.
2. Chasis JA, Mohandas N. Erythroblastic islands: niches for erythropoiesis. Blood 2008;112:470–8.
3. Ramos P, Casu C, Gardenghi S, et al. Macrophages support pathological erythropoiesis in polycythemia vera and beta-thalassemia. Nat Med 2013;19:437–45.
4. Jacobs K, Shoemaker C, Rudersdorf R, et al. Isolation and characterization of genomic and cDNA clones of human erythropoietin. Nature 1985;313:806–10.
5. Lin FK, Suggs S, Lin CH, et al. Cloning and expression of the human erythropoietin gene. Proc Natl Acad Sci U S A 1985;82:7580–4.
6. Bunn HF. Erythropoietin. Cold Spring Harb Perspect Med 2013;3:a011619.
7. Tsai SF, Martin DI, Zon LI, et al. Cloning of cDNA for the major DNA-binding protein of the erythroid lineage through expression in mammalian cells. Nature 1989;339:446–51.
8. D'Andrea AD, Lodish HF, Wong GG. Expression cloning of the murine erythropoietin receptor. Cell 1989;57:277–85.
9. D'Andrea A, Fasman G, Wong G, et al. Erythropoietin receptor: cloning strategy and structural features. Int J Cell Cloning 1990;8(Suppl 1):173–80.
10. Witthuhn BA, Quelle FW, Silvennoinen O, et al. JAK2 associates with the erythropoietin receptor and is tyrosine phosphorylated and activated following stimulation with erythropoietin. Cell 1993;74:227–36.
11. Argetsinger LS, Campbell GS, Yang X, et al. Identification of JAK2 as a growth hormone receptor-associated tyrosine kinase. Cell 1993;74:237–44.
12. Neubauer H, Cumano A, Muller M, et al. Jak2 deficiency defines an essential developmental checkpoint in definitive hematopoiesis. Cell 1998;93:397–409.
13. Wojchowski DM, Gregory RC, Miller CP, et al. Signal transduction in the erythropoietin receptor system. Exp Cell Res 1999;253:143–56.
14. Wojchowski DM, Sathyanarayana P, Dev A. Erythropoietin receptor response circuits. Curr Opin Hematol 2010;17:169–76.
15. Porpiglia E, Hidalgo D, Koulnis M, et al. Stat5 signaling specifies basal versus stress erythropoietic responses through distinct binary and graded dynamic modalities. PLoS Biol 2012;10:e1001383.
16. Libani IV, Guy EC, Melchiori L, et al. Decreased differentiation of erythroid cells exacerbates ineffective erythropoiesis in beta-thalassemia. Blood 2008;112:875–85.
17. Chow A, Huggins M, Ahmed J, et al. CD169(+) macrophages provide a niche promoting erythropoiesis under homeostasis and stress. Nat Med 2013;19:429–36.
18. Saharinen P, Takaluoma K, Silvennoinen O. Regulation of the Jak2 tyrosine kinase by its pseudokinase domain. Mol Cell Biol 2000;20:3387–95.
19. Baxter EJ, Scott LM, Campbell PJ, et al. Acquired mutation of the tyrosine kinase JAK2 in human myeloproliferative disorders. Lancet 2005;365:1054–61.
20. James C, Ugo V, Le Couedic JP, et al. A unique clonal JAK2 mutation leading to constitutive signalling causes polycythaemia vera. Nature 2005;434:1144–8.
21. Kralovics R, Passamonti F, Buser AS, et al. A gain-of-function mutation of JAK2 in myeloproliferative disorders. N Engl J Med 2005;352:1779–90.

22. Levine RL, Wadleigh M, Cools J, et al. Activating mutation in the tyrosine kinase JAK2 in polycythemia vera, essential thrombocythemia, and myeloid metaplasia with myelofibrosis. Cancer Cell 2005;7:387–97.

23. Zhao R, Xing S, Li Z, et al. Identification of an acquired JAK2 mutation in poly-cythemia vera. J Biol Chem 2005;280:22788–92.

24. Atallah E, Verstovsek S. Emerging drugs for myelofibrosis. Expert Opin Emerg Drugs 2012;17:555–70.

25. Hensley B, Geyer H, Mesa R. Polycythemia vera: current pharmacotherapy and future directions. Expert Opin Pharmacother 2013;14:609–17.

26. Tefferi A. Polycythemia vera and essential thrombocythemia: 2013 update on diagnosis, risk-stratification, and management. Am J Hematol 2013;88: 507–16.

27. Ginzburg Y, Rivella S. Beta-thalassemia: a model for elucidating the dynamic regulation of ineffective erythropoiesis and iron metabolism. Blood 2011;118: 4321–30.

28. Rivella S. The role of ineffective erythropoiesis in non-transfusion-dependent thalassemia. Blood Rev 2012;26(Suppl 1):S12–5.

29. Musallam KM, Rivella S, Vichinsky E, et al. Non-transfusion-dependent thalasse-mias. Haematologica 2013;98:833–44.

30. Rivella S. Ineffective erythropoiesis and thalassemias. Curr Opin Hematol 2009; 16:187–94.

31. Rivella S, Rachmilewitz E. Future alternative therapies for beta-thalassemia. Expert Rev Hematol 2009;2:685.

32. Melchiori L, Gardenghi S, Rivella S. Beta-thalassemia: HiJAKing ineffective erythropoiesis and iron overload. Adv Hematol 2010;2010:938640.

33. Gardenghi S, Grady RW, Rivella S. Anemia, ineffective erythropoiesis, and hep-cidin: interacting factors in abnormal iron metabolism leading to iron overload in beta-thalassemia. Hematol Oncol Clin North Am 2010;24:1089–107.

34. Harrison CA, Al-Musawi SL, Walton KL. Prodomains regulate the synthesis, extracellular localisation and activity of TGF-beta superfamily ligands. Growth Factors 2011;29:174–86.

35. Akhurst RJ, Hata A. Targeting the TGFbeta signalling pathway in disease. Nat Rev Drug Discov 2012;11:790–811.

36. Worthington JJ, Klementowicz JE, Travis MA. TGFbeta: a sleeping giant awoken by integrins. Trends Biochem Sci 2011;36:47–54.

37. Tsuchida K, Nakatani M, Hitachi K, et al. Activin signaling as an emerging target for therapeutic interventions. Cell Commun Signal 2009;7:15.

38. Makanji Y, Temple-Smith PD, Walton KL, et al. Inhibin B is a more potent sup-pressor of rat follicle-stimulating hormone release than inhibin a in vitro and in vivo. Endocrinology 2009;150:4784–93.

39. Walton KL, Makanji Y, Robertson DM, et al. The synthesis and secretion of in-hibins. Vitam Horm 2011;85:149–84.

40. Walton KL, Makanji Y, Harrison CA. New insights into the mechanisms of activin action and inhibition. Mol Cell Endocrinol 2012;359:2–12.

41. Matzuk MM, Lu N, Vogel H, et al. Multiple defects and perinatal death in mice deficient in follistatin. Nature 1995;374:360–3.

42. Fields SZ, Parshad S, Anne M, et al. Activin receptor antagonists for cancer-related anemia and bone disease. Expert Opin Investig Drugs 2013;22:87–101.

43. Besa EC. Myelodysplastic syndromes (refractory anemia). A perspective of the biologic, clinical, and therapeutic issues. Med Clin North Am 1992;76:599–617.

44. Ineffective erythropoiesis. Lancet 1973;301:1164–5.

45. Centis F, Tabellini L, Lucarelli G, et al. The importance of erythroid expansion in determining the extent of apoptosis in erythroid precursors in patients with beta-thalassemia major. Blood 2000;96:3624–9.
46. Cappellini MD. The thalassemias. In: Goldman L, Shafer AI, editors. Goldman's Cecil medicine. Philadelphia: Elsevier; 2011. p. 1060–6.
47. Steinberg MH. Sickle cell disease and other hemoglobinopathies. In: Goldman L, Shafer AI, editors. Goldman's Cecil medicine. Philadelphia: Elsevier; 2011. p. 1066–75.
48. Rivella S. Do not super-excess me! Blood 2012;119:5064–5.
49. Bowman WD Jr. Abnormal ("ringed") sideroblasts in various hematologic and non-hematologic disorders. Blood 1961;18:662–71.
50. Tanno T, Miller JL. Iron loading and overloading due to ineffective erythropoiesis. Adv Hematol 2010;2010:358283.
51. Wu CJ, Krishnamurti L, Kutok JL, et al. Evidence for ineffective erythropoiesis in severe sickle cell disease. Blood 2005;106:3639–45.
52. Bohlius J, Schmidlin K, Brillant C, et al. Recombinant human erythropoiesis-stimulating agents and mortality in patients with cancer: a meta-analysis of randomised trials. Lancet 2009;373:1532–42.
53. Steensma DP. Hematopoietic growth factors in myelodysplastic syndromes. Semin Oncol 2011;38:635–47.
54. Perrien DS, Akel NS, Edwards PK, et al. Inhibin A is an endocrine stimulator of bone mass and strength. Endocrinology 2007;148:1654–65.
55. Gaddy-Kurten D, Coker JK, Abe E, et al. Inhibin suppresses and activin stimulates osteoblastogenesis and osteoclastogenesis in murine bone marrow cultures. Endocrinology 2002;143:74–83.
56. Gajos-Michniewicz A, Piastowska AW, Russell JA, et al. Follistatin as a potent regulator of bone metabolism. Biomarkers 2010;15:563–74.
57. Leto G, Incorvaia L, Badalamenti G, et al. Activin A circulating levels in patients with bone metastasis from breast or prostate cancer. Clin Exp Metastasis 2006;23:117–22.
58. Terpos E, Kastritis E, Christoulas D, et al. Circulating activin-A is elevated in patients with advanced multiple myeloma and correlates with extensive bone involvement and inferior survival; no alterations post-lenalidomide and dexamethasone therapy. Ann Oncol 2012;23:2681–6.
59. Vallet S, Mukherjee S, Vaghela N, et al. Activin A promotes multiple myeloma-induced osteolysis and is a promising target for myeloma bone disease. Proc Natl Acad Sci U S A 2010;107:5124–9.
60. Matzuk MM, Finegold MJ, Su JG, et al. Alpha-inhibin is a tumour-suppressor gene with gonadal specificity in mice. Nature 1992;360:313–9.
61. Cipriano SC, Chen L, Kumar TR, et al. Follistatin is a modulator of gonadal tumor progression and the activin-induced wasting syndrome in inhibin-deficient mice. Endocrinology 2000;141:2319–27.
62. Takabe K, Wang L, Leal AM, et al. Adenovirus-mediated overexpression of follistatin enlarges intact liver of adult rats. Hepatology 2003;38:1107–15.
63. Maguer-Satta V, Bartholin L, Jeanpierre S, et al. Regulation of human erythropoiesis by activin A, BMP2, and BMP4, members of the TGFbeta family. Exp Cell Res 2003;282:110–20.
64. Maguer-Satta V, Rimokh R. FLRG, member of the follistatin family, a new player in hematopoiesis. Mol Cell Endocrinol 2004;225:109–18.
65. Johansson BM, Wiles MV. Evidence for involvement of activin A and bone morphogenetic protein 4 in mammalian mesoderm and hematopoietic development. Mol Cell Biol 1995;15:141–51.

66. Li F, Lu S, Vida L, et al. Bone morphogenetic protein 4 induces efficient hemato-poietic differentiation of rhesus monkey embryonic stem cells in vitro. Blood 2001;98:335–42.

67. Shiozaki M, Sakai R, Tabuchi M, et al. In vivo treatment with erythroid differenti-ation factor (EDF/activin A) increases erythroid precursors (CFU-E and BFU-E) in mice. Biochem Biophys Res Commun 1989;165:1155–61.

68. Fuchs O, Simakova O, Klener P, et al. Inhibition of Smad5 in human hematopoi-etic progenitors blocks erythroid differentiation induced by BMP4. Blood Cells Mol Dis 2002;28:221–33.

69. Perry JM, Harandi OF, Paulson RF. BMP4, SCF, and hypoxia cooperatively regu-late the expansion of murine stress erythroid progenitors. Blood 2007;109: 4494–502.

70. Perry JM, Harandi OF, Porayette P, et al. Maintenance of the BMP4-dependent stress erythropoiesis pathway in the murine spleen requires hedgehog signaling. Blood 2009;113:911–8.

71. Schneyer AL, Sidis Y, Gulati A, et al. Differential antagonism of activin, myostatin and growth and differentiation factor 11 by wild-type and mutant follistatin. Endocrinology 2008;149:4589–95.

72. Maguer-Satta V, Bartholin L, Jeanpierre S, et al. Expression of FLRG, a novel ac-tivin A ligand, is regulated by TGF-beta and during hematopoiesis [corrected]. Exp Hematol 2001;29:301–8.

73. Imamura T, Takase M, Nishihara A, et al. Smad6 inhibits signalling by the TGF-beta superfamily. Nature 1997;389:622–6.

74. Zhou L, McMahon C, Bhagat T, et al. Reduced SMAD7 leads to overactivation of TGF-beta signaling in MDS that can be reversed by a specific inhibitor of TGF-beta receptor I kinase. Cancer Res 2011;71:955–63.

75. Liu T, Feng XH. Regulation of TGF-beta signalling by protein phosphatases. Biochem J 2010;430:191–8.

76. Aaron W, Mulivor DB, Kumar R, et al. RAP-011, a soluble activin receptor type IIa murine IgG-Fc fusion protein, prevents chemotherapy induced anemia. Blood 2009. Available at: https://ash.confex.com/ash/2009/webprogram/Paper23536.html.

77. Chantry AD, Heath D, Mulivor AW, et al. Inhibiting activin-A signaling stimulates bone formation and prevents cancer-induced bone destruction in vivo. J Bone Miner Res 2010;25:2633–46.

78. Kim KT, Borgstein NG, Yang Y, et al. ACE-011, a soluble activin receptor type IIa IgG-Fc fusion protein, increases hemoglobin and hematocrit levels in post-menopausal healthy women. Blood 2008. Available at: https://ash.confex.com/ash/2008/webprogram/Paper13363.html.

79. Ruckle J, Jacobs M, Kramer W, et al. Single-dose, randomized, double-blind, placebo-controlled study of ACE-011 (ActRIIA-IgG1) in postmenopausal women. J Bone Miner Res 2009;24:744–52.

80. Iancu-Rubin C, Mosoyan G, Wang J, et al. Stromal cell-mediated inhibition of erythropoiesis can be attenuated by sotatercept (ACE-011), an activin receptor type II ligand trap. Exp Hematol 2013;41:155–66.e17.

81. Rajasekhar NV, Suragani RL, Sako D, et al. RAP-536 promotes terminal erythroid differentiation and reduces anemia in a murine model of myelodysplastic syn-dromes. In 54th ASH Annual Meeting and Exposition. Atlanta, GA. December 8–11, 2012.

82. Lin YW, Slape C, Zhang Z, et al. NUP98-HOXD13 transgenic mice develop a highly penetrant, severe myelodysplastic syndrome that progresses to acute leukemia. Blood 2005;106:287–95.

Modulation of Hepcidin as Therapy for Primary and Secondary Iron Overload Disorders
Preclinical Models and Approaches

Paul J. Schmidt, PhD[a], Mark D. Fleming, MD, DPhil[b],*

KEYWORDS

- Iron metabolism • Ineffective erythropoiesis • Hereditary hemochromatosis
- β-Thalassemia • Hepcidin/minihepcidins • Lipid nanoparticle siRNA/antisense oligonucleotide

KEY POINTS

- Dysregulation of iron metabolism is a primary or secondary cause of morbidity and mortality in many diverse diseases, including hereditary hemochromatosis and β-thalassemia.
- Hepcidin is the central hormonal regulator of iron metabolism.
- Tmprss6 is a serine protease that regulates hepcidin expression by the hepatocyte through a mechanism that involves several of the hereditary hemochromatosis proteins.
- Modulation of hepcidin activity has demonstrated potential as a treatment modality to treat iron overload disorders in preclinical animal models.

INTRODUCTION TO IRON METABOLISM

Because iron is highly toxic when present in excess, mammals have evolved elaborate mechanisms for the regulation of iron acquisition, transport, storage, and utilization. A typical adult human is endowed with approximately 4 g of iron, almost two-thirds of which is distributed in hemoglobin in red blood cells (RBCs). Nearly 25 mg of iron is

Funding Sources: Dr P.J. Schmidt: none. Dr M.D. Fleming: Alnylam Pharmaceuticals, NIH R01 DK087992, and R01 DK100806.
Conflict of Interest: Dr P.J. Schmidt: none. Dr M.D. Fleming receives research funding from Alnylam Pharmaceuticals and has served as a paid consultant to Bayer, Eli Lilly and Co, Novartis, and FerruMax.
[a] Department of Pathology, Boston Children's Hospital, Harvard Medical School, 300 Longwood Avenue, Enders 11, Boston, MA 02115, USA; [b] Department of Pathology, Boston Children's Hospital, Harvard Medical School, 300 Longwood Avenue, Bader 124.1, Boston, MA 02115, USA
* Corresponding author.
E-mail address: Mark.Fleming@childrens.harvard.edu

Hematol Oncol Clin N Am 28 (2014) 387–401
http://dx.doi.org/10.1016/j.hoc.2013.11.004
0889-8588/14/$ – see front matter © 2014 Elsevier Inc. All rights reserved.

required to support erythropoiesis each day, but most of the iron required for erythropoiesis derives from recycling of iron from effete RBCs by macrophages of the reticuloendothelial system. Under normal conditions, only 1 to 2 mg of iron is absorbed each day from the diet; that is only to offset iron losses, which are not regulated, and limited to physiologic and nonphysiologic epithelial cell (eg, skin and intestine) or blood loss. Accordingly, total body iron is regulated entirely at the level of intestinal absorption, which can be modulated according to the body's needs.

The Hepcidin-Ferroportin Iron Regulatory Axis

Hepcidin is a peptide hormone produced predominately by the liver in response to iron stores.[1] As iron levels increase, so does hepcidin,[2,3] which, as a negative regulator of iron release from cells, binds to and causes the internalization and degradation of ferroportin (FPN1), the only known iron exporter.[4] FPN1 is expressed in abundance on macrophages and duodenal enterocytes, the cells that are directly responsible for iron recycling from senescent RBCs and for iron absorption from the intestine (**Fig. 1**). Thus, hepcidin production simultaneously leads to decreased intestinal iron absorption and sequestration of iron in macrophages, limiting its availability for erythropoiesis. Conversely, decreasing hepcidin expression permits more nonheme iron to be taken up from the diet and released from internal stores. A failure of this stores regulator of systemic iron metabolism[5] underlies the pathophysiology of most forms of hereditary hemochromatosis (HH) (see later discussion).

In addition to systemic iron deficiency, hepcidin expression is also suppressed by anemia and hypoxia.[6] Anemias characterized by ineffective erythropoiesis (bone marrow erythroid hyperplasia with premature, intramedullary death of maturing erythroblasts) seem to uniquely potently suppress hepcidin production *even in the presence of systemic iron overload*.[7] The factor or factors that communicate this signal from the bone marrow to the liver to suppress hepcidin have been termed the *erythroid regulator* of iron metabolism.[5] It is the apparent supremacy of the erythroid regulator compared with the stores regulator that underlies the pathogenesis of iron overload in *iron-loading anemias*, such as β-thalassemia intermedia, which are characterized by ineffective erythropoiesis. Importantly, in these anemias, as well as in HH, the regulatory dysfunction leading to iron overload is a *relative if not absolute deficiency in hepcidin for the degree of iron overload.* It is on this theoretical basis that upregulation of hepcidin has been envisioned as a means to treat iron overload in these apparently diverse diseases.

Iron-Responsive Hepcidin Expression by the Hepatocyte

It is now evident that the autosomal recessive forms of HH caused by mutations in *HFE*, *HJV*, or *TFR2* result from a disruption of the hepatocyte's ability to translate systemic iron stores and availability for erythropoiesis represented by the transferrin saturation (or concentration of diferric transferrin) into a signal that promotes hepcidin gene transcription.[8–10] In this way, they are thought to disrupt the stores regulator of systemic iron homeostasis. This pathway has been reviewed comprehensively elsewhere.[11–13] Only elements that are fundamental to the therapeutic innovations discussed later are highlighted here.

There is strong evidence that the bone morphogenetic protein (BMP)–sons of mothers against decapentaplegic (SMAD) signaling pathway plays a key role in the regulation of hepcidin and systemic iron metabolism (**Fig. 2**). Hemojuvelin (HJV), which is mutated in patients with a severe, juvenile onset from of HH,[9] is a BMP coreceptor protein[14] that facilitates signaling through the BMP type I receptors (BMPRIs) ALK2 and ALK3[15,16] in response to BMP6,[17,18] which is itself upregulated in the liver by iron. Activated BMP receptors phosphorylate SMADS1, 5, and 8, which in turn

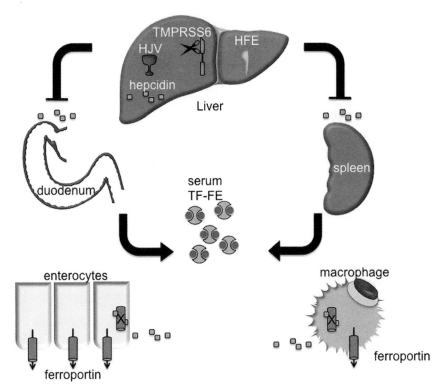

Fig. 1. The role of the liver and hepcidin in iron regulation. Hepcidin, produced in hepato-cytes of the liver, is a soluble regulator of iron metabolism. Classic hereditary hemochroma-tosis gene (HFE) and hemojuvelin (HJV) are necessary for appropriate sensing of transferrin (TF) saturation and, consequently, total body iron burden. TMPRSS6 is a membrane-bound serine protease thought to regulate HJV function by cleaving the bone morphogenetic pro-tein coreceptor HJV at the cell membrane. On release from the liver, hepcidin binds to FPN1 on the surface of duodenal enterocytes and macrophages responsible for recycling iron from RBCs, leading to internalization and degradation of the iron transporter FPN1 and diminution of transferrin-bound iron (TF-FE) in the serum.

phosphorylate SMAD4, which translocates to the nucleus, stimulating transcription by binding to a BMP-response element in the hepcidin promoter.

Although juvenile hemochromatosis is rare, mutations in the classic hereditary hemochromatosis gene (HFE) account for most of the patients with HH in the Western hemisphere.[19] Early work demonstrated that HFE interacts with the transferrin receptor (TFRC or TFR1) in a manner that can be competitively inhibited by diferric transferrin binding to TFR1.[20,21] A second transferrin receptor, TFR2,[22] mutated in a fraction of patients with HH,[23] also interacts with HFE[24,25] in vitro, but it associates with diferric transferrin only very poorly. In this way, there would seem to be a means for hepatocytes to sense the amount of iron in the plasma. It is a matter of debate whether TFR2, HFE, or both directly interact with the HJV-BMPR complex[26,27]; how-ever, inactivation of either protein diminishes the activation of the downstream SMADS as well as hepcidin transcription in response to iron.

Mutations in any of the HH proteins or certain components of the BMP-SMAD signaling cascade in hepatocytes in model organisms lead to hyporesponsiveness of hepcidin transcription in response to iron. In contrast, mutations in TMPRSS6,

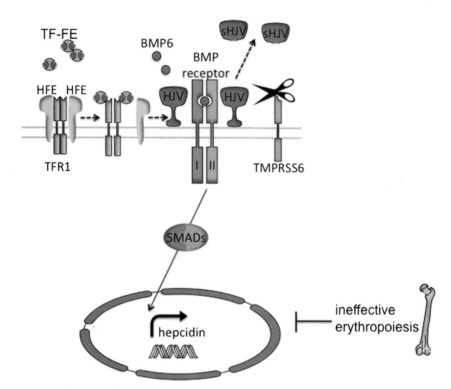

Fig. 2. Involvement of the BMP/hemojuvelin (HJV)/SMAD signaling pathway in the regulation of hepatocyte-generated hepcidin. Hepcidin expression is increased in response to elevated iron and decreased because of ineffective erythropoiesis such as is found in β-thalassemia intermedia. Mutations in the classic hereditary hemochromatosis gene (HFE) and hemojuvelin (HJV) cause hereditary hemochromatosis. HJV, a BMP coreceptor, plays a central role in hepcidin regulation through an SMAD signaling cascade. BMP6 expression increases with elevated iron conditions and acts as a ligand, binding to hemojuvelin (HJV) and initiating hepcidin expression. Diferric transferrin (TF-FE) displaces HFE from transferrin receptor-1 (TFR1) likely leading to interaction with the HJV/BMP receptor complex or a possibly separate signaling pathway. The membrane-bound serine protease TMPRSS6 cleaves HJV from the cell surface, forming a soluble protein (sHJV).

a membrane associated protease expressed solely in the liver, cause the opposite phenotype: excessively high hepcidin levels in response to a given iron status, and the clinical phenotype of congenital iron deficiency.[28–31] Work in vitro suggests that TMPRSS6 regulates HJV protein levels at the cell membrane by cleaving it to generate a soluble form (see **Fig. 2**).[32,33] It seems that iron, BMP6, and hypoxia are all able to induce TMPRSS6 transcription in vivo.[34,35] In toto, TMPRSS6 activity and expression are coordinated to inhibit hepcidin transcription mediated by the BMP-SMAD pathway and in doing so may ordinarily help to prevent excessive hepcidin induction and prevent iron deficiency.

PRECLINICAL INVESTIGATION OF HEPCIDIN MIMETIC AND HEPCIDIN-INDUCTION THERAPIES IN MURINE MODELS OF HH

As described earlier, because of the relative hepcidin deficiency seen in both HH and in the iron-loading anemias associated with ineffective erythropoiesis, manipulation of hepcidin levels either through exogenous administration or endogenous stimulation has been envisioned as a potential pharmacologic approach to these disorders (**Box 1**). In many ways, because of the safety, efficacy, and low cost of phlebotomy for the treatment of HH, many have seen using animal models of HH as the proof of principle for these therapies as a prelude to the more complicated secondary hepcidin suppression seen in the iron-loading anemias.

Transgenic Hepcidin Overexpression in HFE HH

Hepcidin therapy was first attempted by Nicolas and colleagues[36] in a murine model of HH. This group showed that $Hfe^{-/-}$ animals[37] have inappropriately low hepcidin expression that does not change as the animals age and load iron (**Fig. 3**A). Earlier work in this laboratory had generated a transgenic animal that overexpressed the mouse hepcidin gene under control of the liver-specific transthyretin promoter.[38] These transgenic animals are extremely pale; have diminished whole body iron stores and a severe hypochromic, microcytic anemia; and, on a C57BL/6 background, die within a few hours of birth. Transgenic mice on a mixed 129Sv-C57BL/6 background are viable, and the anemia eventually subsides as the endogenous hepcidin normalizes at approximately 9 weeks of life. More severely affected founder animals require treatment with exogenous iron to survive past weaning. As one would expect, overexpression of hepcidin in $Hfe^{-/-}$ animals (see **Fig. 3**B) greatly decreased iron loading in whole embryos and also in the livers of 1- and 2-month-old HH animals.[36] In fact, in many animals, the correction of the hepcidin deficiency was too great, leading to iron deficiency anemia. In toto, this work was the proof in principle for hepcidin therapy in iron overload diseases, but it equally illustrated the potential complications of an inability to titer the therapy to the physiologic state of the animal.

Exogenous BMP6 for the Treatment of HFE HH

Mice lacking Hfe, although iron overloaded, do not have detectable elevations in hepatic Bmp-Smad pathway signaling.[39,40] Furthermore, Bmp6 expression is appropriately upregulated in comparison with the increased tissue iron found in $Hfe^{-/-}$ mice, suggesting that Hfe is not necessary for Bmp6 regulation. As a result, Corradini and colleagues[41] hypothesized that treatment of $Hfe^{-/-}$ mice with supraphysiologic levels of Bmp6 could compensate for the defect in Smad-mediated hepcidin regulation (see **Fig. 3**C). To evaluate this possibility, they administered BMP6 to $Hfe^{-/-}$ mice twice daily for 10 days and found that treatment increased liver hepcidin mRNA expression

Box 1	
Experimental preclinical models focused on repressing iron absorption and utilization	
Genetic ablation of Tmprss6 ($Tmprss6^{-/-}$)[43,57]	Murine β-thalassemia intermedia ($Hbb^{th3/+}$), murine HH ($Hfe^{-/-}$)
Transferrin (Tf) therapy[54]	Murine β-thalassemia intermedia ($Hbb^{th1/th1}$)
Transgenic overexpression of hepcidin ($Hamp1$)[36,55]	Murine β-thalassemia intermedia ($Hbb^{th3/+}$) and murine HH ($Hfe^{-/-}$)
Dietary iron restriction[55]	Murine β-thalassemia intermedia ($Hbb^{th3/+}$)
Pharmacologic repression of Tmprss6 expression (siRNA, antisense oligonucleotide)	Murine β-thalassemia intermedia ($Hbb^{th3/+}$), murine HH ($Hfe^{-/-}$)
Treatment with hepcidin mimetic (minihepcidin)[48,49]	Murine juvenile HH ($Hamp1^{-/-}$)
BMP6 therapy[41]	Murine HH ($Hfe^{-/-}$)

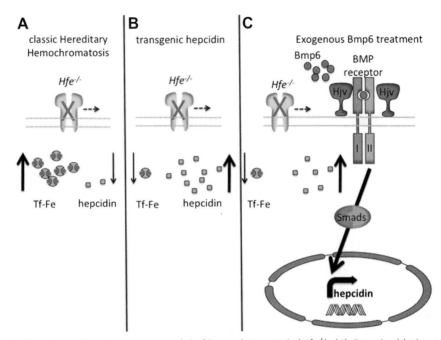

Fig. 3. Interventions in a mouse model of hemochromatosis ($Hfe^{-/-}$). (*A*) Genetic ablation of the Hfe protein ($Hfe^{-/-}$) leads to diminished hepcidin production and elevated iron uptake and distribution. Transgenic overexpression of hepcidin (*B*) greatly diminishes tissue iron loading and leads to a microcytic, hypochromic anemia. Application of supraphysiologic amounts of BMP6 (*C*) initiates hepcidin production through stimulation of the Bmp/Hjv/Smad signaling pathway, leading to diminished available iron. Transferrin-bound iron, Tf-Fe.

by almost 2-fold. This resulted in reduced serum iron, transferrin saturation, and elevated nonheme iron deposition in the spleen. Improvement of liver, heart, and pancreas iron levels was not observed, almost certainly because of the relatively short treatment regimen, which was necessitated by dysplastic calcification at the injection site. This study clearly demonstrated the limitations of systemic BMP6 treatment of iron overload but equally pointed out the potential for therapeutic efficacy if local, hepatic expression of BMP6 is achieved.

Genetic and Pharmacologic Inhibition of Tmprss6 in HFE HH

Mice lacking Tmprss6 overexpress hepcidin because of the constitutive hyperactivation BMP-SMAD signaling pathway, leading to an iron-refractory iron deficiency anemia (IRIDA) phenotype.[28,42] A similar IRIDA phenotype occurs in humans with biallelic mutations in TMPRSS6. Current models postulate that TMPRSS6 cleaves HJV from the cell membrane, dampening BMP-SMAD signaling and consequently hepcidin expression, particularly when ambient iron levels are low. As a result, genetic or pharmacologic targeting of TMPRSS6 may be beneficial in disorders of iron regulation dependent on physiologically upstream of HJV (**Fig. 4**A). As a genetic proof of principle, Finberg and colleagues[43] showed that deletion of a single *Tmprss6* allele greatly diminished iron loading in $Hfe^{-/-}$ animals. Complete loss of Tmprss6 ameliorated the iron overload phenotype but also caused a hypochromic, microcytic iron deficiency anemia on the $Hfe^{-/-}$ background, indicating that a delicate balance must be struck between too much and too little hepcidin.

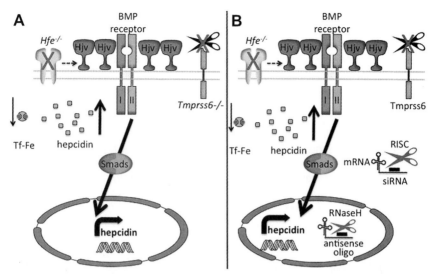

Fig. 4. Modulation of hepcidin expression through genetic or pharmacologic targeting of Tmprss6. Loss of all endogenous Tmprss6 protein (*A*) leads to elevated levels of Hjv, the Bmp coreceptor, on the cell membrane. Significant hepcidin expression causes suppressed iron levels and a hypochromic, microcytic anemia, even in a mouse lacking Hfe. (*B*) Targeting of Tmprss6 through pharmacologic means. Targeting of Tmprss6 siRNA to the liver in lipid nanoparticle–formulated siRNAs, or by antisense oligonucleotide technology, leads to diminished *Tmprss6* mRNA expression through classic RNA-induced silencing complex (RISC)-mediated (cytoplasmic) or RnaseH-mediated (nucleus) suppression, respectively. Suppression of Tmprss6 causes elevated levels of Hjv to remain on the cell membrane, triggering heightened hepcidin expression and ameliorating the *Hfe*[-/-] phenotype.

Two research groups have subsequently sought to promote hepcidin expression by targeting Tmprss6 mRNA for degradation in vivo (see **Fig. 4**B). Schmidt and colleagues[44,45] tested an siRNA targeting *Tmprss6* mRNA encapsulated in lipid nanoparticles (LNP) composed of an ionizable lipid, disteroylphosphatidyl choline, cholesterol, and polyethylene glycol-dimyristoylglycerol (PEG-DMG). Because they are taken up by the chylomicron scavenger receptors, these vesicles can be injected into a peripheral vein and are avidly taken up by hepatocytes relatively specifically, where they induce *Tmprss6* mRNA degradation through a mechanism involving the RNA-induced silencing complex. Treatment of wild-type animals with Tmprss6 siRNA decreased liver expression of *Tmprss6* mRNA in a dose-dependent manner, leading to prolonged hepcidin induction and suppression of the transferrin (Tf) saturation and liver nonheme iron levels.[45] Silencing *Tmprss6* in *Hfe*[-/-] mice had similar effects. Furthermore, siRNA treatment also increased total spleen iron, indicating that hepcidin induction also caused splenic macrophages to sequester iron from senescent RBCs. As might be expected, even in *Hfe*[-/-] animals, chronic suppression of Tmprss6 has a cumulative effect on erythropoiesis, leading to a hypochromic, microcytic anemia.

Guo and colleagues[46] used a related antisense oligonucleotide (ASO) approach to suppressing Tmprss6 expression.[47] Here, antisense oligonucleotides form an RNA-DNA hybrid that is then degraded through a nuclear RNaseH-mediated mechanism. As is true of the siRNA approach, Tmprss6 ASO treatment decreased hepatic expression of *Tmprss6* mRNA in a dose-dependent manner, leading to elevated hepcidin production, eventuating in a decrease in serum iron and transferrin saturation.

Likewise, treatment of Hfe$^{-/-}$ mice also suppressed serum and liver iron parameters and increased spleen iron concentration, indicating, as before, a redistribution of iron from hepatocytes to recycling macrophages in the spleen. As noted with siRNA treatment, ASO manipulation of hepcidin also leads to a hypochromic, microcytic anemia.

Minihepcidins Correct Hepcidin Deficiency in HH

As in other hormone deficiency disorders (eg, type I diabetes mellitus and hypothyroidism), the iron loading in HH could equally be treated by hormone replacement therapy. The relative abundance of hepcidin, which is one of the most highly expressed RNAs in the liver, as well as its short plasma half-life caused by proteolysis and renal clearance, however, severely limits the potential for direct hormone replacement. To address the pharmacologic shortcomings of the natural peptide, Preza and colleagues[48] developed a series of orally bioavailable, long-acting minihepcidins for the treatment of iron overload disorders. In cell-based assays, they showed that the 7–9 N-terminal amino acids of hepcidin seem to be the minimal sequence able to induce FPN1 degradation. Chemically synthesized N-terminal peptides assembled from D-amino acids in the reverse orientation (so-called retro-inverso peptides) are equally active as the natural L-amino acid N-terminal peptides but are resistant to proteases. Further modification of the retro-inverso peptides with C-terminal carboxyamide-linked PEG and palmitic acid groups produced biologically active molecules that are both orally bioavailable and have a longer plasma half-life. Indeed, daily intraperitoneal injection of minihepcidins was able to reverse iron loading in mice deficient in hepcidin. Subsequent work by Ramos and colleagues[49] used an optimized minihepcidin, containing only L-amino acids, to treat hepcidin deficient animals that were either dietarily iron loaded or depleted. Most notably, minihepcidin administration to iron-depleted hepcidin null animal mice prevented liver iron loading, decreased heart iron levels, and caused iron retention in splenic macrophages. However, treatment of already iron-loaded knockout animals caused a significant increase in spleen iron but only small changes in liver, heart, and serum iron measurements. As expected, very high doses of the peptides lead to anemia because of iron restriction, once again highlighting the very narrow therapeutic window for manipulating this pathway.

Small Molecule Modulation of Hepcidin Expression

Other recent work has sought to generate small molecules that induce hepcidin. Genistein, a member of the isoflavone family of organic molecules related to estrogens, was found to induce hepcidin transcription in a zebra fish model system.[50] This modulation was shown to be both BMP and Stat3 mediated, but does not require estrogen receptor signaling, in an in vitro cell culture system. Further research will be necessary to determine if this potential treatment modality is viable in a mammalian animal model of iron metabolism.

PRECLINICAL INVESTIGATION OF HEPCIDIN-INDUCTION THERAPIES IN MURINE MODELS OF β-THALASSEMIA INTERMEDIA

Unlike in HH, phlebotomy is not an approach that can be applied to mitigate the iron overload in all but the most mildly anemic patients with ineffective erythropoiesis and secondary iron overload (eg, some patients with sideroblastic anemia). Consequently, if intervention in the hepcidin-FPN1 axis to limit iron absorption is to find a clinical application, it is most likely in untransfused patients with chronic anemia and iron overload. To this end, several of the strategies described earlier, as well as several others (see **Box 1**), have been applied to mouse models of non–transfusion-dependent β-thalassemia (ie, β-thalassemia intermedia), which display many of the key characteristics of the human disease. Specifically, 2 mutant genotypes, $Hbb^{th3/+}$ and $Hbb^{th1/th1}$,[51,52] have transfusion-independent, moderately severe anemia associated with ineffective erythropoiesis, splenomegaly, and secondary iron overload.

Transferrin Therapy to Modulate Iron Metabolism in β-Thalassemia Intermedia

Despite the systemic iron overload, caused by the massive erythroid demand and plasma iron turnover, thalassemic erythroblasts are actually functionally iron deficient. Indeed, Ginzburg and colleagues[53] observed that treatment of $Hbb^{th1/th1}$ thalassemic animals with iron improves the anemia but comes at the expense of more marked iron overload. Reasoning that Tf therapy could improve iron delivery to the erythron without adding additional iron to the system, this same group of investigators treated thalassemic mice with chronic Tf injections. They observed that Tf treatment increased the hemoglobin and decreased the reticulocytosis, splenomegaly, and plasma erythropoietin as well as decreased the membrane-associated α-globin precipitates and normalized the RBC half-life.[54] Treatment with either apo or holo Tf significantly increased hepcidin expression in comparison with untreated animals and demonstrated an increase in comparison with wildtype (WT) littermates. Iron staining in treated spleen was decreased, but there was no difference in other tissues.

Despite the rationale leading to its investigation, it is unclear if Tf therapy is effective because it *promotes* or *inhibits* iron delivery to the erythron. Some data would suggest that the latter is the case. For example, dietary iron restriction has similar effects on anemia and ineffective erythropoiesis in the $Hbb^{th3/+}$ mouse model.[55] Furthermore, RBC parameters in both of these models change in a manner that would suggest more severe iron deficiency: both Tf-treated $Hbb^{th1/th1}$ and iron-deficient $Hbb^{th3/+}$ mice respond to the treatment by making more RBCs with a smaller mean corpuscular volume (MCV) and a lower mean corpuscular hemoglobin (MCH) and mean corpuscular hemoglobin concentration (MCHC), all characteristics of RBC iron deficiency. These observations provided the seminal insight that actual or functional iron deficiency had the potential to modify the disease phenotype in these β-thalassemia models, suggesting that targeting the hepcidin-FPN1 axis to restrict iron availability would effect not only iron loading but also the primary disease itself.

Genetic and Pharmacologic Induction of Hepcidin in β-Thalassemia Intermedia

Based on the effect of dietary iron deficiency, it was recognized that limiting iron absorption and macrophage iron recycling with hepcidin might equally mitigate the thalassemic and iron overload phenotypes. To test this possibility, Gardenghi and colleagues[55] transplanted $Hbb^{th3/+}$ hematopoietic stem cells into mice transgenically expressing hepcidin in a tetracycline-inducible manner.[56] Here, moderate overexpression of hepcidin in the $Hbb^{th3/+}$ model reduces iron overload, improves anemia, and decreases splenomegaly. Importantly, in several animals, the anemia actually became worse. These rare individuals, it was found, expressed higher levels of hepcidin than their counterparts that experienced improvement in the anemia, once again illustrating the delicate balance between iron restriction and desirable effects.

Similar to previous work that validated *Tmprss6* as a target to moderate murine $Hfe^{-/-}$ HH, Nai and colleagues[57] showed that targeted deletion of *Tmprss6* not only decreases iron loading but also *uniformly* ameliorates the anemia and ineffective erythropoiesis in $Hbb^{th3/+}$ mice (see **Fig. 4**A). Importantly, this would suggest that, unlike the induction of endogenous hepcidin through other means or potentially the administration of hepcidin mimetics, complete inhibition of this target should not have the untoward effect of excessively iron-restricted erythropoiesis.

Using methodologies described earlier, Schmidt and colleagues[45] and Guo and colleagues[46] used LNP-formulated siRNAs and ASOs, respectively, targeted against *Tmprss6* mRNA to enhance hepcidin expression in the *Hbb*[th3/+] thalassemia model. Both groups had qualitatively similar results, demonstrating that suppression of Tmprss6 expression in *Hbb*[th3/+] mice significantly induces liver-expressed hepcidin and diminishes tissue and serum iron levels. More importantly, both treatments substantially improved the anemia by altering RBC survival and ineffective erythropoiesis. This improvement in RBC survival was likely a consequence of a decrease in accumulated erythrocyte membrane-associated α-globin precipitates. A reduction in splenomegaly and ineffective erythropoiesis was confirmed by the restoration of proper splenic architecture and diminution of serum erythropoietin.

SUMMARY AND FUTURE DIRECTIONS

Although it is quite evident that iron restriction through either dietary limitation or elevating serum hepcidin activity improves anemia in the *Hbb*[th3/+] mouse model of β-thalassemia intermedia, the mechanism by which this occurs has not yet been defined. At least in the case of hepcidin and hepcidin mimetics, it is possible that intervening in the hepcidin-FPN1 axis itself may play a direct role in the maturation of erythroblasts. For example, work by Zhang and colleagues[58] showed that Fpn1 is highly expressed on the cell membrane in erythroblasts, which may modulate iron availability in early erythroid cells by exporting the metal.[59] Nevertheless, as noted earlier, the same effect is observed when thalassemic animals are placed on a low-iron diet alone, suggesting that iron-restricted erythropoiesis is the critical factor.[55]

In humans, it is well documented that induction of γ-globin (and thus hemoglobin F) can mitigate the clinical phenotype of the β-hemoglobinopathies (reviewed in[60,61]). However, this cannot be the mechanism in rodents because they lack a γ-globin equivalent, switching directly from embryonic to adult β-globins. Similarly, much the same as coinheritance of an α-thalassemia allele mitigates a β-thalassemia genotype,[62] it is possible that the suppression of available iron decreases the α/β globin synthesis ratio, leading to fewer free α-chains and diminishing the damage caused by membrane-associated α-globin. However, this does not seem to be the case either in this mouse model (Paul J. Schmidt and Mark D. Fleming, unpublished data). The stability of free α-globin might equally be increased through the elevation of AHSP,[63] the α-hemoglobin stabilizing protein whose expression is increased in iron deficiency.[64] However, although theoretically possible, this is unlikely because transgenic overexpression of AHSP does not improve the anemia in *Hbb*[th3/+] animals.[65] Another, still unconfirmed, hypothesis is that erythroid iron deficiency causes a global decrease in globin protein synthesis, which, because of the absolute decrease in α-chains, would lead to less membrane damage and increased intramedullary and extramedullary RBC survival. A potential mechanism for this decrease could be through the heme-regulated eIF2α kinase (*HRI*).[66] HRI is an erythroid-specific translational elongation factor 2a kinase that, in the absence of heme, is a potent inhibitor of protein synthesis.[67–69] Although *Hri*[-/-] mice have no baseline phenotype, these animals develop a paradoxic hyperchromic, macrocytic anemia with reduced RBC numbers in the setting of iron deficiency.[70] Hri deficiency increases the abundance of α-globin aggregates and in doing so exacerbates the phenotype of the *Hbb*[th1/th1] thalassemia.[71] Determining whether this or another mechanism underlies the phenotypic improvement in each of the preclinical models discussed earlier will most certainly contribute to further refinement of therapeutics designed to enhance these effects.

The application of these experimental therapies has, thus far, been limited to HH and β-thalassemia intermedia mouse models. It is possible, however, that they may eventually find application in transfusion-dependent β-thalassemia major patients, in which the hepcidin levels are at baseline grossly elevated but may, nonetheless, still be inappropriately low for the systemic iron burden.[72] Although chronic transfusion therapy is meant to suppress ineffective erythropoiesis and its complications, the episodic nature of transfusions leads to gradually increasing erythropoietic drive pre-transfusion, punctuated by periods of maximal suppression immediately following a transfusion. A recent analysis of β-thalassemia major patients pretransfusion and posttransfusion demonstrated an increase in hepcidin and a decrease in both erythro-poietin and growth differentiation factor-15 (GDF15). Dimished GDF15 is thought to indicate ineffective erythropoiesis is decreased after transfusion.[73] Thus, although the primary source of iron in transfused β-thalassemia is from transfused RBCs, intes-tinal iron absorption may, nonetheless, be relatively stimulated, particularly as the he-moglobin approaches a nadir. Thus, in this situation, when ongoing erythropoiesis is entirely undesirable, a compromise between erythropoiesis and iron absorption need not be struck, and maximal suppression of the pathway, as might be achieved with a hepcidin mimetic, in particular, is a desirable goal. Furthermore, combination of these therapies with state-of-the-art iron chelation strategies may further decrease the burden of iron and iron-related complications in transfusion-dependent and -inde-pendent β-thalassemias.

REFERENCES

1. Krause A, Neitz S, Magert HJ, et al. LEAP-1, a novel highly disulfide-bonded human peptide, exhibits antimicrobial activity. FEBS Lett 2000;480(2–3): 147–50.
2. Pigeon C, Ilyin G, Courselaud B, et al. A new mouse liver-specific gene, encod-ing a protein homologous to human antimicrobial peptide hepcidin, is overex-pressed during iron overload. J Biol Chem 2001;276(11):7811–9.
3. Park CH, Valore EV, Waring AJ, et al. Hepcidin, a urinary antimicrobial peptide synthesized in the liver. J Biol Chem 2001;276(11):7806–10.
4. Nemeth E, Tuttle MS, Powelson J, et al. Hepcidin regulates cellular iron efflux by binding to ferroportin and inducing its internalization. Science 2004;306(5704): 2090–3.
5. Finch C. Regulators of iron balance in humans. Blood 1994;84(6):1697–702.
6. Nicolas G, Chauvet C, Viatte L, et al. The gene encoding the iron regulatory pep-tide hepcidin is regulated by anemia, hypoxia, and inflammation. J Clin Invest 2002;110(7):1037–44.
7. Adamsky K, Weizer O, Amariglio N, et al. Decreased hepcidin mRNA expres-sion in thalassemic mice. Br J Haematol 2004;124(1):123–4.
8. Nemeth E, Roetto A, Garozzo G, et al. Hepcidin is decreased in TFR2 hemo-chromatosis. Blood 2005;105(4):1803–6.
9. Papanikolaou G, Samuels ME, Ludwig EH, et al. Mutations in HFE2 cause iron overload in chromosome 1q-linked juvenile hemochromatosis. Nat Genet 2004;36(1):77–82.
10. Bridle KR, Frazer DM, Wilkins SJ, et al. Disrupted hepcidin regulation in HFE-associated haemochromatosis and the liver as a regulator of body iron homoeo-stasis. Lancet 2003;361(9358):669–73.

11. Schmidt P. Molecular basis of hemochromatosis. In: Culotta VC, Scott RS, editors. Metals in cells. Chichester (United Kingdom): John Wiley & Sons, Ltd; 2013. p. 361–72.

12. Corradini E, Babitt JL, Lin HY. The RGM/DRAGON family of BMP co-receptors. Cytokine Growth Factor Rev 2009;20(5–6):389–98.

13. Babitt JL, Lin HY. The molecular pathogenesis of hereditary hemochromatosis. Semin Liver Dis 2011;31(3):280–92.

14. Babitt JL, Huang FW, Wrighting DM, et al. Bone morphogenetic protein signaling by hemojuvelin regulates hepcidin expression. Nat Genet 2006; 38(5):531–9.

15. Yu PB, Hong CC, Sachidanandan C, et al. Dorsomorphin inhibits BMP signals required for embryogenesis and iron metabolism. Nat Chem Biol 2008;4(1): 33–41.

16. Steinbicker AU, Bartnikas TB, Lohmeyer LK, et al. Perturbation of hepcidin expression by BMP type I receptor deletion induces iron overload in mice. Blood 2011;118(15):4224–30.

17. Andriopoulos B Jr, Corradini E, Xia Y, et al. BMP6 is a key endogenous regulator of hepcidin expression and iron metabolism. Nat Genet 2009;41(4):482–7.

18. Meynard D, Kautz L, Darnaud V, et al. Lack of the bone morphogenetic protein BMP6 induces massive iron overload. Nat Genet 2009;41(4):478–81.

19. Feder JN, Gnirke A, Thomas W, et al. A novel MHC class I-like gene is mutated in patients with hereditary haemochromatosis. Nat Genet 1996;13(4):399–408.

20. Feder JN, Penny DM, Irrinki A, et al. The hemochromatosis gene product complexes with the transferrin receptor and lowers its affinity for ligand binding. Proc Natl Acad Sci U S A 1998;95(4):1472–7.

21. West AP Jr, Giannetti AM, Herr AB, et al. Mutational analysis of the transferrin receptor reveals overlapping HFE and transferrin binding sites. J Mol Biol 2001;313(2):385–97.

22. Kawabata H, Yang R, Hirama T, et al. Molecular cloning of transferrin receptor 2. A new member of the transferrin receptor-like family. J Biol Chem 1999;274(30): 20826–32.

23. Camaschella C, Roetto A, Cali A, et al. The gene TFR2 is mutated in a new type of haemochromatosis mapping to 7q22. Nat Genet 2000;25(1):14–5.

24. Goswami T, Andrews NC. Hereditary hemochromatosis protein, HFE, interaction with transferrin receptor 2 suggests a molecular mechanism for mammalian iron sensing. J Biol Chem 2006;281(39):28494–8.

25. Gao J, Chen J, Kramer M, et al. Interaction of the hereditary hemochromatosis protein HFE with transferrin receptor 2 is required for transferrin-induced hepcidin expression. Cell Metab 2009;9(3):217–27.

26. Schmidt PJ, Fleming MD. Transgenic HFE-dependent induction of hepcidin in mice does not require transferrin receptor-2. Am J Hematol 2012;87(6):588–95.

27. D'Alessio F, Hentze MW, Muckenthaler MU. The hemochromatosis proteins HFE, TfR2, and HJV form a membrane-associated protein complex for hepcidin regulation. J Hepatol 2012;57(5):1052–60.

28. Du X, She E, Gelbart T, et al. The serine protease TMPRSS6 is required to sense iron deficiency. Science 2008;320(5879):1088–92.

29. Finberg KE, Heeney MM, Campagna DR, et al. Mutations in TMPRSS6 cause iron-refractory iron deficiency anemia (IRIDA). Nat Genet 2008;40(5):569–71.

30. Folgueras AR, de Lara FM, Pendas AM, et al. Membrane-bound serine protease matriptase-2 (Tmprss6) is an essential regulator of iron homeostasis. Blood 2008;112(6):2539–45.

31. Melis MA, Cau M, Congiu R, et al. A mutation in the TMPRSS6 gene, encoding a transmembrane serine protease that suppresses hepcidin production, in familial iron deficiency anemia refractory to oral iron. Haematologica 2008;93(10): 1473–9.

32. Silvestri L, Pagani A, Nai A, et al. The serine protease matriptase-2 (TMPRSS6) inhibits hepcidin activation by cleaving membrane hemojuvelin. Cell Metab 2008;8(6):502–11.

33. Maxson JE, Chen J, Enns CA, et al. Matriptase-2- and proprotein convertase-cleaved forms of hemojuvelin have different roles in the down-regulation of hepcidin expression. J Biol Chem 2010;285(50):39021–8.

34. Meynard D, Vaja V, Sun CC, et al. Regulation of TMPRSS6 by BMP6 and iron in human cells and mice. Blood 2011;118(3):747–56.

35. Maurer E, Gutschow M, Stirnberg M. Matriptase-2 (TMPRSS6) is directly up-regulated by hypoxia inducible factor-1: identification of a hypoxia-responsive element in the TMPRSS6 promoter region. Biol Chem 2012;393(6):535–40.

36. Nicolas G, Viatte L, Lou DQ, et al. Constitutive hepcidin expression prevents iron overload in a mouse model of hemochromatosis. Nat Genet 2003;34(1): 97–101.

37. Levy JE, Montross LK, Cohen DE, et al. The C282Y mutation causing hereditary hemochromatosis does not produce a null allele. Blood 1999;94(1):9–11.

38. Nicolas G, Bennoun M, Porteu A, et al. Severe iron deficiency anemia in transgenic mice expressing liver hepcidin. Proc Natl Acad Sci U S A 2002;99(7): 4596–601.

39. Kautz L, Meynard D, Besson-Fournier C, et al. BMP/Smad signaling is not enhanced in Hfe-deficient mice despite increased Bmp6 expression. Blood 2009;114(12):2515–20.

40. Corradini E, Garuti C, Montosi G, et al. Bone morphogenetic protein signaling is impaired in an Hfe knockout mouse model of hemochromatosis. Gastroenterology 2009;137(4):1489–97.

41. Corradini E, Schmidt PJ, Meynard D, et al. BMP6 treatment compensates for the molecular defect and ameliorates hemochromatosis in Hfe knockout mice. Gastroenterology 2010;139(5):1721–9.

42. Finberg KE, Whittlesey RL, Fleming MD, et al. Down-regulation of Bmp/Smad signaling by Tmprss6 is required for maintenance of systemic iron homeostasis. Blood 2010;115(18):3817–26.

43. Finberg KE, Whittlesey RL, Andrews NC. Tmprss6 is a genetic modifier of the Hfe-hemochromatosis phenotype in mice. Blood 2011;117(17):4590–9.

44. Semple SC, Akinc A, Chen J, et al. Rational design of cationic lipids for siRNA delivery. Nat Biotechnol 2010;28(2):172–6.

45. Schmidt PJ, Toudjarska I, Sendamarai AK, et al. An RNAi therapeutic targeting Tmprss6 decreases iron overload in Hfe(-/-) mice and ameliorates anemia and iron overload in murine beta-thalassemia intermedia. Blood 2013;121(7): 1200–8.

46. Guo S, Casu C, Gardenghi S, et al. Reducing TMPRSS6 ameliorates hemochromatosis and beta-thalassemia in mice. J Clin Invest 2013;123(4):1531–41.

47. Bennett CF, Swayze EE. RNA targeting therapeutics: molecular mechanisms of antisense oligonucleotides as a therapeutic platform. Annu Rev Pharmacol Toxicol 2010;50:259–93.

48. Preza GC, Ruchala P, Pinon R, et al. Minihepcidins are rationally designed small peptides that mimic hepcidin activity in mice and may be useful for the treatment of iron overload. J Clin Invest 2011;121(12):4880–8.

49. Ramos E, Ruchala P, Goodnough JB, et al. Minihepcidins prevent iron overload in a hepcidin-deficient mouse model of severe hemochromatosis. Blood 2012; 120(18):3829–36.

50. Zhen AW, Nguyen NH, Gibert Y, et al. The small molecule, genistein, increases hepcidin expression in human hepatocytes. Hepatology 2013;58(4):1315–25.

51. Skow LC, Burkhart BA, Johnson FM, et al. A mouse model for beta-thalassemia. Cell 1983;34(3):1043–52.

52. Yang B, Kirby S, Lewis J, et al. A mouse model for beta 0-thalassemia. Proc Natl Acad Sci U S A 1995;92(25):11608–12.

53. Ginzburg YZ, Rybicki AC, Suzuka SM, et al. Exogenous iron increases hemoglobin in beta-thalassemic mice. Exp Hematol 2009;37(2):172–83.

54. Li H, Rybicki AC, Suzuka SM, et al. Transferrin therapy ameliorates disease in beta-thalassemic mice. Nat Med 2010;16(2):177–82.

55. Gardenghi S, Ramos P, Marongiu MF, et al. Hepcidin as a therapeutic tool to limit iron overload and improve anemia in beta-thalassemic mice. J Clin Invest 2010; 120(12):4466–77.

56. Roy CN, Mak HH, Akpan I, et al. Hepcidin antimicrobial peptide transgenic mice exhibit features of the anemia of inflammation. Blood 2007;109(9):4038–44.

57. Nai A, Pagani A, Mandelli G, et al. Deletion of TMPRSS6 attenuates the phenotype in a mouse model of beta-thalassemia. Blood 2012;119(21):5021–9.

58. Zhang DL, Hughes RM, Ollivierre-Wilson H, et al. A ferroportin transcript that lacks an iron-responsive element enables duodenal and erythroid precursor cells to evade translational repression. Cell Metab 2009;9(5):461–73.

59. Zhang DL, Senecal T, Ghosh MC, et al. Hepcidin regulates ferroportin expression and intracellular iron homeostasis of erythroblasts. Blood 2011;118(10): 2868–77.

60. Bauer DE, Orkin SH. Update on fetal hemoglobin gene regulation in hemoglobinopathies. Curr Opin Pediatr 2011;23(1):1–8.

61. Sankaran VG. Targeted therapeutic strategies for fetal hemoglobin induction. Hematology Am Soc Hematol Educ Program 2011;2011:459–65.

62. Winichagoon P, Fucharoen S, Weatherall D, et al. Concomitant inheritance of alpha-thalassemia in beta 0- thalassemia/Hb E disease. Am J Hematol 1985; 20(3):217–22.

63. Kihm AJ, Kong Y, Hong W, et al. An abundant erythroid protein that stabilizes free alpha-haemoglobin. Nature 2002;417(6890):758–63.

64. Yu X, Kong Y, Dore LC, et al. An erythroid chaperone that facilitates folding of alpha-globin subunits for hemoglobin synthesis. J Clin Invest 2007;117(7): 1856–65.

65. Nasimuzzaman M, Khandros E, Wang X, et al. Analysis of alpha hemoglobin stabilizing protein overexpression in murine beta-thalassemia. Am J Hematol 2010; 85(10):820–2.

66. Chen JJ, Throop MS, Gehrke L, et al. Cloning of the cDNA of the heme-regulated eukaryotic initiation factor 2 alpha (eIF-2 alpha) kinase of rabbit reticulocytes: homology to yeast GCN2 protein kinase and human double-stranded-RNA-dependent eIF-2 alpha kinase. Proc Natl Acad Sci U S A 1991; 88(17):7729–33.

67. Chen JJ, Pal JK, Petryshyn R, et al. Amino acid microsequencing of internal tryptic peptides of heme-regulated eukaryotic initiation factor 2 alpha subunit kinase: homology to protein kinases. Proc Natl Acad Sci U S A 1991;88(2):315–9.

68. Chen JJ, Crosby JS, London IM. Regulation of heme-regulated eIF-2 alpha kinase and its expression in erythroid cells. Biochimie 1994;76(8):761–9.

69. Chen JJ. Regulation of protein synthesis by the heme-regulated eIF2alpha kinase: relevance to anemias. Blood 2007;109(7):2693–9.
70. Han AP, Yu C, Lu L, et al. Heme-regulated eIF2alpha kinase (HRI) is required for translational regulation and survival of erythroid precursors in iron deficiency. EMBO J 2001;20(23):6909–18.
71. Han AP, Fleming MD, Chen JJ. Heme-regulated eIF2alpha kinase modifies the phenotypic severity of murine models of erythropoietic protoporphyria and beta-thalassemia. J Clin Invest 2005;115(6):1562–70.
72. Origa R, Galanello R, Ganz T, et al. Liver iron concentrations and urinary hepcidin in beta-thalassemia. Haematologica 2007;92(5):583–8.
73. Pasricha SR, Frazer DM, Bowden DK, et al. Transfusion suppresses erythropoiesis and increases hepcidin in adult patients with beta-thalassemia major: a longitudinal study. Blood 2013;122(1):124–33.

Index

Note: Page numbers of article titles are in **boldface** type.

A

Acute chest syndrome, as clinical example of sickle ischemia-reperfusion injury, 190–191

Adenosine, as cytoprotective mediator in sickle cell disease, 270

Adenosine 2A receptor ($A_{2A}R$), role in sickle cell disease, 289–293

Adenosine 2A receptor ($A_{2A}R$) agonist, and inflammation in sickle cell disease, 277–278

Adenosine 2B receptor ($A_{2B}R$), role in sickle cell disease, 293–294

Adenosine signaling, role in sickle cell therapeutics, **287–299**

    future directions in, 296

    limitations of adenosine therapeutics, 296

    pathway, 288–289

    protective and deleterious roles, 294–295

    role of adenosine A_{2A} receptor ($A_{2A}R$) in, 289–293

    role of adenosine A_{2B} receptor ($A_{2B}R$) in, 293–294

Adhesion. *See* Cellular adhesion.

Aes-103 (5-HMF), clinical development of, to treat sickle cell disease, 224–225

Allosteric modifiers, of hemoglobin, development of to treat sickle cell disease, 220–224

Allosteric states, of hemoglobin and sickle cell disease, 218–219

Anti-P-selectin aptamer, and inflammation in sickle cell disease, 276

Anti-P-selectin monoclonal antibody (SelG1), and inflammation in sickle cell disease, 275

Anticoagulant level, physiologic, reduction of in sickle cell disease, 358

Anticoagulant therapy, for sickle cell disease, 364–366

Arginase, increased activity in sickle cell disease, 305–306

Arginine metabolome, alterations of, in sickle cell disease, **301–321**

    altered arginine homeostasis, 304–306

    altered nitric oxide homeostasis, 303–304

    arginine coadministration with hydroxyurea, 307–308

    arginine therapy for clinical complications, 308–313

        leg ulcers, 308

        priapism, 311

        pulmonary hypertension risk, 308–311

        vaso-occlusive pain episodes, 311–313

    impact of arginine therapy on nitric oxide production, 304–305

    rationale for, 314

    safety data for arginine supplementation, 313–314

Arginine therapy, for sickle cell disease, coadministration with hydroxyurea, 307–308

    for clinical complications of, 308–313

        leg ulcers, 308

        priapism, 311

        pulmonary hypertension risk, 308–311

        vaso-occlusive pain episodes, 311–313

    impact on nitric oxide production, 304–305

Hematol Oncol Clin N Am 28 (2014) 403–413

http://dx.doi.org/10.1016/S0889-8588(14)00011-2

0889-8588/14/$ – see front matter © 2014 Elsevier Inc. All rights reserved.

hemonc.theclinics.com